Epidermolysis Bullosa

Andrew N. Lin   D. Martin Carter

Editors

Epidermolysis Bullosa
Basic and Clinical Aspects

With 51 Illustrations

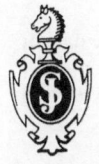

Springer-Verlag
New York Berlin Heidelberg London Paris
Tokyo Hong Kong Barcelona Budapest

Andrew N. Lin, M.D.
Laboratory for Investigative Dermatology
The Rockefeller University
1230 York Avenue
New York, NY 10021–6399
USA

D. Martin Carter, M.D., Ph.D.
Laboratory for Investigative Dermatology
The Rockefeller University
1230 York Avenue
New York, NY 10021–6399
USA

Library of Congress Cataloging-in-Publication Data
Epidermolysis bullosa : basic and clinical aspects / [edited by]
  Andrew N. Lin, D. Martin Carter..
      p. cm.
    Includes bibliographical references and index.
    ISBN-13: 978-1-4612-7717-0   e-ISBN-13: 978-1-4612-2914-8
    DOI: 10.1007/978-1-4612-2914-8

    1. Epidermolysis bullosa.   I. Lin, Andrew N.   II. Carter, D. Martin
  (David Martin), 1936–
    [DNLM: 1. Epidermolysis Bullosa.   WR 200 E64]
  RL793.E65   1992
  616.5—dc20
  DNLM/DLC
  for Library of Congress   92-2141

Printed on acid-free paper.

Production managed by Ellen Seham; Manufacturing supervised by Robert Paella.
Typeset by Asco Trade Typesetting Ltd., Hong Kong.

9 8 7 6 5 4 3 2 1

To epidermolysis bullosa patients the world over, and their families, friends, and relatives, who are their real care-givers.

Preface

Because skin blisters are the initial manifestation of epidermolysis bullosa (EB), patients invariably present to the dermatologist for diagnosis and treatment. However, EB is a systemic disease whose management requires input from clinicians in virtually all fields of medicine, including pediatricians, surgeons, dentists, gastroenterologists, hematologists, otorhinolaryngologists, dietitians, and physical therapists, to name a few. Because EB is a rare disease, few clinicians are familiar with it, and many recoil at the prospect of caring for individuals covered with blisters caused by a disease they know little about. For patients, insult is thus added to injury and they feel abandoned, neglected, and frustrated. One way to remedy this deplorable situation is to provide clinicians with a compact source of information detailing the principles of EB diagnosis and treatment. This text seeks to fulfill this role.

From 1986–1991, The Rockefeller University Hospital has been the coordinating center of the National EB Registry. Supported by The National Institutes of Health, this Registry consists of four university centers* committed to collecting clinical data concerning diagnosis, treatment, and epidemiology on all American EB patients. As of April 1992, nearly 1,799 EB patients have enrolled nationwide. The Registry is now in its second five-year phase of operation. In this text, scientists actively involved in the forefront of EB research review our current understanding of EB pathology and pathogenesis, and clinicians who have served as Registry consultants in the evaluation and treatment of EB patients present their experience. We have included a chapter on EB acquisita even though it is a non-heritable disorder believed to be autoimmune in nature. We did this because by its very name EB acquisita is automatically included in the EB family of disorders, and we feel

---

* The Rockefeller University (D.M. Carter, M.D., Ph.D., principal investigator); Stanford University (E.A. Bauer, M.D., principal investigator); University of North Carolina at Chapel Hill (J.-D. Fine, M.D., principal investigator); and University of Washington (V.P. Sybert, M.D., principal investigator).

any comprehensive volume on EB should not ignore it but should clarify its relation with heritable forms of EB. We hope this text will serve as a handy reference for scientists seeking to understand EB pathology, and for clinicians faced with practical problems in the daily management of EB patients.

We thank Joan Hofmann, David Wesolowski, and Andrea Seelall, members of the secretarial staff of The Laboratory for Investigative Dermatology at The Rockefeller University for their expert assistance in editing the manuscripts.

Andrew N. Lin, M.D.
D. Martin Carter, M.D., Ph.D.

Contents

Contributors

EUGENE A. BAUER, M.D. Professor and Chairman, Department of Dermatology, Stanford University School of Medicine, Stanford, California; Chief of Dermatology, Stanford University Medical Center, Stanford, CA, USA.

SHELLEY R. BERSON, M.D. Assistant Attending Surgeon, Manhattan Eye, Ear and Throat Hospital, New York, NY; Good Samaritan Hospital, Suffern, NY, Nyack Hospital, Nyack, NY, USA

ROBERT A. BRIGGAMAN, M.D. Professor and Chairman, Department of Dermatology, School of Medicine, The University of North Carolina at Chapel Hill, Chapel Hill, North Carolina; Chief of Dermatology Service, North Carolina Memorial Hospital, Chapel Hill, NC, USA

SCOTT BRODIE, M.D. Assistant Professor of Ophthalmology, Mount Sinai School of Medicine, New York, NY; Visiting Associate Physician, The Rockefeller University Hospital, New York, NY, USA

DOROTHEA CALDWELL-BROWN, B.S.N., M.P.H. Clinical Coordinator (formerly: Project Coordinator), The National Epidermolysis Bullosa Registry, The Rockefeller University, New York, NY, USA

D. MARTIN CARTER, M.D., PH.D. Professor and Senior Physician, The Rockefeller University, New York, NY; Professor of Medicine (Dermatology), Cornell University Medical College; Attending Physician, New York Hospital, New York, NY, USA

ROBIN A.J. EADY, M.B., F.R.C.P. Professor of Experimental Dermatopathology and Consultant Dermatologist, St. John's Institute of Dermatology, St. Thomas's Hospital, London SE1 7EH, England

ERVIN H. EPSTEIN JR., M.D. Research Dermatologist and Clinical Professor of Dermatology, University of California, San Francisco; San Francisco General Hospital, San Francisco, CA, USA

GULCHIN ERGUN, M.D.   Assistant Professor of Medicine, Northwestern University Medical School, Chicago, Illinois; Attending Physician, Northwestern Memorial Hospital, VA Lakeside Medical Center, Chicago, IL, USA

JO-DAVID FINE, M.D.   Associate Professor of Dermatology, University of North Carolina at Chapel Hill, Chapel Hill, North Carolina; Attending Dermatologist, North Carolina Memorial Hospital, Chapel Hill, NC, USA

W. RAY GAMMON, M.D.   Professor of Dermatology, School of Medicine, University of North Carolina at Chapel Hill, Chapel Hill, North Carolina; Attending Dermatologist, North Carolina Memorial Hospital, Chapel Hill, NC, USA

PATRICIA J. GIARDINA, M.D.   Associate Professor of Clinical Pediatrics, Cornell University Medical College; Associate Attending Pediatrician, New York Hospital, New York, NY, USA

SHEILA GIBBONS, L.V.N.   Nurse Administrator, Department of Dermatology, Stanford University School of Medicine, Stanford, CA, USA

ROSALIND A. GRYMES, PH.D.   Research Scientist, Life Science Division, NASA–Ames Research Center, Moffett Field, CA, USA

KAREN A. HOLBROOK, PH.D.   Associate Dean for Scientific Affairs, Professor of Biological Structure, Adjunct Professor of Medicine (Medicine), University of Washington School of Medicine, Seattle, WA, USA

ROBERT E. KELLY, M.D.   Assistant Professor of Anesthesiology, Cornell University Medical College, New York, NY; Assistant Attending Anesthesiologist, The New York Hospital, New York, NY, USA

ANNEMARIE KRONBERGER, PH.D.   Senior Research Associate, Department of Dermatology, Stanford University School of Medicine, Stanford, CA, USA

THOMAS J.A. LEHMAN, M.D.   Associate Professor of Pediatrics, Cornell University Medical College; Chief, Division of Pediatric Rheumatology, Hospital for Special Surgery, New York, NY, USA

ANDREW N. LIN, M.D.   Assistant Professor and Associate Physician, The Rockefeller University, New York, NY; Adjunct Assistant Professor of Medicine (Dermatology), Cornell University Medical College, New York, NY, USA

REBECCA L. LIPNICK, B.S., O.T.R.   Coordinator of Occupational Therapy, Therapy Services Department, St. Louis Children's Hospital, St. Louis, MO, USA

N. SCOTT MCNUTT, M.D.   Professor of Pathology, Cornell University Medical College, New York, NY; Attending Pathologist and Chief, Dermatopathology Division, New York Hospital, New York, NY, USA

MICHAEL J. PAGNANI, M.D.   Resident Physician (Orthopedic Surgery), Hospital for Special Surgery, New York, NY, USA

JOHN J. PUTNAM, D.D.S.   Clinical Associate Professor of Surgery (Dentistry), Cornell University Medical College, New York, NY; Attending Dentist and Director of General Dentistry, New York Hospital, New York, NY, USA

MIGDALIA REID, B.S.N., M.P.H.   Clinical Coordinator, The National Epidermolysis Bullosa Registry, The Rockefeller University, New York, NY, USA

KENNETH O. ROTHAUS, M.D.   Clinical Assistant Professor of Surgery, Cornell University Medical College, New York, NY; Assistant Attending Surgeon, New York Hospital and Hospital for Special Surgery, New York, NY; Visiting Associate Physician, The Rockefeller University Hospital, New York, NY, USA

ROBERT A. SCHAEFER, M.D.   Clinical Associate Professor of Medicine, Cornell University Medical College, New York, NY; Associate Attending Physician, New York Hospital, New York, NY, USA

GEORGE W. SFERRA, JR, D.D.S.   Clinical Instructor of Surgery, Cornell University Medical College, New York, NY; Assistant Attending Dentist (Periodontist), New York Hospital, New York, NY, USA

BARBARA S. STANERSON, B.S., P.T.   Child Development Center, St. John's Mercy Hospital, St. Louis, MO, USA

VIRGINIA P. SYBERT, M.D.   Associate Professor of Pediatrics (Medical Genetics), Adjunct Associate Professor of Medicine (Dermatology), University of Washington School of Medicine, Children's Hospital and Medical Center, Seattle, WA, USA

DONNA TESI, R.D.   Medical Student, State University of New York/Health Science Center of Brooklyn, New York, NY. Formerly: Research Dietitian, The Rockefeller University Hospital, New York, NY, USA

ELKE VOGES, M.D.   Research Fellow, Department of Dermatology, Stanford University School of Medicine, Stanford, CA, USA

ROBERT F. WARD, M.D.   Assistant Professor of Otorhinolaryngology, Cornell University Medical College; Assistant Attending Otorhinolaryngologist, New York Hospital, New York, NY, USA

DAVID T. WOODLEY, M.D.   Professor and Associate Chairman, Department of Dermatology, Stanford University School of Medicine, Stanford, California; Attending Dermatologist, Stanford University Medical Center, Stanford, CA, USA

I
Current Perspectives

1
Current Perspectives and Differential Diagnosis in Epidermolysis Bullosa

Robin A.J. Eady

Definition and Historical Perspective

Epidermolysis bullosa is the name given to a number of genetically determined diseases that share the major characteristic of a tendency to develop
blisters and erosions in the skin, and sometimes the mucous membranes, after
mild trauma. These hereditary disorders should be distinguished from other
genetic and acquired diseases (see below) and should not be confused with
epidermolysis bullosa acquisita.

Several historical reviews[1-4] illustrate the evolution of ideas and descriptions relating to a very heterogeneous group of disorders. The classical literature will provide an important insight into how modern classifications of
epidermolysis bullosa have developed. The three main discriminants were:
a) the clinical features, including the presence of nail dystrophy, scars and
epidermal cysts (milia), and involvement of mucous membranes, b) the mode
of inheritance, and c) rather primitive histology. Early accounts of familial
bullous disorders can be attributed to von Hebra,[5] Fox,[6] and Goldscheider,[7]
but the term "epidermolysis bullosa" was coined by Köbner[8] in 1886. For
years, two major forms of epidermolysis bullosa (EB) were recognized: the
simplex (nonscarring) form, in which the lesions arose within the epithelium,
and the dystrophic form, associated with subepidermal lesions and the presence of scars and milia. As can be seen in Cockayne's monograph,[1] many
published reports contained details of isolated cases. Even now, eponyms are
commonly used for several of the major types of EB and if they are to
continue to be used equitably, more authors should share the honors, than
those whose names are in customary use today. To get around this problem,
and generally simplify the system, it would be preferable eventually to avoid
eponyms altogether.

EB Simplex

The name of the recurrent seasonal eruption affecting the hands and feet is
attributed to Weber[9] and Cockayne.[1,10] Cockayne[1] also points out that

blisters may occur elsewhere such as "the line of garters and the waist." The fact that a more widespread involvement may be found in the classical Weber-Cockayne EB is often not stressed in contemporary reviews: and it is possible that Weber-Cockayne disease may be confused with other forms of EB simplex, including perhaps the Köbner[8] and Dowling-Meara[11] types.

EB Dystrophica

Hallopeau[12] distinguished between the "forme bulleuse simple" of Köbner, and Siemens[13] underlined the association between dystrophic skin changes, subepidermal bulla formation, and recessive inheritance.

Cockayne,[1] on reviewing accounts of some 20 families with the dominant form of EB dystrophica, noted that "the majority of those affected were strong and well grown, and have good teeth and hair. Some of the nails may be absent or nearly so, but more often they are greatly thickened and sometimes claw-like." Regarding the recessive form, he wrote "in this form the scars, epidermal cysts and lesions of the mucous membranes are commoner than in the dominant form, and the nails are invariably absent or deformed..., in many cases the teeth are abnormal, deficient in number, irregularly implanted..., and liable to decay early."

Touraine[14] reviewed cases from more than 300 families with dystrophic EB and concluded that hypertrophic or hyperplastic changes (onychogryphosis and hyperkeratosis) were characteristic of the dominant form, whereas atrophic "polydysplasique" changes characterized the recessive type. Pasini[15] described a single family with a relatively mild form of dominant dystrophic EB associated with small hypopigmentated papules or plaquelike areas on the trunk, the so-called albopapuloid lesions. The Pasini or "albopapuloid" variant of dystrophic EB has since become entrenched as a distinct entity in most modern classifications of EB.

EB Letalis

In 1935, Herlitz[16] described a hereditary bullous disease that was lethal in early infancy, and thus different from the other major forms of EB, although we now recognize that infants can die with widespread involvement of both severe dystrophic and simplex (especially Dowling-Meara) forms of EB. The term "junctional EB" is now commonly favored as an alternative for "EB letalis." However, "EB atrophicans" (atrophic EB) is also widely used to describe this major form of EB.

Current Perspectives and Classification of EB

Gedde-Dahl[2] made several original observations and described the "inverse" form of dystrophic EB and the so-called neurotrophic variant. Pearson[17] showed that the lethal or Herlitz form could be distinguished from the dystrophic form on the basis of ultrastructural differences in the level of blistering within the skin. He found that the Herlitz (or junctional) EB blisters formed in the "intermembrane space" (lamina lucida) of the epidermal basement membrane, and that lesions in recessive dystrophic EB were just beneath the basement membrane (sublamina densa) and associated with disintegration of collagen.

Electron microscopy has since become recognized as the most reliable means for diagnosis—at least for the delineation of the major types of EB—even though other techniques, especially immunofluorescence using monoclonal antibodies, now have a valuable role in the diagnosis of certain subtypes of EB[18,19] (see Chapter 3).

Various criteria have been proposed for classifying patients for treatment, genetic counseling, and prognosis.[20-26] None of the schemes is either ideal or comprehensive and, in certain cases, diagnostic criteria may still be considered somewhat arbitrary. The establishment of a federally funded national registry within the United States[27] has had an important role, not only in recruiting patients for both clinical and laboratory studies but also for determining the optimal methods for diagnosis and classification. A subcommittee on Diagnosis and Classification[28] has been formed and has recently published a consensus report on "revised clinical and laboratory criteria for subtypes of inherited epidermolysis bullosa." Table 1.1 details a classification largely based on the proposals of the subcommittee. Similar national registries are also being set up in the United Kingdom and South Africa.[29]

It is implicit that the lesions in EB are induced by trauma (hence the term "mechanobullous"). Nevertheless, not all blisters or erosions in EB are overtly trauma related, and there are other genetic diseases, characterized by skin fragility and trauma-induced bullae (porphyria, for example) that are not considered to be a form of EB. Mendes da Costa disease,[30,31] an exceptionally rare X-linked recessive disorder that has been identified in a single Dutch kindred, is characterized by a blistering tendency that is not typically posttraumatic.[2,31] Should this disorder therefore be regarded, as it often is, as a form of EB simplex?

A recent review[32] listed at least 17 forms of the simplex or epidermolytic subgroup of EB including epidermolytic hyperkeratosis (congenital bullous ichthyosiform erythroderma) and pachyonychia congenita. Neither of these disorders is usually regarded as a form of EB, even though blistering in these conditions may be trauma associated. Dowling-Meara disease[11,33,34] has recently become recognized as a respectable form of EB simplex. It is especially distinguished by the occurrence of a herpetiform distribution of the blisters, but otherwise shares two characteristics with epidermolytic hyperkeratosis. The first is clumping of tonofilaments (keratin filaments) leading to keratinocyte disruption and intraepidermal blistering,[33,34] and the second is palmoplantar hyperkeratosis. However, the keratin filament clumping occurs at different intraepidermal levels in the two disorders, and the hyperkeratosis is more localized in Dowling-Meara disease. It might therefore

TABLE 1.1. Classification of epidermolysis bullosa (based on proposal by Subcommittee of National EB Registry[28], modified with permission of the publisher).

Eb Simplex, localized
  EBS of hands and feet (Weber-Cockayne)
  EBS with hypodontia (Kallin's syndrome)
EB simplex, generalized
  EBS, Köbner
  EBS herpetiformis (Dowling-Meara)
  EBS superficialis
  EBS, Ogna
  EBS with mottled pigmentation
  EBS with (or without) associated neuromuscular disease
  EBS, Mendes da Costa
Junctional EB, localized
  JEB inverse
  JEB acral
  JEB progressive (neurotrophic)
  JEB localized (other)
Junctional EB, generalized
  JEB gravis (Herlitz)
  JEB mitis (non-Herlitz; generalized atrophic benign)
  JEB cicatricial
Dystrophic EB, localized
  DEB inverse
  DEB acral
  DEB pretibial
  DEB centripetal
  DEB localized (other)
Dystrophic EB, generalized
  Dominant forms of dystrophic EB (DDEB)
    DDEB albopapuloidea (Pasini)
    DDEB hyperplasique (Cockayne-Touraine)
    Transient bullous dermolysis of the newborn
  Recessive forms (RDEB)
    RDEB gravis (Hallopeau-Siemens)
    RDEB mitis

---

seem logical to group the Dowling-Meara subtype of EB together with congenital bullous ichthyosiform erythroderma rather than include the latter with other forms of ichthyosis. In both, a disorder of the keratin filament network may be central to the pathogenesis.[35]

Congenital absence of skin in a localized distribution has been used as the major criterion for Bart's syndrome, which originally referred to a large kindred with an autosomal dominant mode of inheritance.[36,37] The disorder has been included in numerous classifications as a form of EB simplex. Since both junctional and dystrophic EB may present with very similar features, it is questionable whether Bart's syndrome should be retained as a distinct entity.[38,39]

It should also be questioned whether there are clear divisions between the so-called Cockayne-Touraine and Pasini forms of dominant dystrophic EB. A hallmark of the Pasini variant is the presence of albopapuloid lesions. In addition, variations in the onset and severity of the disease and distribution of the lesions have been reported.[20,24,40] Differences in ultrastructural and biochemical findings have also been described,[41-43] but not confirmed by others,[44,45] suggesting possible heterogeneity. It is also possible that albopapuloid lesions are nonspecific.[22,46,47]

Newly Described Forms of EB

This group includes various forms of autosomal recessive EB simplex, such as the "lethal" form,[48] that associated with neuromuscular defects,[49,50] and Kallin syndrome.[51] EB simplex superficialis,[52] mimicking the peeling skin syndrome, is autosomal dominant.

Transient Bullous Dermolysis of the Newborn: Relationship to Retained Type VII Collagen

In 1985, Hashimoto et al.[53] described a newborn who developed blisters on the extremities and in other friction areas soon after birth. The bullae resolved rapidly without the formation of scars or milia. No new lesions appeared after 4 months. Ultrastructurally, the blisters formed beneath the lamina densa and were associated with lysis of dermal collagen and altered anchoring fibrils. Basal epidermal keratinocytes contained dilated rough endoplasmic reticulum enclosing electron-dense stellate bodies. One year after the patient's birth, only slight pigmentary changes remained in the previously affected sites. Subsequently, the same author[54] reported two additional cases with similar features. In one of these cases, acral erosions were present at birth, and generalized blisters including oral involvement appeared soon afterward. In three other patients, and one of the original cases,[55] the intracellular inclusions were shown to express type VII collagen (or at least part of the molecule) and to have other features consistent with dystrophic EB. Another patient,[56] with similar morphological and immunohistochemical findings, had a more severe form of recessive dystrophic EB, and died in infancy. Schofield et al.[57] have since identified three additional patients. These cases not only reinforce the association between an abnormality of a basement membrane component (type VII collagen) and a form of EB, but also raise interesting questions concerning the synthesis and assembly of type VII collagen. Another aspect of this relationship is illustrated in the inverse form of recessive dystrophic EB.[58]

Frequency of EB

Modern diagnostic criteria will have a large influence on determining relative frequencies of different forms of EB. Existing data were collected without the benefit of all these diagnostic aids. In Norway,[2] the prevalence (per million population) was estimated as 14.2 for the Ogna form of EB, 9 for Weber-Cockayne, about 1 for Köbner, and 1.4 for the dominant dystrophic forms. In Finland,[59] the frequency of the recessive dystrophic form was calculated to be much less than in Norway, and in England,[60] the frequency of recessive EB was given as 1 per 300,000.

Differential Diagnosis

For practical purposes, it is useful to consider those conditions that may present at birth or during the first few days of life and second, those that arise subsequently—usually during infancy or in later childhood (Table 1.2). Essentially, there are no conditions that can mimic EB in every respect, and the main problem usually is to differentiate one form of EB from another. However, diagnostic difficulties may occur, especially in the neonatal period.

Neonatal Period

Congenital Bullous Ichthyosiform Erythroderma

This is probably the most frequent congenital abnormality that must be distinguished from EB. The disorder presents at birth with blisters and/or erosions that may be extensive and occur on an erythrodermic background. The mucosae are usually not involved. Histological examination shows changes of epidermolytic hyperkeratosis (see above).

TABLE 1.2. Disorders that may be included in the differential diagnosis of epidermolysis bullosa.

Neonatal period
  Congenital bullous ichthyosiform erythroderma (bullous ichthyosis; epidermolytic hyperkeratosis)
  Bullous impetigo
  Scalded skin syndrome
  Congenital neonatal herpes simplex
  Incontinentia pigmenti
  Mastocytosis
  Aplasia cutis
  Congenital erythropoietic porphyria
  Kindler's syndrome
Childhood
  Autoimmune acquired blistering disorders
  Pachyonychia congenita
  Peeling skin syndrome

Lesions may be induced by trauma or by infection. As the child develops, erythema and blistering tend to diminish and verrucous thickenings appear, often in a ridgelike pattern affecting the major flexures.

The disorder is transmitted in an autosomal dominant mode, but is often sporadic. The underlying abnormality is unknown and the gene has not been mapped.

Incontinentia Pigmenti (Bloch-Sulzberger Syndrome)

This disorder is inherited as an X-linked dominant trait and is thought to be generally lethal for males. Ninety-five percent of cases are female. Evolution of the disease may occur in three stages: vesicular, warty, and pigmentary. However, there is often overlap among the different stages. At birth, vesicles and erythema occur in a linear distribution on the limbs and trunk. The lesions are not overtly induced by trauma. The primary lesions tend to diminish during infancy and are followed by warty thickenings, and eventually by characteristic hyperpigmented arcs or whorls, especially on the trunk. There may be associated abnormalities of the teeth, eyes, bones, and central nervous system.

Histopathology of the blisters shows an eosinophilic infiltration of both dermis and epidermis. The gene for incontinentia pigmenti has been mapped to Xq28.[61]

Mastocytosis

A form of mastocytosis may present in the neonate. More often the disorder first appears in older children or in adult life. The lesions are flesh colored or slightly pigmented macules or papules and widespread (urticaria pigmentosa) or nodular and often solitary (mastocytoma). Rubbing the skin causes erythema and wealing, and occasionally bulla formation. A skin biopsy will show increased numbers of dermal mast cells.

Bullous Impetigo

The lesions result from an infection with phage group II *Staphylococcus aureus* and are not primarily related to trauma. The blisters contain clear yellow or turbid fluid and occur at the subcorneal level within the epidermis.

Staphylococcal Scalded Skin Syndrome

This disorder, resulting from the action of a staphylococcus-derived toxin, presents with areas of denuded skin rather than blisters. However, it may be necessary to distinguish it from those forms of EB that can also cause extensive loss of skin in the neonate. The child will be pyrexial and often "toxic." Histologically, the level of the lesion is within the upper part of the epidermis.

Neonatal Herpes Simplex

This infection is usually contracted from the mother during birth, but rarely may arise in utero. The eruption can be widespread with vesicles and erosions, mimicking EB.[62]

Aplasia Cutis

The majority of these congenital lesions are solitary and arise in the scalp.[63] They do not form blisters but appear as a circumscribed defect involving the full thickness of the skin.

Kindler's Syndrome

A recent review[64] of this rare syndrome[65] indicated that in most cases blisters are either congenital or arise in the early neonatal period. The mainly acral blisters often follow trauma or sun exposure. The lesions diminish in later childhood. Diffuse atrophy and poikiloderma are cardinal features that are not congenital.

Palmar/plantar hyperkeratosis and mucosal involvement are frequent findings. The blisters are usually intraepidermal, but may also occur at other levels. The etiology is unknown; many cases are sporadic.

Porphyria

Congenital erythropoietic porphyria (Gunter's disease) may appear in the neonatal period with distressing photosensitivity and bullae in the light-exposed skin. The bullae are associated with skin fragility and will heal with scarring. There is red discoloration of the urine and, in older children, erythrodontia.

Later Childhood

Acquired Autoimmunobullous Diseases

A few years ago these diseases might not have been included in the differential diagnosis of blistering disorders before the age of about 5 years, but examples of many of these diseases occurring in younger children have recently been described. Generally they do not cause difficulty in differentiation from EB. However, linear IgA disease (chronic bullous disease of childhood) can manifest as clusters of blisters on an inflammatory base—similar, perhaps, to EB simplex herpetiformis (Dowling-Meara). Second, pemphigus and herpes gestationis may rarely occur in the neonatal period, presumably as a result of transplacental transfer of maternal antibodies.[66]

Pachyonychia Congentia

At least two forms of this disorder have been described. An autosomal dominant inheritance is most frequent. There is precocious eruption of the teeth, oral leukokeratosis, and discoloration and thickening of the nails associated with subungual hyperkeratosis. Hyperkeratosis of the soles, hyperhidrosis, and blistering may, in certain ways, resemble EB simplex.

Peeling Skin Syndrome

This disorder, which seems to be heterogeneous, is characterized by continuous focal shedding of stratum corneum.[67] True blistering is not a feature. The condition may be worse in winter than summer. Autosomal recessive inheritance has been reported.

Impact on Health Care and Research

Of all the genodermatoses, or at least those that one might presume result from single gene mutations, EB has aroused an extraordinary amount of interest, as shown in a recent review of the literature on EB[68] that included at least 1300 titles that span just over 100 years up to the end of 1986, and cover a wide range of disciplines including dermatology, surgery, pediatrics, pathology, gastroenterology, dentistry, clinical genetics, radiology, anesthesiology, general medicine, nursing, and basic science. The number of specialties involved in managing the diverse medical problems of EB is brought into focus; physicians operating clinical centers that offer a comprehensive service to EB sufferers and their families also need the direct help of nurse specialists, clinical psychologists, social workers, physiotherapists, occupational therapists, dietitians, and many others.

The establishment of national registries will provide accurate data on the incidence and prevalence of EB and will help to generate new research on diagnostic methods, pathogenesis, and treatment.

Organizations such as the Dystrophic Epidermolysis Bullosa Research Association (DEBRA), which now exists in many countries and is dedicated to helping EB sufferers and their families, can and do have a crucial role not only in promoting and funding research, but also in informing the public, politicians, and health workers of the special needs of EB patients.

Morphology, biochemistry, and applied immunology (especially immunohistochemistry) have each had an important part in the investigation of various aspects of EB, but future research, aimed at improving knowledge of causation and pathogenesis, must surely concentrate on molecular biological approaches. Recent studies including the production of a transgenic mouse carrying a mutant keratin gene and expressing a disorder phenotypically similar to the Dowling-Meara form of EB simplex,[69] in addition to linkage[70,71] and mutational[71-73] data in EB simplex and linkage in dominant dystrophic EB,[74] might encourage one to predict that several of the genes relevant to the molecular pathology of EB will soon be cloned and sequenced and new probes will become available for diagnosis (including early prenatal diagnosis) and screening.

References

1. Cockayne EA. *Inherited Abnormalities of the Skin and its Appendages.* London: Oxford University Press; 1933:118–133.
2. Gedde-Dahl Jr T. *Epidermolysis bullosa. A clinical, genetic and epidemiological study.* Universitets Forlaget. (Oslo). Baltimore: The Johns Hopkins Press; 1971.
3. Pearson RW. The machanobullous diseases (epidermolysis bullosa). In: Fitzpatrick TB, Arndt KA, Clark WH et al., eds. *Dermatology in General Medicine.* New York: McGraw-Hill; 1971:621–647.
4. Holubar R. Historical background. In: Wojnarowska F, Briggaman RA, eds. *Management of Blistering Diseases.* London: Chapman and Hall; 1990:1–12.
5. von Hebra F. Pemphigus. Artzlicher berict des KK. Allgemeinen krankenhausen zu Wien vom Jahre 1870. Vienna; 362–364.
6. Fox T. Notes on unusual or rare forms of skin disease. IV. Congenital ulceration of skin (two cases) with pemphigus eruption. *Lancet.* 1897;1:766–767.
7. Goldscheider A. Hereditare neigung zur blasenbildung. *Monatsch Prakt Dermatol.* 1882:1:163–164.
8. Köbner H. Hereditare anlage zur blasenbildung (epidermolysis bullosa hereditaria). *Dtsch Med Wschr.* 1886;12:21–22.
9. Weber FP. Recurrent bullous eruption on the feet of a child. *Proc R Soc Med.* 1926;19:72.
10. Cockayne EA. Recurrent bullous eruption of the feet. *Br J Dermatol.* 1938;50:358–362.
11. Dowling GB, Meara RH. Epidermolysis bullosa resembling juvenile dermatitis herpetiformis. *Br J Dermatol.* 1954;66:139–143.
12. Hallopeau H. Sur la dermatose bulleuse hereditaire et traumatique. *Ann Derm Syph (Paris).* 1898;9:721–728.
13. Siemens HW. Zur klinik histologie und atiologie der sog. Epidermolysis bullosa traumatica (bullosis mechanica) mit klinische—experimentellen studien uber die erzeugung von reibungsblasen. *Arch Derm Syph.* 1921;134:454–447.
14. Touraine MA. Classification des epidermolyses bulleuses. *Ann Derm Syph (Paris).* 1942;8:138–144.
15. Pasini A. Dystrophie cutanée bulleuse atrophiante et albo-papuloide. *Ann Derm Syph (Paris).* 1928;10:1044–1065.
16. Herlitz G. Kongenitaler, nicht syphilitischer pemphigus: Eine ubersicht nebst beschreibung einer neuen krankheitsform (epidermolysis bullosa hereditaria letalis). *Acta Pediatr.* 1935;17:315–371.
17. Pearson RW. Studies on the pathogenesis of epidermolysis bullosa. *J Invest Dermatol.* 1962;39:551–575.
18. Fine J-D. Altered skin basement membrane antigenicity in epidermolysis bullosa. *Curr Probl Dermatol.* 1987;17:111–126.
19. Eady RAJ, Tidman MJ, Heagerty AHM, Kennedy AR. Approaches to the study of epidermolysis bullosa. *Curr Probl Dermatol.* 1987;17:127–141.
20. Gedde-Dahl Jr T. Sixteen types of epidermolysis bullosa: their clinical discrimination, therapy and prenatal diagnosis. *Acta Derm Venereol (Stockh).* 1981;95 (suppl):74–87.
21. Briggaman RA. Hereditary epidermolysis bullosa with special emphasis on newly recognized syndromes and complications. *Dermatol Clin.* 1983;1:263–280.
22. Eady RAJ, Tidman MJ. Diagnosing epidermolysis bullosa. *Br J Dermatol.* 1983;108:621–628.

23. Cooper TW, Bauer EA. Epidermolysis bullosa: a review. *Pediatr Dermatol*. 1984; 1:181–188.
24. Haber RM, Hanna W, Ramsay CA, Boxall LB. Hereditary epidermolysis bullosa. *J Am Acad Dermatol*. 1985;13:252–275.
25. Fine J-D. Epidermolysis Bullosa. Clinical aspects, pathology and recent advances in research. *Int J Dermatol*. 1986;25:143–157.
26. Kero M, Niemi KM. Epidermolysis bullosa. *Int J Dermatol*. 1986;25:75–82.
27. Carter DM, Caldwell-Brown D. The national epidermolysis bullosa registry. In: Priestley GC, Tidman MJ, Weiss JB, Eady RAJ, eds. *Epidermolysis Bullosa: A Comprehensive Review of Classification, Management and Laboratory Studies.* Crowthorne UK: Dystrophic Epidermolysis Bullosa Research Association; 1990:173–175.
28. Fine J-D, Bauer EA, Briggaman RA, et al. Revised clinical and laboratory criteria for subtypes of inherited epidermolysis bullosa. *J Am Acad Dermatol*. 1991; 24:119–135.
29. Winship IM. Epidermolysis bullosa in South Africa: formation of a national registry. In: Priestley GC, Tidman MJ, Weiss JB, Eady RAJ, eds. *Epidermolysis Bullosa: A Comprehensive Review of Classification, Management and Laboratory Studies.* Crowthorne UK: Dystrophic Epidermolysis Bullosa Research Association; 1990:134–136.
30. Mendes da Costa S, van der Valk JW. Typus maculatus der bullosen hereditaren dystrophie. *Arch Derm Syph (Berlin)*. 1908;91:1.
31. Woerdeman MJ. Dystrophia bullosa hereditaria typus maculatus. *Acta Derm Venereol (Stockh)*. 1957;111:678–686.
32. Pearson RW. Clinicopathologic types of epidermolysis bullosa and their non-dermatological complications. *Arch Dermatol*. 1988;124:718–725.
33. Anton-Lamprecht I, Schnyder UW. Epidermolysis bullosa herpetiformis Dowling-Meara. Report of a case and pathomorphogenesis. *Dermatologica*. 1982;164:221–235.
34. Niemi K-M, Kero M, Kanerva L, Mattila R. Epidermolysis bullosa simplex: a new histologic subtype. *Arch Dermatol*. 1983;119:138–141.
35. Ishida-Yamamoto A, McGrath JA, Chapman SJ, Leigh IM, Lane EB, Eady RAJ. Epidermolysis bullosa simplex (Dowling-Meara Type) is a genetic disease characterized by an abnormal keratin filament network involving keratins K5 and K14. *J Invest Dermatol*. 1991;97:959–968.
36. Bart BJ, Gorlin RJ, Elving Anderson V, Lynch FW. Congenital localized absence of skin and associated abnormalities resembling epidermolysis bullosa. *Arch Dermatol*. 1966;93:296–304.
37. Bart BJ. Epidermolysis bullosa and congenital localized absence of the skin. *Arch Dermatol*. 1970;101:68–81.
38. Wojnarowska F, Eady RAJ, Wells RS. Dystrophic epidermolysis bullosa presenting with congenital localized absence of skin: report of four cases. *Br J Dermatol*. 1983;108:477–483.
39. Bouwes Bavinck JN, Van Haeringen A, Rutter D, van Der Schroeff JG. Autosomal dominant epidermolysis bullosa dystrophic: are the Cockayne-Touraine, the Pasini and the Bart-types different expressions of the same mutant gene. *Clin Genet*. 1987;31:416–424.
40. Schachner LA, Press S. Vesicular, bullous and pustular disorders. In: Schachner LA, Hansen RC, eds. *Pediatric Dermatology*. New York: Churchill Livingstone; 1988:775–835.

41. Hashimoto I, Anton-Lamprecht I, Gedde-Dahl Jr T, et al. Ultrastructural studies in epidermolysis bullosa herediteria: 1. Dominant dystrophic type of Pasini. *Arch Derm Forsch.* 1975;252:167–178.
42. Sasai Y, Saito N, Seiji M. Epidermolysis bullosa dystrophica et albopapuloidea. *Arch Dermatol.* 1973;108:554–557.
43. Bauer EA, Fiehlek WK, Esterly NB. Increased glycosominoglycan accumulation as a genetic characteristic in cell cultures of one variety of dominant dystrophic epidermolysis bullosa. *J Clin Invest.* 1979;64:32–39.
44. Tidman MJ, Eady RAJ. Evaluation of anchoring fibrils and other components of the dermal epidermal junction in dystrophic epidermolysis bullosa by a quantative ultrastructural technique. *J Invest Dermatol.* 1985;84:374–377.
45. Priestley GC. Glycosaminoglycans production from the Pasini and Cockayne-Touraine forms of dominant dystrophic epidermolysis bullosa. *J Invest Dermatol.* 1991;96:168–169.
46. Ramelet A-A, Boillat C. Epidermolysis bulleuse dystrophique albopapuloide autosomique recessive. *Dermatologica.* 1985;171:397–406.
47. Kemmett D, Spencer M-J, Tidman MJ. An unusual pedigree of dystrophic epidermolysis bullosa. In: Priestley GC, Tidman MJ, Weiss JB, Eady RAJ, eds. Epidermolysis bullosa: a comprehensive review of classification, management and laboratory studies, Crowthorne, UK. Dystrophic Epidermolysis Bullosa Research Association; 1990:89–92.
48. Salih MAA, Lake BD, el Hag MA, Atherton DJ. Lethal epidermolysis bullosa: a new autosomal recessive type of epidermolysis bullosa. *Br J Dermatol.* 1985;113:135–145.
49. Niemi K-M, Sommer H, Kero M, Kanerva L, Haltia M. Epidermolysis bullosa simplex associated with muscular dystrophy with recessive inheritance. *Arch Dermatol.* 1988;124:551–554.
50. Fine J-D, Steen J, Johnson L, et al. Autosomal recessive epidermolysis bullosa simplex: generalized phenotypic features suggestive of junctional or dystrophic epidermolysis bullosa, and association with neuromuscular diseases. *Arch Dermatol.* 1989;125:931–938.
51. Nielsen PG, Sjölund E. Epidermolysis bullosa simplex localisata associated with anodontia, hair and nail disorders: a new syndrome. *Acta Derm Venereol (Stockh).* 1985;65:526–530.
52. Fine J-D, Johnson L, Wright T. Epidermolysis bullosa simplex superficialis: a new variant of epidermolysis bullosa characterized by subcorneal skin cleavage mimicking peeling skin syndrome. *Arch Dermatol.* 1989;125:633–638.
53. Hashimoto K, Matsumoto M, Iacobelli D. Transient bullous dermolysis of the newborn. *Arch Dermatol.* 1985;121:1429–1438.
54. Hashimoto K, Burk J, Bale GF, et al. Transient bullous dermolysis of the new born: two additional cases. *J Am Acad Dermatol.* 1989;21:708–713.
55. Fine J-D, Horiguchi Y, Stein D, Esterly NB, Leigh IM. Intraepidermal type VII collagen. Evidence for abnormal intracytoplasmic processing of a major basement membrane protein in rare patients with dominant and possibly localized recessive forms of dystrophic epidermolysis bullosa. *J Am Acad Dermatol.* 1990;22:188–195.
56. Smith LT, Sybert VP. Intraepidermal retention of type VII collagen in a patient with recessive dystrophic epidermolysis bullosa. *J Invest Dermatol.* 1990;94:261–264.

57. Schofield OMV, Yamamoto A, McGrath J, et al. Transient bullous dermolysis of the newborn: a disorder of type VII collagen secretion. *Br J Dermatol.* 1991;125 (suppl 38):89.
58. Bruckner-Tuderman L, Niemi K-M, Kero M, Schnyder UW, Reunala T. Type VII collagen is expressed but anchoring fibrils are defective in dystrophic epidermolysis bullosa inversa. *Br J Dermatol.* 1990;122:383–339.
59. Kero M. Occurrence of epidermolysis bullosa in Finland. *Acta Derm Venereol (Stockh).* 1984;64:57–62.
60. Davison BCC. Epidermolysis bullosa. *J Med Genet.* 1965;2:233–242.
61. Sefiani A, Abel L, Henertz S, et al. The gene for incontinentia pigmentia is assigned to Xq28. *Genomics.* 1989;4:427–429.
62. Honig PJ, Brown D. Congenital herpes simplex virus infection initially resembling epidermolysis bullosa. *J Pediatr.* 1982;101:958–960.
63. Freiden IJ. Aplasia cutis congenita: a clinical review and proposal for classification. *J Am Acad Dermatol.* 1986;14:646–660.
64. Hovnainen A, Blanchet-Bardon C, de Prost Y. Poikiloderma of Theresa Kindler. Report of a case with ultrastructural study, and review of the literature. *Pediatr Dermatol.* 1989;6:82–90.
65. Kindler T. Congenital poikiloderma with traumatic bulla formation and progressive cutaneous atrophy. *Br J Dermatol.* 1954;66:104–111.
66. Atherton DA. The Neonate. In: Champion RH, Burton JA, Ebling FJJ, eds. Blackwell; Oxford: *Textbook of Dermatology.* 1992. Vol 1, Chapter 11, pp 381–443.
67. Levy SB, Goldsmith LA. The peeling skin syndrome. *J Am Acad Dermatol.* 1982;7:606–613.
68. Priestley GC. A bibliography of epidermolysis bullosa. *Acta Derm Venereol (Stockh).* 1987 (suppl 133).
69. Vassar R, Coulombe PA, Degenstein L, Albers K, Fuchs E. Mutant keratin expression in transgenic mice causes marked abnormalities resembling a human genetic disease. *Cell.* 1991;64:365–380.
70. Humphries MM, Pheils D, Lawler M, et al. Epidermolysis bullosa: evidence for linkage to genetic markers on chromosome 1 in a family with the autosomal dominant simplex form. *Genomics.* 1990:7:377–381.
71. Bonifas JM, Rothman AL, Epstein Jr EH. Epidermolysis bullosa simplex: evidence in two families for keratin gene abnormalities. *Science.* 1991;254:1202–1205.
72. Coulombe PA, Hutton ME, Letain A, Herbert A, Paller AS, Fuchs E. Point mutation in human keratin 14 genes of epidermolysis bullosa simplex patients: genetic and functional analysis. *Cell.* 1991;66:1301–1311.
73. Lane EB, Rugg EL, Navsaria et al. A mutation in the conserved helix termination peptide of keratin 5 in hereditary skin blistering. *Nature.* 1992;356:244–246.
74. Ryynanen M, Knowlten RG, Parente MG, Chung LC, Chu M-L, Uitto J. Human type VII collagen: genetic linkage of gene (Col7A) on chromosome 3 to dominant dystrophic epidermolysis bullosa. *Amer J Hum Gen.* 1991;49:797–803.

II
Basic Science Aspects

2
The Basement Membrane Zone at the Dermal–Epidermal Junction of Human Skin

DAVID T. WOODLEY and SCOTT MCNUTT

The epidermal basement membrane is an important interface between the cells of epidermis and the connective tissues.[1-3] A variety of nutrients and signals must pass through this interface, carrying some messages from the blood to the epidermis and other messages from the epidermis to other structures. The basement membrane region must also function well in the attachment of the delicate cells of the epidermis to the strong fibers in the dermis. During embryogenesis and wound healing, the basement membrane acts as a scaffold affecting the organization of cell growth.

There are basement membranes at the interface between other cellular regions and the dermal connective tissues (e.g., the epidermal appendages, including the hair follicles and sweat glands). There are substantial differences between these various basement membranes. Also certain components of the basement membrane are present at the interface between the dermis and blood vessels, nerves, and muscle cells. Each of these regions is specialized and different from the dermal–epidermal junction. We have restricted our discussion of the basement membrane regions to the dermal–epidermal junction because of its importance in the pathogenesis of epidermolysis bullosa. An overview of the structure and biochemistry of this region is given to provide a background for subsequent chapters on the pathogenesis of epidermolysis bullosa.

Structure of the Dermal–Epidermal Junction

The initial structural investigations of the dermal–epidermal junction (DEJ) have led to the frequent consideration of the basement membrane as a rigid, static structural barrier instead of the dynamic structure that it is. There is turnover of the components at various rates and there must be dynamic changes in the structure of the region as epidermal cells undergo mitoses and certain daughter cells lose contact with the basement membrane. There also must be dynamic changes in the structure when Langerhans' cells and lymphocytes move from the dermis into the epidermis and then back again carrying out immunosurveillance. In the following discussion, the reader should keep in mind that the DEJ is dynamic and that we are presenting the structures found at the DEJ where the average basal keratinocyte contacts the dermis. There are indications that there is heterogeneity in basal keratinocyte function and basement membrane structure reflecting different proliferative states of the basal cells[4]. The DEJ also serves melanocytes and Merkel cells in the basal layers of the epidermis, and there are differences in the structure of the DEJ beneath these cells that are beyond the scope of this chapter.

In routine paraffin sections stained with hematoxylin and eosin and examined by light microscopy, the DEJ appears as a very thin eosinophilic band just beneath the epidermis. This band tends to exclude the nuclei of dermal cells, but does not exclude their dendritic processes or exclude the small extensions of the collagen and elastic fibers of the dermis. The application of the periodic acid Schiff (PAS) stain led to the demonstration of abundant neutral carbohydrates in the DEJ[2]. This PAS-positive zone was initially considered to be the basement membrane. Differentiated regions within the basement membrane were not appreciated. At high magnification, in paraffin sections stained with the PAS method, the basal keratinocytes could be seen to form small cytoplasmic projections into the basement membrane.

Electron microscopy revealed that this PAS-positive basement membrane region contained a variety of structures (Fig. 2.1). This discovery required subdivision of the region into at least four layers, as described by Briggaman and Wheeler[2] (Fig. 2.2). Some of the layers are contributed by the epidermal cells themselves and other layers are from the dermal cells. The layers derived from the epidermis begin at the plasma membrane of the basal keratinocyte, which is layer #1. Immediately beneath the plasma membrane is an electron-lucent layer, named the lamina lucida (layer #2), which lies between the plasma membrane and an electron-dense layer, the lamina densa (layer #3). The fourth layer is a zone derived from dermal fibroblasts[5]. It contains many small filaments and is named the subbasal lamina fibrous zone. The mechanical strength of the DEJ depends on the internal strength of each of these layers as well as how well they are attached to each other.

The basal plasma membrane of the keratinocytes forms a vital link between the cytoskeleton of the keratinocyte and the lamina lucida and lamina densa.[6] The central morphological feature of this linkage is the hemidesmosome, which is an electron-dense plaque approximately 500 to 1000 nm in diameter. Cytokeratin filaments approximately 10 nm in diameter attach to each other in the cytoplasm of the keratinocytes and attach to the desmosomes on the lateral surfaces of the cells and to the hemidesmosomes at the bases of the cells.[6, 7] This structural filamentous network limits the deformability of the cells. The cytokeratin filaments bind to the dense material at the cytoplasmic surface of the basal plasma membrane, which defines the hemidesmosome. At the hemidesmosome, the trilaminar plasma membrane appears to be continuous, at least without interruption of the hydrophobic

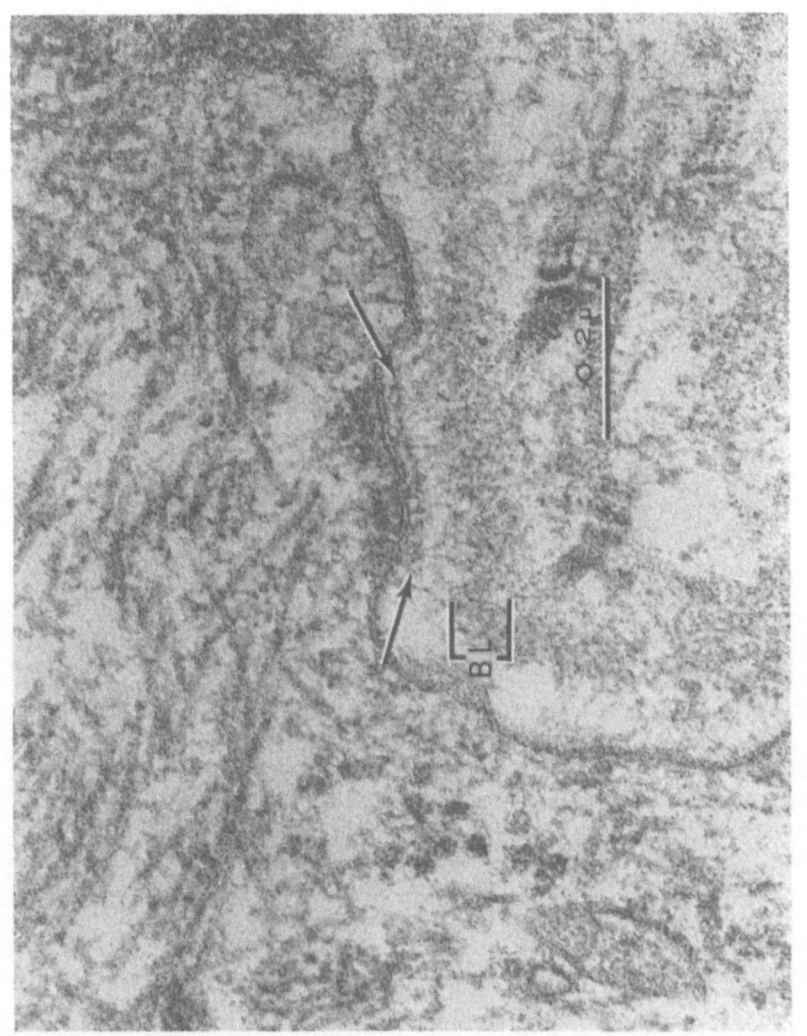

FIGURE 2.1. Basement membrane zone of human skin in an electron micrograph at high magnification. BL is the lamina densa. Arrows point to the subbasal dense plaque, which contains anchoring filaments. The cytoplasmic density attached to the plasma membrane is the hemidesmosome plaque. Below this region, anchoring fibrils are frequent and are seen here as the dense, banded structure below the lamina densa.

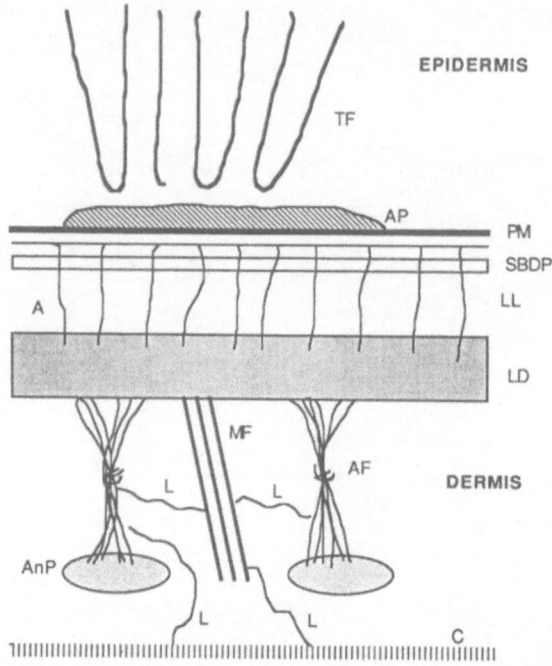

FIGURE 2.2. A schematic diagram of the basement membrane zone of human skin and the region of the hemidesmosomes. TF, tonofilaments; AP, attachment plaque; PM, plasma membrane; SBDP, subbasal dense plaque; LL, lamina lucida; A, anchoring filaments that course vertically through the subbasal dense plaque; LD, lamina densa; AF, anchoring fibrils; AnP, anchoring plaques within the upper papillary dermis; MF, microfibrils; L, linkin and microthreadlike fibers; C, interstitial collagen fibers. Modified, with permission, from a schematic created by Dr. Yves Sarret in Briggaman RA, Wheeler CE. The epidermal–dermal junction. *J Invest Dermatol.* 1975;65:71–84.

character of the interior of the membrane. It is clear that hydrophobic proteins form an important part of the structure of the membrane at this site rather than just a lipid bilayer since simple lipid extraction does not cleave the membrane at this site. Fine anchoring filaments, in the size range of 2 to 4 nm in diameter, pass from the hemidesmosome plasma membrane into the lamina lucida and attach to the lamina densa part of the basement membrane.[2,8] Within the lamina lucida, these filaments attach to a region called the subbasal dense plaque, which forms a dense line just beneath the plasma membrane of the hemidesmosome in routine electron micrographs.[7] The function of this small plaque is unknown. It is a distinctive component of the hemidesmosome, when compared with the adjacent plasma membrane, from which small anchoring filaments can pass without a subbasal dense plaque. The greatest concentration of anchoring filaments is at the hemidesmosome.

Except for these anchoring filaments and subbasal dense plaques, the lamina lucida appears as an empty layer often 30 to 40 nm thick. However, from the use of immunostains for electron microscopy and alternative staining and fixation procedures, we know that this lamina lucida contains components of glycoproteins, which stain poorly in routine preparations. Morphometric studies have shown that the normal human epidermis has approximately 50% to 60% of its basal surface covered with hemidesmosomes.[9] The anchoring filaments form the weakest segment mechanically in the basement membrane zone, and are easily lysed by salt solutions.[10]

In the routine thin section electron micrographs, there are densities in the cytoplasm adjacent to the basal plasma membrane that are intermediate between a fully formed hemidesmosome and the electron-lucent background cytoplasm.[5] They are generally slightly smaller than hemidesmosomes (in the range of 400 to 600 nm in diameter) and have fewer intermediate filaments attached to them in the keratinocyte cytoplasm.[11] They may represent a heterogeneous population of specialized attachment sites, for example, sections near the periphery of the fully formed hemidesmosomes, intermediate stages in the formation or degradation of hemidesmosomes, and attachment sites where actin filaments attach to the membrane.[9] Such intermediate densities may form up to 15% of the basal surface of the normal keratinocyte and are increased in wound healing and some pathologic conditions.[9] During normal wound healing, actin filament bundles appear in the cytoplasm adjacent to the basal plasma membrane.[12] These actin bundles attach to the basal plasma membrane at intermediate densities that lack a subbasal dense plaque in the lamina lucida and have a lower density at the cytoplasmic surface of the keratinocyte plasma membrane. These attachment plaques are associated with epidermal cell motility during wound healing; the anchoring fibrils are not regenerated until months after the wound is closed.[13,14]

The lamina densa appears in routine electron microscopy preparations as a continuous finely filamentous layer approximately 30 to 50 nm in thickness. The fine filaments are at the level of resolution of the electron microscopy preparations and have a granular appearance in many photographs. The substructure of the lamina densa is difficult to resolve but there are several components, such as type IV collagen and heparan sulfate proteoglycan, that are the main components. The lamina densa, or basal lamina, is much thinner than the PAS-stained basement membrane as seen by light microscopy, and thus should not be referred to as the basement membrane. Although collagen is a component of the lamina densa, a cross-banding pattern is not seen.

Type IV collagen is the principal component of the lamina densa that is resolved in electron micrographs. The side-to-side or lateral associations between the type IV collagen filaments in vivo resemble ultrastructurally those formed in matrices from type IV collagen in vitro.[15]

The subbasal lamina fibrous zone, or sublamina densa fibrous zone, is a complex layer containing small banded fibrils,[16–18] named anchoring fibrils, that attach directly to the lamina densa and may form the principal attachment mechanism for all of the fibrous components of the dermis.[10] These short anchoring fibrils form looping arrays, with one or both ends of the fibrils attached to the lamina densa. These looping arrays entrap small type III collagen to larger type I collagen fibers. The elastin microfibrils attach to the larger elastin fibers in the dermis.

The substructure of the anchoring fibrils is complex. The central portion of the anchoring fibril has a symmetric banding pattern.[17] Their length is variable and may be from 30 to 100 nm. The ends of the fibrils are splayed and the centers are condensed, which resembles the shape of sheaves of wheat bundled together. In contrast, the elastin microfibrils are straight, have a regular beaded pattern in longitudinal sections, and in cross sections have a hollow-appearing tubular profile with a diameter of approximately 9 nm. Small type I collagen fibers often have a characteristic 64-nm periodicity that is visible in longitudinal sections.

Recently, two new structures have been described in the subbasal lamina fibrous zone. One of these is named anchoring plaques[19] and consists of 200×170 nm, electron-dense globules. These form attachment sites for the anchoring fibrils in the region below the lamina densa. Both the lamina densa and the anchoring plaques contain type IV collagen. The other new component is named microthreadlike fibers. These fibers are the thin strands of material that link together the anchoring fibrils, elastin microfibrils, and the small collagen fibers.[20-22] The microthreadlike fibers stain with the ruthenium red stain similar to glycoproteins and contain the noncollagenous protein linkin. They are located not only in the subbasal lamina fibrous zone but also high in the papillary dermis.[22]

Two other components have been identified in the basement membrane region. Fine and Couchman[23] identified a proteoglycan containing chondroitin-6-sulfate in the lamina densa by immunoelectron microscopy. This was present along the DEJ and within vascular and adnexal basement membranes. Basic fibroblast growth factor has also been shown to be stored or at least bound within the basement membrane. This important growth factor has been found to be bound to heparan sulfate and is released by heparin or by heparanase.[24,25]

During normal fetal development, the basement membrane zone converts from a flattened to an interdigitated morphology by the third month of fetal life.[26] The lamina densa can be detected ultrastructurally in the first month of life. However, hemidesmosomes are not found until the third month. This is important for prenatal diagnosis, for example, of epidermolysis bullosa of the junctional type in which hemidesmosomes are decreased in number.[27] Anchoring fibrils are present by the third month so that their decrease can be appreciated in fetal skin biopsies of recessive dystrophic epidermolysis bullosa at that time.[26,27]

Biochemical detection of basement membrane components during fetal life indicated that type IV collagen, laminin, and fibronectin are all present in the basement membrane in the first month of life. By the third to fourth month, the bullous pemphigoid antigen, associated with the hemidesmosomes, can be detected. By the ninth week, type VII collagen and banded anchoring fibrils appear.[26,27] Anchoring fibrils are more abundant in the region of the hemidesmosomes than in the intervening regions of the lamina densa.[28] Knowledge concerning the biology of developing fetal skin is important in prenatal diagnosis of certain genetic skin diseases.[29]

Biochemistry of the Cutaneous Basement Membrane

Until the late 1970s, the cutaneous basement membrane zone (BMZ) was defined only by light and electron microscopy. During the early 1980s, great strides were made in defining the biochemical nature of the BMZ due to the discovery of a murine, transplantable tumor called the Engelbreath Holm Susarm (EHS) sarcoma that synthesized large amounts of native BMZ components that could be extracted in native form. Most of these components have been well characterized such as laminin, heparan sulfate proteoglycan, nidogen-entactin, type IV collagen, and type VII collagen.[30,31] In addition, with the advent of monoclonal antibody technology, there has been a proliferation of pure antibodies that bind to specific components of the BMZ but are not well characterized biochemically. These include AF1, AF2, GB3, KF1, and AA3.[32] Although the biochemical targets for these antibodies are often poorly understood, many of these antibodies have proven useful for the diagnosis of blistering diseases and have a practical utility. In this chapter, only the well-characterized BMZ components will be discussed. These include the bullous pemphigoid antigen, laminin, nidogen-entactin, type IV collagen, heparan sulfate proteoglycan, and type VII collagen (the EBA antigen).

The Bullous Pemphigoid Antigen

Bullous pemphigoid (BP) is a subepidermal blistering disease in which patients have a tissue-bound and plasma antibody against a component of normal skin called the bullous pemphigoid antigen (BPA). These antibodies are immunoglobulin G (IgG) antibodies that fix complement.[33] Recently, Regnier et al.,[34] Westgate et al.,[35] and Klatte et al.,[36] and Mutasim et al.[37] demonstrated that BPA is associated with the basal keratinocyte hemidesmosome. Therefore, the BPA has both intracellular and extracellular components since part of the molecule has been detected within the lamina lucida zone of the BMZ.[38,39] BPA is synthesized by human keratinocytes[40-43] and the number of keratinocytes that stain positive with BP antibodies is identical to the number of basal keratinocytes in the culture.[43] When keratinocytes are maintained in the basal state by keeping the calcium in the cultures very low, there is high expression of BPA by the cells when compared with parallel cultures kept in high calcium.[44] This is because the low calcium culture conditions select for the growth and maintenance of basal keratinocytes over more differentiated keratinocytes. Stanley et al.[42] demonstrated that the BPA can be immunoprecipitated from cell culture with sera from BP patients and demonstrated that the BPA is a noncollagenous glycoprotein with a molecular weight of 220 to 230 kDa. In a second report, Stanley et al.[45] demonstrated that the BPA product synthesized in culture was identical to the BPA extracted from the suction blister roofs from the skin of normal patients. In addition to the 220- to 230-kDa BPA, some BP sera also react with another protein band extracted from keratinocytes with a molecular size between 160 and 180 kDa.[46]. The relationship betweens the 230-kDa antigen and the 180-kDa antigen is unclear. The lower molecular weight species may be a breakdown product from the 230-kDa molecule, or they may be completely distinct entities.

Recently, Stanley and colleagues[47] have identified the gene for the BP antigen. A human keratinocyte cDNA library was made and screened with BP sera. The fusion protein from a clone was labeled with the antibody and this clone was isolated and amplified. The fusion protein from this amplified clone was labeled by all other BP sera tested. When whole BP sera were allowed to absorb to lawns of phage-plaques expressing the BP-fusion protein and then the bound IgG eluted off, affinity purified IgG was recovered with specific affinity to the BP-fusion protein. This IgG stained the DEJ of human skin and immunoprecipitated the 230-kDa BP antigen from keratinocyte cultures. When the cDNA insert that coded for the BP fusion protein was characterized, fragments of 680 and 1500 base pairs were identified. Riboprobes were made to these fragments and Northen analysis performed on total keratinocyte RNA. Both probes hybridized to a 9-kB fragment of mRNA, a fragment large enough to code for a 230-kDa protein. When the cDNA was sequenced, a 1922 base pair reading frame was found. The amino acid sequence deduced from this open reading frame characterized a 76-kDa protein fragment of the BP antigen near the carboxyl terminus that lacks homology with all other proteins.[47] This means that the BPA is a unique constituent of stratified sqamous epithelium. This new probe will be helpful in further studies that are designed to understand the regulation of BP antigen. Hemidesmosomes have been found to be abnormal in some forms of junctional EB.[48] It is conceivable that hemidesmosomal proteins such as BPA may be abnormal in this disease.

Laminin

The BPA shares the lamina lucida space with laminin, another large glycoprotein.[49] Ten to 15 percent of the weight of laminin is made up of carbohydrate.[50] Laminin consists of two chains: a single A chain of 400 kDa and two B chains of about 200 kDa.[51] These chains align themselves into a cruciate structure. The amino acid sequence of each chain is known. Laminin in its native state is about 800 kDa and about 80 nm long.[51] Unlike the BPA, which exists only beneath stratified squamous epithelium, laminin is a component of all BMZs including those around vessels, in the liver, and in the kidney.[1] Laminin is synthesized by both human keratinocytes and fibroblasts.[52,53]

Laminin is a highly biologically active molecule.[30] One of its primary roles is to link other components of the BMZ together in order to form a true tissuelike structure. Laminin has affinity for both type IV collagen (i.e., that collagen within the lamina densa zone, vide infra) and BMZ-specific heparan sulfate proteoglycan.[54] It also binds to nidogen-entactin, another major BMZ glycoprotein discussed in detail below.[55] This affinity for other BMZ components may mean that laminin has a central role in holding together the BMZ structure. In addition to its affinity for other connective tissue components, laminin binds to cell surfaces and laminin receptors have been identified on certain malignant cell lines.[56] Laminin may mediate attachment of certain cells to type IV basement membrane collagen.[57] It appears that a site on the B1 chain of laminin has a specific peptide sequence [-tyrosine-isoleucine-glycine-serine—arginine (YIGSR)] that supports cell attachment.[58] This peptide has been used in a melanoma mouse model to suppress metastasis.[58] When melanoma cells are injected into the tail vein of a mouse, pulmonary metastasis readily occurs. However, if the melanoma cells are first incubated with YIGSR and then injected into the mouse, pulmonary metastases are depressed.[58] It is thought that this is due to the YIGSR peptide binding to the melanoma cell receptor for laminin and covering the receptor. This would render the cell unable to attach to laminin within the BMZ of blood vessels of the mouse host. Without attaching to the BMZ around blood vessels, it is thought that the melanoma cells cannot invade the blood vessels and metastasize into new tissues.[58] In addition to the YIGSR cell attachment site on the B1 chain of laminin, a second cell attachment site has been identified that is an arginine glycine d-aspartic acid (RGD) "integrin" type of sequence.[51]

Laminin may also play a role in stabilizing epidermis on the BMZ.[59] In a guinea pig wound healing models Clark et al.[60] demonstrated that laminin was not reexpressed beneath the reepithelializing epidermis until it had stopped migrating over the wound. Using a human keratinocyte locomotion assay, it was found recently that laminin inhibits keratinocyte locomotion but actually slightly promotes keratinocyte proliferation.[59] In contrast to laminin, fibronectin and collagen markedly enhance keratinocyte locomotion. Laminin is capable of inhibiting "collagen-driven" locomotion.[59] In normal unwounded skin, the keratinocyte rests on a laminin-rich lamina lucida that places the plasma membrane of the basal cell at least 35 nm away from the nearest collagen. Our current hypothesis is that collagens promote keratinocyte migration while laminin inhibits it. These phenomena may play a role in gestational development of the skin and in wound healing. Apposition of the cell to collagen signals the basal keratinocyte to migrate and maintain an undifferentiated "basal" phenotype capable of locomotion and cell division. Apposition to laminin signals the phenotypically identical cell to be stationary and set up a stable epithelium.[59]

Nidogen-entactin

Entactin was described by Carlin et al.[61] and nidogen was discovered by Timpl et al.[62] It turns out that they are the same BMZ component. This component is a noncollagenous glycoprotein that is highly sulfated. About 5% of its molecular mass is carbohydrate. Nidogen-entactin is shaped like a dumbbell with two globular ends separated by a 17-nm rodlike central domain. This component has marked affinity for laminin with which it forms a complex in vitro in addition to some affinity for type IV collagen.[4] Therefore, like laminin, nidogen-entactin may play a role in holding together the BMZ in a unified structure. Caughman et al.[63] have shown by immunoelectron microscopy that nidogen is localized to the lamina densa zone where laminin and type IV collagen meet.

The function of nidogen-entactin is unknown. It has been sequenced and found to have epidermal growth factor (EGF)-like repeats.[61] However, cell growth–promoting properties of the component have not been described. It also has an RGD (arginine-glycine-d-aspartic acid) sequence in the central rodlike domain so it may interact with certain cells.[51] Human keratinocytes have been shown to be able to use nidogen-entactin as a substrate adhesion molecule.[64]

Type IV Collagen

Type IV collagen is a type of collagen found only in BMZs.[1,51] Like laminin, it is found in all BMZs, and like other BMZ components it is a large macromolecule with a molecular mass of about 550 kDa.[1,65] On SDS-polyacrylamide gels run under reducing conditions, two alpha chains (Mr = 185,000 and Mr = 172,000) are identified. Ultrastructural studies have shown that type IV collagen is specifically localized to the lamina densa zone[66] and to anchoring plaques.[19] Human keratinocytes synthesize both laminin and type IV collagen.[52,67] Recently, it was shown that type IV collagen can serve as a substrate attachment factor, a cell spreading factor, and a mitogenic factor for human keratinocytes.[68] In addition, type IV collagen markedly promotes keratinocyte locomotion.[59] All of these studies point to the concept that keratinocytes interact with type IV collagen and likely have a putative "type IV collagen receptor." Second, it should be appreciated that keratinocytes are capable of creating their own BMZ matrix and then interact with this matrix as the particular set of circumstances dictates.

Type IV collagen molecules are shaped like a hockey stick with a ball on one end.[1,69] The ball represents a noncollagen NCI domain at the carboxyl terminus and the blade of the hockey stick represents a 7S collagen domain at the amino terminus that is completely resistant to degradation by collagenase.[70] The 7S domain serves as an aggregation site where four type IV collagen molecules aggregate together like-end to like-end.[69] This alignment creates a series of spider-shaped aggregations that link together into a "chicken wire" scaffold. Side-to-side molecular linking has also been described.[71] This lattice arrangement probably serves to give the lamina densa both tensile strength but yet allows for some flexibility.[1]

Heparan Sulfate Proteoglycan

Proteoglycans are composed of a protein core to which polysaccharide sugar chains (glycosaminoglycans) are covalently attached. Although these molecules are found in the dermis and on the cell surfaces of many cell types, a BMZ-specific heparan sulfate proteoglycan (HSPG) has been described by Hassel and colleagues.[72] Both high density and low density forms of HSPG have been isolated from basement membrane.[51,72,73] The localization of HSPG within the BMZ of skin is a little more diffuse that the other components. The bulk of HSPG is seen within the lamina densa, but some appears to be in the lamina lucida and sublamina densa spaces.[63]

The function of HSPG within the skin BMZ is unknown. Its affinity to other BMZ components may suggest that it plays a role in holding together the BMZ.[54] It is known that HSPG carries a strong anionic charge.[72–74] Moreover, when kidney BMZs are treated with heparinase or heparitinase that degrade HSPG, there are marked alterations in protein filtration. Taken together, it is likely that HSPG within BMZs acts as a charge-dependent permeability barrier for proteins. This would allow some selectivity of what proteins are allowed to traverse the BMZ and come into contact with the basal keratinocytes. This function may determine the growth-promoting or -inhibiting factors from plasma that ultimately influence the avascular epidermis.

Type VII Collagen/EBA Antigen

Anchoring fibrils are rich in type VII collagen,[75,76] the molecular target for autoantibodies in the sera of patients with epidermolysis bullosa acquisita (EBA).[77–79] Type VII collagen chains are 290 kDa in size and align themselves into a triple helix. Therefore, the native type VII collagen molecule is about 900 kDa. About half of the molecule is collagen and about half a noncollagen glycoprotein that is resistant to collagenase degradation.[79,80]

The noncollagen domain is the carboxyl terminus, which is the major antigenic site for EBA antibodies. Both human keratinocytes and dermal fibroblasts synthesize type VII collagen.[81-83] It is not clear if all or part of the type VII collagen molecule is missing in dystrophic epidermolysis bullosa.[84,85] Rusenko et al.[85] showed that the carboxyl domain of the molecule was readily detected by immunofluorescent staining of skin from RDEB with a monoclonal antibody that is specific for the carboxyl domain. Despite this result, it appears that anchoring fibrils are depressed in the skin of patients with RDEB.[86] It may be that some synthesis of type VII collagen occurs but that it is not aligned properly into anchoring fibril structures. Conversely, a molecule that is more susceptible to collagenase degradation may be synthesized by these patients, which again mitigates against the normal number of anchoring fibrils in RDEB skin.

A major protein in the papillary dermis is a large glycoprotein called fibronectin (Mr = 440,000).[50] It has been shown that type VII collagen binds to fibronectin and that this affinity is mediated by the gelatin-binding domain on the fibronectin molecule.[87] Although not directly proven, it has been thought that anchoring fibrils serve literally to "anchor" the epidermis and its BMZ to the papillary dermis. The evidence for this is largely circumstantial and indirect. For example, when burn wounds are covered with transplanted keratinocyte autografts, the healed wounds exhibit fragility and spontaneous blister formation for months at a time when anchoring fibrils within the DEJ are depressed.[13] Likewise, patients with RDEB and EBA have depressed anchoring fibril numbers and associated blistering.[86,88-90] It may be that anchoring fibrils serve to attach the lamina densa structure to the papillary dermis and do this via the affinity of type VII collagen for fibronectin within the papillary dermis.

Type VII collagen is limited to basement membranes beneath stratified squamous epithelium and therefore has the same distribution as BPA. Type VII collagen is aligned within the BMZ into anchoring fibril structures in a precise fashion: one type VII molecule has its noncollagenous carboxyl terminus lodged within the lamina densa. The triple helical collagen portion is aligned perpendicularly within the lamina densa. The distal amino terminus is linked to the amino terminus of a second type VII collagen molecule.[19,76] So, like the type IV collagen lattice, type VII molecules are aligned like-end to like-end. The second molecule's globular carboxyl terminus is lodged within an anchoring plaque.[19] Numerous dimeric forms of type VII collagen are aligned perpendicularly to the lamina densa and laterally aggregated near the amino termini contacts of each dimer.[19,76] This probably accounts for the cross-banded "wheat stack" appearance of anchoring fibrils. This arrangement plus the additional contacts between components created by microthreadlike fibers (vide infra) makes the sublamina densa space very resistant to fracture. We know of no in vitro method to consistently create a sublamina densa separation between the epidermis and dermis. In contrast, this area may be fractured in certain disease states such as RDEB and EBA.

Linkin

Microthreadlike fibers have been described recently in human skin.[20-22] These fibers stain with ruthenium red and have a delicate wispy appearance within the papillary dermis when viewed with an electron microscope. Each fiber is about 90 nm in length and can be seen traversing the spaces between anchoring fibrils, single collagen fibrils, and elastic microfibrils. A new monoclonal antibody to microthreadlike fibers has been developed.[20-22] Using this antibody, two microthreadlike fiber proteins have been identified by immunoprecipitation from fibroblast cultures and by Western blot analysis of proteins extracted from human skin BMZ. These two noncollagenous proteins are 83 kDa and 73 kDa in size and have been termed "linkin." The role of linkin in human skin is unknown. The expression of linkin is usually confined to the upper papillary dermis in normal skin but is found diffuse in the "neodermis" beneath a healing wound.[91] It may be that linkin acts as a kind of "glue" that holds connective tissue components together within a healing wound bed.

Summary

It must be realized that the BMZ is a tissue composite of multiple different connective tissue molecules. Each component of the BMZ discussed above has its own literature. An understanding of the biology and biochemistry of each component will give us insight into the pathomechanisms of subepidermal blistering diseases. Although not proven, it is likely that some of the hereditary subepidermal bullous diseases are the result of perturbed or poorly developed BMZ components.

References

1. Stanley JR, Woodley DT, Katz SI, Martin GR. The structure and function of basement membrane. *J Invest Dermatol.* 1982;79:69–72.
2. Briggaman RA, Wheeler CE. The epidermal–dermal junction. *J Invest Dermatol.* 1975;65:71–84.
3. Woodley DT. The importance of the dermal-epidermal junction and recent advances. *Dermatologica.* 1987;174:1–10.
4. Lavker RM, and Sun TT. Heterogeneity in epidermal basal keratinocytes: morphological and functional correlations. *Science.* 1982;215:1239–1241.
5. Delvoye P, Pierard D, Noel A, Nusgens B, Foidart JM, Lapiere CM. Fibroblasts induce assembly of the micromolecules of the basement membrane. *J Invest Dermatol.* 1988;90:276–282.
6. Kelly DE. Fine structure of desmosomes, hemidesmosomes, and an adepidermal globular layer in developing newt epidermis. *J Cell Biol.* 1966;28:51–72.
7. Shienvold FL, Kelly DE. The desmosome: new fine structural features revealed by freeze-fracture techniques. *Cell Tissue Res.* 1976;172:289–307.

8. Ellison J, Garrod DR. Anchoring filaments of the amphibian epidermal–dermal junction traverse the basal lamina entirely from the plasma membrane of hemidesmosomes to the dermis. *J Cell Sci.* 1984;72:163–172.

9. McNutt NS. Ultrastructural comparison of the interface between epithelium and stroma in basal cell carcinoma and control human skin. *Lab Invest.* 1976;35:132–142.

10. Heaphy MR, Winkelmann RK. The human cutaneous basement membrane-anchoring fibril complex: preparation and ultrastructure. *J Invest Dermatol.* 1977;68:177–186.

11. Krawczyk WS, Wilgram GF. Hemidesmosome and desmosome morphogenesis during epidermal wound healing. *J Ultrastruct Res.* 1973;45:93–101.

12. Gabbiani G, Chapponnier C, Huttner I. Cytoplasmic filaments and gap junctions in epithelial cells and myofibroblasts during wound healing. *J Cell Biol.* 1978;76:561–568.

13. Woodley DT, Peterson HD, Herzok SR, et al. Burn wounds resurfaced by cultured epidermal autografts show abnormal reconstitution of anchoring fibrils. *JAMA.* 1988;259:2566–2571.

14. Compton CC, Gill JM, Bradford DA, Regauer S, Gallico GG, O'Connor NE. Skin regenerated from cultured epithelial autografts on full-thickness burn wounds from 6 days to 5 years after grafting. A light, electron microscope and immunohistochemical study. *Lab Invest.* 1989;60:600–612.

15. Yurchenco PD, Ruben GC. Basement membrane structure in situ: evidence for lateral associations in the type IV collagen network. *J Cell Biol.* 1987;105:2559–2568.

16. Palade GE, Farquhar MG. A special fibril of the dermis. *J Cell Biol.* 1965;27:215–214.

17. Bruns RR. A symmetrical extracellular fibril. *J Cell Biol.* 1969;42:418–430.

18. Kawanami O, Ferrans VJ, Roberts WC, Crystal RG, Fulmer JD. Anchoring fibrils: a new connective tissue structure in fibrotic lung disease. *Am J Pathol.* 1978;92:389–410.

19. Keene DR, Sakai LY, Lunstrum GP, Morris NP, Burgeson RE. Type VII collagen forms an extended network of anchoring fibrils. *J Cell Biol.* 1987;104:611–621.

20. Yoshiike T, Briggaman RA, Woodley DT, Gammon WR, Cronce DJ. Identification and partial characterization of a microthread-like filamentous network beneath human skin basement membrane zone. *J Invest Dermatol.* 1988;90:620.

21. Yoshiike T, Briggaman RA, Woodley DT, Gammon WR, Cronce DJ. Linkin, a newly recognized component of extracellular matrix associated with microthread-like filamentous network beneath stratified squamous epithelium. *J Invest Dermatol.* 1992 (in press).

22. Briggaman RA, Yoshiike T, Woodley DT, Gammon WR, Cronce DJ. Linkin, a newly recognized component of extracellular matrix associated with microthread-like filamentous network beneath stratified squamous epithelium. *J Cell Biol.* 1988;107:590a.

23. Fine JD, Couchman JR. Chondroitin-6-sulfate-containing proteoglycan: a new component of human skin dermoepidermal junction. *J. Invest Dermatol.* 1988;90:283–288.

24. Folkman, J, Klagsbrun M, Sasse J, Wadzinski M, Ingber D, Vlodavsky I. A heparin-binding angiogenic protein—basic fibroblast growth factor—is stored within basement membrane. *Am J Pathol.* 1988;130:393–400.

25. Gonzalez A-M, Buscaglia M, Ong M, Baird A. Distribution of basic fibroblast growth factor in the 18-day rat fetus: localization in the basement membranes of diverse tissues. *J Cell Biol*. 1990;110:753–765.
26. Smith LI, Sakai LY, Burgeson RE, Holbrook KA. Ontogeny of structural components at the dermal–epidermal junction in human embryonic and fetal skin: the appearance of anchoring fibrils and type VII collagen. *J Invest Dermatol*. 1988; 90:480–485.
27. Lane AT, Helm KF, Goldsmith LA. Identification of bullous pemphigoid, pemphigus, laminin and anchoring fibril antigens in human fetal skin. *J Invest Dermatol*. 1985;84:27–30.
28. Eady RAJ. The basement membrane. Interface between the epithelium and the dermis: structural features. *Arch Dermatol*. 1988;124:709–712.
29. Holbrook KA. The biology of human fetal skin at ages related to prenatal diagnosis. *Pediatr Dermatol*. 1983;1:97–111.
30. Kleinman HK, Klebe RJ, Martin GR. Role of collagenous matrices in the adhesion and growth of cells. *J Cell Biol*. 1981;88:473–485.
31. Timpl R, Martin GR: Components of basement membranes. In: Furthmayr H, ed. *Immunochemistry of the Extracellular Matrix*. vol. II. Fla: Boca Raton; CRC Press.
32. Fine JD. The skin basement membrane zone. In: Callen JP, ed. *Advances in Dermatology*. vol 2. Chicago: Year Book Medical Publisher; 1987:283–304.
33. Jordon RE, Beutner EH, Witebsy E, Blumental G, Hale WL, Lever WF. Basement membrane zone antibodies in bullous pemphigoid. *JAMA*. 1967;200:751–756.
34. Regnier M, Vaigot P, Michel S, Prunieras M. Localization of bullous pemphigoid antigen in isolated human keratinocytes. *J Invest Dermatol*. 1985;85:187–190.
35. Westgate GE, Weaver AC, Couchman JR. Bullous pemphigoid antigen localization suggests an intracellular association with hemidesmosomes. *J Invest Dermatol*. 1985;84:218–244.
36. Klatle DH, Kurpakus MA, Grelling KA, Jones JCR. Immunochemical characterization of three components of the hemisdesmosomes and their expression in cultured epithelial cells. *J Cell Biol*. 1989;109:3377–3390.
37. Mutasim DF, Takahashi Y, Ramzy LS, Anhalt GJ, Patel HP, Diaz LA. A pool of bullous pemphigoid antigen(s) is intracellular and associated with the basal cell cytoskeleton-hemidesmosome complex. *J Invest Dermatol*. 1985;84:47–53.
38. Schaumburg-Lever G, Rule RA, Schmidt-Ullrich B, Lever WF. Ultrastructural localization of *in vivo* bound immunoglobulins in bullous pemphigoid: a preliminary report. *J Invest Dermatol*. 1975;64:47–49.
39. Holubar K, Wolff K, Konrad K, Beutner EH. Ultrastructural localization of immunoglobulins in bullous pemphigoid skin. *J Invest Dermatol*. 1975;64:220–227.
40. Woodley DT, Regnier M. Bullous pemphigoid antigen deposited on a millipore filter. *Arch Dermatol Res*. 1979;266:319–322.
41. Woodley DT, Didierjean L, Regnier M, Saurat JH, Prunieras M. Bullous pemphigoid antigen synthesized in vitro by human epidermal cells. *J Invest Dermatol*. 1980;75:148–151.
42. Stanley JR, Hawley-Nelson P, Yuspa SH, Shevach EM, Katz SI. Characterization of bullous pemphigoid antigen: a unique basement membrane protein of stratified squamous epithelia. *Cell*. 1981;24:897–904.

43. Woodley DT, Saurat JH, Prunieras M, Regnier M. Pemphigoid, pemphigus, and Pr antigens in human keratinocytes grown on nonviable substrates. *J Invest Dermatol.* 1982;79:23–29.

44. Stanley JR, Yuspa SH. Specific epidermal protein markers are modulated during calcium-induced terminal differentiation. *J Cell Biol.* 1983;96:1809–1814.

45. Stanley JR, Woodley DT, Katz SI. Identification and partial characterization of pemphigoid antigen extracted from normal skin. *J Invest Dermatol.* 1984;82:108–111.

46. Labib RS, Anhalt GJ, Patel HP, Mutasim DF, Diaz LA. Molecular heterogeneity of the bullous pemphigoid antigens as detected by immunoblotting. *J Immunol.* 1986;136:1231–1234.

47. Stanley JR, Tanaka T, Mueller S, Klaus-Kovtun V, Roop D. Isolation of complementary DNA for bullous pemphigoid antigen by use of patients' autoantibodies. *J Clin Invest.* 1988;82:1864–1870.

48. Tidman MJ, Eady RAF. Hemidesmosome heterogeneity in junctional epidermolysis bullosa revealed by morphometric analysis. *J Invest Dermatol.* 1986;86:51–56.

49. Timpl R, Rohde H, Gehron-Robey P, Rennard SI, Foidart J-M, Martin GR. Laminin—a glycoprotein from basement membrane. *J Biol Chem.* 1979;254:9933–9937.

50. Yamada KM. Fibronectin and other structural proteins, In: Hay ED, ed. *Cell Biology of Extracellular Matrix.* New York: Plenum Press, 1983:95–110.

51. Timpl R. Structure and biological activity of basement membrane proteins. *Eur J Biochem.* 1989;180:487–502.

52. Stanley JR, Hawley-Nelson P, Yaar M, Martin GR, Katz SI. Laminin and bullous pemphigoid antigen are distinct basement membrane proteins synthesized by epidermal cells. *J Invest Dermatol.* 1982;78:456–459.

53. Woodley DT, Stanley JR, Reese MJ, O'Keefe EJ. Human dermal fibroblasts synthesize laminin. *J Invest Dermatol.* 1988;90:679–683.

54. Woodley DT, Rao CN, Hassell JR, Liotta LA, Martin GR, Kleinman HK. Interactions of basement membrane components. *Biochim Biophys Acta.* 1983;761:278–283.

55. Paulsson M, Aumailley M, Deutzmann R, Timpl R, Beck K, Engel J. Laminin-nidogen complex: extraction with chelating agents and structural characterization. *Eur J Biochem.* 1987;166:11–19.

56. Gehlsen KR, Dillner L, Engvall E, Ruoslahti E. The human laminin receptor is a member of the integrin family of cell adhesion receptors. *Science.* 1988;241:1228–1229.

57. Terranova VP, Rohrbach DH, Martin GR. Role of laminin in the attachment of PAM 212 (epithelial) cells to basement membrane collagen. *Cell.* 1980;22:719–726.

58. Iwamoto Y, Robey FA, Graf J, Sasaki M, Kleinman HK, Yamada Y, Martin GR. YIGSR, a synthetic laminin pentapeptide, inhibits experimental metastasis formation. *Science.* 1987;238:1132–1134.

59. Woodley DT, Bachmann PM, O'Keefe EJ. Laminin inhibits human keratinocyte migration. *J Cell Physiol.* 1988;136:140–146.

60. Clark RAF, Lanigan JM, Della Pelle P, Manseau E, Dvorak HF, Colvin RB. Fibronectin and fibrin provide a provisional matrix for cell migration during wound re-epithelialization. *J Invest Dermatol.* 1982;70:264–269.

61. Carlin B, Jaffe R, Binder B: Entactin, a novel basal lamina-associated sulfated glycoprotein. *J Biol Chem.* 1981;256:5209–5214.
62. Timpl R, Dziadek M, Fujiwara W, Nowack H, Wick H. Nidogen: a new self-aggregating basement membrane protein. *Eur J Biochem.* 1983;137:455–465.
63. Caughman SW, Krieg T, Timpl R, Hintner H, Katz SI. Nidogen and heparan sulfate proteoglycan: detection of newly isolated basement membrane components in normal and epidermolysis bullosa skin. *J Invest Dermatol.* 1987;89:547–550.
64. Alstadt SP, Hebda PA, Chung AE, Eaglstein WH. The enhancement of epidermal cell attachment by basement membrane entactin. *J Invest Dermatol.* 1985;84:353.
65. Timpl R, Martin GR, Bruckner P, Wick G, Wiedmann H. Nature of the collagenous proteins in a tumor basement membrane. *Eur J Biochem.* 1978;84:43–52.
66. Yaoita H, Foidart JM, Katz SI. Localization of the collagenous component of skin basement membrane. *J Invest Dermatol.* 1978;70:191–193.
67. Petersen MJ, Woodley DT, O'Keefe EJ. Cultured human keratinocytes synthesize and secrete type IV procollagen. *Clin Res.* 1988;36:378A.
68. Woodley DT, Wynn KC, O'Keefe EJ. Type IV collagen and fibronectin enhance human keratinocyte thymidine incorporation and spreading in the absence of soluble growth factors. *J Invest Dermatol.* 1990;94:130–143.
69. Timpl R, Wiedemann H, Van Delden V, Furthmayr H, Kuhn K. A network model for the organization of type IV collagen molecules in basement membranes. *Eur J Biochem.* 1981;120:203–211.
70. Timpl R, Risteli J, Bachinger HP: Identification of a new basement membrane collagen by the aid of a large fragment resistant to bacterial collagenase. *FEBS Lett.* 1979;101:265–268.
71. Yurchenko PD, Furthmayr H. Self-assembly of basement membrane collagen. *Biochemistry.* 1984;23:1839–1850.
72. Hassel JR, Gehron Robey P, Barrach HJ, Wilczer J, Rennard SI, Martin GR. Isolation of a heparan sulfate containing proteoglycan from basement membrane. *Proc Natl Acad Sci USA.* 1980;77:4494–4498.
73. Hassel JR, Leyshon WC, Ledbetter SR, et al. Isolation of two forms of basement membrane proteoglycans. *J Biol Chem.* 1985;260:8098–8105.
74. Farquhar MG, Courtoy PJ, Lemkin MC, Kanwar YS: In: Kuhn K, Shoene HH, Timpl R, eds. *New Trends in Basement Membrane Research.* New York: Raven Press; 1982:9–29.
75. Sakai LY, Keene DR, Morris NP, Burgeson RE. Type VII collagen is a major structural component of anchoring fibrils. *J Cell Biol.* 1986;103:1577–1586.
76. Lunstrum GP, Sakai LY, Keene DR, Morris NP, Burgeson RE. Large complex globular domains of type VII procollagen contribute to the structure of anchoring fibrils. *J Biol Chem.* 1986;261:9042–9048.
77. Woodley DT, Briggaman RA, O'Keefe EJ, Inman AO, Queen LL, Gammon WR. Identification of the skin basement membrane antoantigen in epidermolysis bullosa acquisita. *N Eng J Med.* 1984;310:1007–1013.
78. Woodley DT, Burgeson RE, Lundstrum G, Bruckner-Tuderman L, Reese MJ, Briggaman RA. The epidermolysis bullosa acquisita antigen is the globular carboxyl terminus of type VII procollagen. *J Clin Invest.* 1988;81:683–687.
79. Yoshiike T, Woodley DT, Briggaman RA. Epidermolysis bullosa acquisita antigen; relationship between the collagenase-sensitive and -insensitive domains. *J Invest Dermatol.* 1988;90:127–133.

80. Woodley DT, O'Keefe EJ, Reese MJ, Mechanic GL, Briggaman RA, Gammon WR. Epidermolysis bullosa acquisita antigen, a new major component of cutaneous basement membrane, is a glycoprotein with collagenous domains. *J Invest Dermatol.* 1986;86:668–672.
81. Woodley DT, Briggaman RA, Gammon WR, O'Keefe EJ. Epidermolysis bullosa acquisita antigen is synthesized by human keratinocytes cultured in serum-free medium. *Biochem Biophys Res Commum.* 1985;130:1267–1272.
82. Woodley DT, Briggaman RA, Falk RJ, et al. Epidermolysis bullosa acquisita antigen, a major cutaneous basement membrane component, is synthesized by human dermal fibroblasts and other cutaneous tissues. *J Invest Dermatol.* 1986; 87:227–231.
83. Stanley JR, Rubinstein N, Klaus-Kortun V. Epidermolysis bullosa acquisita antigen is synthesized by both human keratinocytes and human dermal fibroblasts. *J Invest Dermatol.* 1985;85:542–545.
84. Bruckner-Tuderman L, Ruegger S, Odermatt B, Mitsuhashi Y, Schnyder UW. Lack of type VII collagen in unaffected skin of patients with severe recessive dystrophic epidermolysis bullosa. *Dermatologica.* 1988;176:57–64.
85. Rusenko KW, Gammon WR, Fine JD, Briggaman RA. The carboxyl-terminal domain of type VII collagen is present at the basement membrane in recessive dystrophic epidermolysis bullosa. *J Invest Dermatol.* 1989;92:623–627.
86. Briggaman RA, Wheeler CE. Epidermolysis bullosa dystrophica-recessive: a possible role of ancoring fibrils in the pathogenesis. *J Invest Dermatol.* 1975;65:203–211.
87. Woodley DT, O'Keefe EJ, McDonald JA, Reese MJ, Briggaman RA, Gammon WR. Specific affinity between fibronectin and the epidermolysis bullosa acquisita (EBA) antigen. *J Clin Invest.* 1987;79:1826–1830.
88. Hashimoto I, Schnyder UW, Anton-Lamprecht I, et al. Ultrastructural studies in epidermolysis bullosa hereditaria: III. Recessive dystrophic types with dermolytic blistering (Hallopeau-Siemens types and inverse types). *Arch Dermatol Res.* 1976;256:137–150.
89. Tidman MJ, Eady RA. Evaluation of anchoring fibrils and other components of the dermal-epidermal junction in dystrophic epidermolysis bullosa by a quantitative ultrastructural technique. *J Invest Dermatol.* 1985;84:374–376.
90. Briggaman RA. Is there any specificity to defects of anchoring fibrils in epidermolysis bullosa dystrophica, and what does this mean in terms of pathogenesis? *J Invest Dermatol.* 1985;84:371–373.
91. Woodley DT, Briggaman RA, Herzog SR, Meyers AA, Peterson HD, O'Keefe EJ. Characterization of neo-dermis formation beneath cultured human epidermal autografts transplanted on muscle fascia. *J Invest Dermatol.* 1990;95:20–26.

3
Pathology and Pathogenesis of Epidermolysis Bullosa

Jo-David Fine

At least 23 distinctive phenotypes of inherited epidermolysis bullosa (EB) have now been reported; more undoubtedly exist.[1-5] Despite that, each can be separated into one of three broad groups—simplex, junctional, and dystrophic EB—based on shared pathologic features. These specific ultrastructural findings are in some forms of EB accompanied by selective defects in expression of basement membrane or epidermal cell surface antigens or epitopes.

In this chapter, effort will be made to describe the pathologic features in each of the major forms of inherited EB and to discuss these findings in the context of other studies that have been performed to address pathogenesis of mechanical fragility and blister formation in this disease.

Pathology

The classification of each of the three major forms of inherited EB is based on differences in the ultrastructural levels in skin within which blisters develop after minor or seemingly insignificant mechanical trauma.[6,7] Such levels can be determined by either transmission electron microscopy or a specialized indirect immunofluorescence technique ("immunofluorescence antigenic mapping").

Light and Transmission Electron Microscopy

Even in clinically more localized forms of EB, the entire skin surface has potential mechanical fragility due to inherent structural abnormalities. As such, characteristic cleavage planes can be produced in clinically uninvolved skin from patients with more severe forms of EB during the course of harvesting the biopsy itself. In milder or more localized forms, skin cleavage planes can still be visualized if the biopsy site is first gently subjected to mild rotary traction. In general, biopsies obtained in the above manner are preferred to those taken from lesional sites since additional artifactual clefts at other ultrastructural levels occasionally may be observed if the lesion is old, due to the release of proteases from injured keratinocytes.

The findings by routine light microscopy are often misleading or uninterpretable. For example, whereas lower intraepidermal vesicle formation may be detectable in some lesional specimens from patients with EB simplex, especially when disease activity is more generalized, cleavage may appear to be subepidermal in other specimens later proven to be intraepidermal by transmission electron microscopy. Similarly, although light microscopy correctly suggests subepidermal cleavage in specimens from patients with junctional and dystrophic forms of EB, conventional special stains do not permit accurate differentiation of intralamina lucida from sublamina densa clefts. As such, routine light microscopic examination is not recommended in the diagnostic evaluation of patients with any of the inherited forms of EB.

As summarized in Table 3.1, various subsets of EB can be distinguished by their ultrastructural level of skin separation and the presence or absence of associated structural features.[7] Intraepidermal cleavage occurs in all forms of EB simplex.[8] In the most localized form, the Weber-Cockayne variant,

TABLE 3.1. Ultrastructural features of inherited epidermolysis bullosa.

Type of inherited EB	Site of skin cleavage	Associated morphologic finding
EB simplex (except EB simplex superficialis)	Within or just above the level of the basilar keratinocytes	Basilar or suprabasilar keratinocyte cytolysis
EB simplex superficialis	Within or just beneath the level of the stratum granulosum	None
EB herpetiformis (Dowling-Meara variant)	Within the level of the basilar keratinocytes	Clumped tonofilaments (within basilar keratinocytes)
Junctional EB, generalized, Herlitz variant	Intralamina lucida	Rudimentary appearing and/or markedly reduced (or even undetectable) hemidesmosomes (HD) Reduced number or absence of subbasal dense plates (SBDP)
Junctional EB, generalized, non-Herlitz variant	Intralamina lucida	Normal or reduced numbers of HD and SBDP
Dominant dystrophic EB, generalized	Sublamina densa	Normal or reduced numbers of anchoring fibrils (AF)
Dominant dystrophic EB, transient bullous dermolysis of the newborn variant	Sublamina densa	Reduced numbers of AF Perinuclear intracytoplasmic electron dense inclusion ("stellate") bodies (primarily within basilar and suprabasilar keratinocytes) Amorphous perinuclear deposits of type VII collagen
Recessive dystrophic EB, generalized	Sublamina densa	Markedly reduced numbers of absence of AF

cytolysis occurs within suprabasilar or basilar keratinocytes; with time, lesions exhibit suprabasilar or basilar clefting, with scattered intact keratinocytes still attached to the basement membrane zone. Similarly, in one of the more generalized forms of EB simplex, the Köbner variant, blisters begin with basilar keratinocyte cytolysis; when extensive blistering occurs, only occasional remnants of cell membranes may be detectable on an otherwise denuded basement membrane, explaining the frequent false light microscopic appearance of subepidermal cleavage in such specimens. In addition to intraepidermnal vesiculation, in one of the rarer and more severe forms of EB simplex (EB herpetiformis; generalized EB simplex of the Dowling-Meara variant), diagnostic clumping of tonofilaments has been observed.[9,10] Although an apparently specific finding in the Dowling-Meara variant, the sensitivity (i.e., frequency of occurrence) in random biopsies from such patients is as yet unknown.

Skin cleavage occurs within the level of the lamina lucida in all forms of junctional Eb.[11-15] As such, an intact epidermis forms the roof and a lamina densa–covered dermis comprises the base of an induced or spontaneous blister. In more severe forms, such as the gravis variant (EB atrophicans generalisata gravis; Herlitz disease; EB letalis), hemidesmosomes may be rudimentary in appearance, markedly diminished in number, or even absent. Subbasal dense plates may be correspondingly undetectable. In contrast, in more attenuated forms of junctional EB the hemidesmosomes may appear normal and/or be present in apparent normal numbers, although there may be considerable variability in these latter findings.

Blisters develop beneath the level of the lamina densa in both dominant and recessive dystrophic EB.[16-20] In the former, anchoring fibrils may be reduced in numbers whereas they may be virtually absent in recessive dystrophic EB skin.[20,21] Associated dermal collagenolysis may also be observed in some dystrophic EB skin specimens. In one rare variant of dominant dystrophic EB ("transient bullous dermolysis of the newborn") characterized by a tendency for cessation of blister activity within the first year of life, an additional feature is the presence of electron-dense stellate-shaped bodies in perinuclear array within primarily basilar keratinocytes.[22,23]

Diagnostic Immunopathology

Direct immunofluorescence is negative in all specimens from patients with inherited EB, consistent with the lack of significant autoimmunity in this disease.[24]

Several years ago an indirect immunofluorescence staining technique ("immunofluorescence or antigenic mapping") was described using polyclonal antibodies to three well characterized skin basement membrane components—bullous pemphigoid antigen, laminin, and type IV collagen—which differ from one another not only by their biochemical composi-

TABLE 3.2. Patterns of antibody binding in immunofluorescence mapping studies.

| | Site of binding of antibodies (within induced cleft) to: | | |
EB type	Bullous pemphigoid antigen	Laminin	Type IV collagen
EB simplex	Base	Base	Base
Junctional EB	Roof	Base	Base
Dystrophic EB	Roof	Roof	Roof

tion but also by their ultrastructural localization in normal human skin.[25] Bullous pemphigoid antigen is closely associated with hemidesmosomes,[26,27] whereas laminin[28-31] and type IV collagen[32] reside within the lower lamina lucida and/or lamina densa, and lamina densa, respectively. Due to these latter spatial differences, it is possible to differentiate intraepidermal, intra-lamina lucida, and sublamina densa cleavage planes rapidly, and therefore the type of EB present, in unfixed skin specimens stained with combinations of these antibodies. Results of such a study are summarized in Table 3.2 and are schematically illustrated in Figure 3.1. When this simple diagnostic technique was originally reported in 14 patients, correlation was 100% accurate with electron microscopic findings.[25] Since that time our laboratory has performed more than 450 immunofluorescence mapping studies, and has yet to find discordance with electron microscopy.

The major advantages of immunofluorescence mapping over electron microscopy are cost and rapidity. In addition, such unfixed tissue specimens may be later evaluated by more specialized monoclonal antibodies that are capable of generating additionally useful diagnostic information, as will be discussed elsewhere in this chapter. Although inherent technical difficulties related to specificities of some of the antibodies currently commercially available and occasional subtleties in interpretation suggest that mapping studies be best performed in only a few selected laboratories having extensive experience in this technique, the widespread availability of routine immunofluorescence transport media should make these studies available to any physician familiar with obtaining biopsies for routine diagnostic direct immunofluorescence. In contrast, quality transmission electron microscopy is costly, labor intensive, and dependent on specimens that have been properly preserved and forwarded in specialized fixatives to laboratories experienced in their processing and interpretation. Despite that, transmission electron microscopy is the only technique by which certain associated features, particularly clumped tonofilaments and stellate inclusion bodies. can be directly visualized. Furthermore, morphometric analysis of specific basement membrane–associated structures (i.e., anchoring fibrils, subbasal dense plates, hemidesmosomes) [20,21,33,34] can be obtained only through transmission electron microscopy.

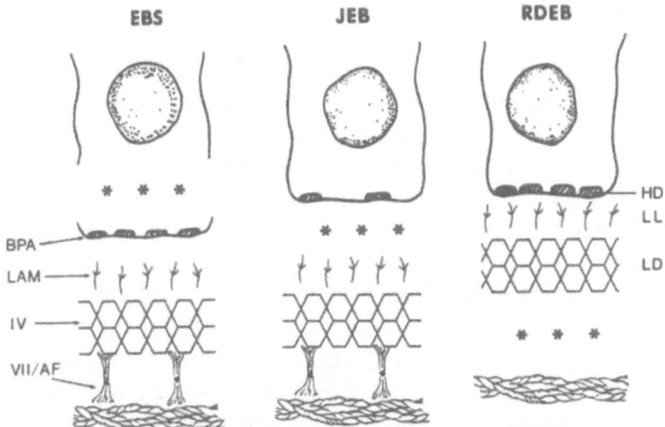

FIGURE 3.1. Schematic diagram of lesional skin in EB simplex (*EBS*), junctional EB (*JEB*), and recessive dystrophic EB (*RDEB*). Asterisks denote the ultrastructural level of blister formation in each of these major EB subtypes [i.e., within the basilar keratinocyte in EBS, within the lamina lucida (*LL*) in JEB, and beneath the lamina densa (*LD*) in RDEB]. AF, anchoring fibrils; note their absence in RDEB skin. Four of the most commonly assessed basement membrane components—bullous pemphigoid antigen (*BPA*), laminin (*LAM*), type IV collagen (*IV*), and type VII collagen (*VII*)—are schematically illustrated within their site of localization in normal skin.

Pathogenesis

Role of Collagenase

The first reported in vitro functional abnormality in inherited EB was the presence of elevated levels of whole skin- and dermal fibroblast-derived collagenase; this was convincingly demonstrated to be the result of enhanced synthesis of this enzyme.[35-41] Initially observed only in recessive dystrophic EB, similar findings have now also been described in occasional patients with junctional EB.[42,43] As will be discussed more comprehensively elsewhere in this volume (chapter 4), this enzyme has increased thermolability and decreased calcium affinity. Such elevated collagenase synthesis can be reduced in vitro and in vivo by phenytoin, correlating with the clinical improvement seen in some[44] but not all[45] patients following administration of this drug. This particular collagenase appears to degrade only selective types of skin collagen, possibly explaining why type IV collagen appears to be present in normal amounts in recessive dystrophic EB skin basement membrane, whereas anchoring fibrils, composed primarily of type VII collagen,[46] are virtually absent.

Role of Other Tissue-derived Enzymes

The in vitro activity of a second fibroblast-derived enzyme, gelatinolytic protease, has been studied in each of the three forms of EB.[47] In the original report on this enzyme, markedly reduced levels were detected in fibroblast culture supernatants from patients with generalized EB simplex and in about half of the cultures from patients with localized EB simplex. Other investigators, unfortunately, have reported normal gelatinolytic protease levels in all major types of EB.[48] Based on these collective data, it is unclear what role, if any, reduced levels of gelatinolytic protease play in the pathogenesis of EB simplex. For example, it is highly unlikely that altered expression of a matrix-degrading protease directly results in intraepidermal blister formation. However, it is possible that these findings may represent linkage to another cellular defect, such as glycosylation, which may contribute to enhanced keratinocyte dysadhesion.

Other investigators have reported that incubation in tissue culture of normal human skin explants in the presence of blister fluids from patients with simplex, junctional, and dystrophic forms of EB results in the production of intraepidermal, intralamina lucida, and sublamina densa cleavage planes, respectively, thereby reproducing each form of EB in vitro.[49-53] Such findings were not seen if protease inhibitors were added, suggesting the presence of proteases in EB blister fluid that possess remarkable specificity for their ultrastructural site of action. These experiments suggested that the level of blister formation that occurs in each of the forms of EB is the result of the presence and release of specific enzymes, rather than inherent structural defects within such skin. As possible support of the latter, elevated levels of neutral proteases have been detected in skin and blister fluid in some patients.[54] More rigorously performed in vitro studies, however, have not confirmed these former findings.[55] When examined in blinded fashion, multiple levels of skin cleavage were seen with blister fluids from each type of EB, as well as with control blister fluid (including thermal burns). Therefore, it must be concluded that whereas proteases are present in EB blister fluids and may contribute secondarily in a nonspecific manner to the propagation of blisters following injury to the skin, their presence and release do not necessarily define the characteristic level of skin cleavage in any of the forms of inherited EB.

Altered Skin Basement Membrane Antigenicity and EB

At least 17 distinct antigens or antigenic epitopes have been defined in human skin basement membrane zone (dermal–epidermal junction) through the generation of a series of polyclonal and monoclonal antibodies.[56-58] One result of such efforts has been the development of the immunofluorescence mapping technique.[25] More recently, studies have been performed to determine whether any of these epitopes is abnormally expressed in EB skin and

TABLE 3.3. Reported alterations in the expression of specific basement membrane-associated antigens in inherited EB.

Antigen	EBS	JEB	DDEB	RDEB
Type VII collagen				
LH 7:2 epitope	Normal	Normal	Normal	Absent (normal in inversa)
L3d epitope	Normal	Normal	Normal	Reduced
C6-SPG	Normal	Normal	Absent or reduced	Absent
KF-1	Normal	Normal	Reduced	Absent
AF1 and AF2	Normal	Normal	Normal	Absent
AA3	Normal	Reduced or absent	Normal	Normal
GB3 (BM600)	Normal	Variable[a]	Normal	Normal
19-DEJ-1	Normal	Absent	Normal	Absent in 25%

[a] Reduced or absent in Herlitz variant; normal, reduced or absent in non-Herlitz forms.

EBS, EB simplex; JEB, junctional EB; DDEB, dominant dystrophic EB; RDEB, recessive dystrophic EB; C6-SPG, chondroitin 6-sulfate proteoglycan. All other notations refer to names of antigens and their corresponding monoclonal or polyclonal antibodies.

if so, whether the known sites of localization of such epitopes in non-EB skin correlate with either level of skin cleavage or associated morphological findings in any of the forms of EB.[57,59,60] The results of these studies are summarized in Table 3.3. It should be noted that each of the studies described was performed using clinically uninvolved skin from patients with EB, so as to avoid potential artifacts resulting from the release of proteases from injured keratinocytes.

Five ubiquitous antigens—laminin, type IV collagen, entactin-nidogen, heparan sulfate proteoglycan, and LDA-1—have been shown to be expressed normally in the skin of all inherited EB patients.[59,61-63] Similarly, type V collagen appears to be expressed normally in all the major forms of inherited EB.[64] In contrast, several other antigens are abnormally expressed in skin from patients with selected forms of EB, suggesting a possible primary or secondary role of altered basement membrane antigenicity in the pathogenesis of mechanical fragility and blister formation.

KF-1 is a noncollagenous primate- and dermal–epidermal junction (DEJ)-specific antigen defined by monoclonal antibody technique.[65] KF-1 monoclonal antibody was produced by immunization with intact viable human keratinocytes. Its corresponding antigen has been ultrastructurally localized to the lamina densa of normal human skin and the epithelial–connective tissue interface of other stratified squamous epithelial tissues. In human fetal skin, KF-1 is first detectable at approximately 16 gestational weeks.[66] Using this antibody, it has been suggested that a 72-kD molecular weight protein can be identified from a human squamous cell carcinoma cell line[67]; similar findings have not as yet been demonstrated from any other normal or transformed human or primate cell line or tissue extract. KF-1 appears to be normally expressed in the lamina densa of skin from all patients with simplex or junctional forms of EB, consistent with the normal integrity of the lamina densa in skin from such patients.[68] In contrast, clinically normal-appearing skin from patients with dominant and recessive dystrophic EB have been shown to have either reduced amounts or absence of KF-1, as assessed by indirect immunofluorescence technique over a range of antibody titers. However, obligate heterozygote carriers for recessive dystrophic EB could not be identified by this same technique.

At essentially the same time that KF-1 was reported to be aberrantly expressed in dystrophic EB skin, similar work was presented with two monoclonal antibodies, AF1 and AF2, which were produced from extracts of either human stratum corneum or human cervical carcinoma cells.[69] Similar to KF-1, AF1 and AF2 have been shown to be primate- and stratified squamous epithelial–specific, and have been noted to bind exclusively along the DEJ of such tissue. In contrast to KF-1, however, AF1 and AF2 recognize epitopes along the anchoring fibrils rather than a portion of the lamina densa itself. These epitopes are not detectable in human fetal skin until approximately 26 gestational weeks.[70] Similar to KF-1, both AF1 and AF2 are normally expressed in skin from all patients with simplex and junctional EB. In contradistinction to KF-1, however, AF1 and AF2 are absent in recessive dystrophic but are normally expressed in dominant dystrophic EB skin. As such, it is likely that AF1 and AF2 recognize antigens truly distinct from that identified by KF-1 monoclonal antibody.

More recently a monoclonal antibody, referred to as LH 7:2, has been generated that binds along the DEJ and along adnexal but not vascular basement membranes in human skin and selected other squamous epithelial-lined organs.[71] This particular antigen is detectable in the human fetus at approximately 7 to 8 gestational weeks.[72] Ultrastructurally, this antigen appears to reside within the lower portion of the lamina densa. Very recently it has been shown that this monoclonal antibody recognizes a portion of the carboxy terminus of type VII collagen.[73] This epitope is normally expressed in simplex, junctional, and dominant dystrophic EB skin. In contrast, some epitopes of type VII collagen are usually undetectable in skin from patients with generalized recessive dystrophic EB (i.e., gravis variant) and detectable in reduced intensity in specimens from patients with the generalized mitis or more localized forms of recessive dystrophic EB.[72,74-77] The only major exception to the latter is in patients with the inversa variant of recessive dystrophic EB, in whom type VII collagen expression appears to be indistinguishable from that noted in normal control skin.[75,78] Similar lack of staining has been noted with an antibody to a collagenous domain of type VII collagen; immunoblots of extracts from recessive dystrophic EB skin are reportedly negative with the latter antibody probe, suggesting lack of type VII collagen within such skin.

An important finding has been reported recently using a monoclonal antibody (L3d) that recognizes another epitope on the carboxy terminus of type VII collagen.[79] In contrast to findings with LH 7:2 monoclonal antibody and a polyclonal antibody to the helical collagenous domain of type VII collagen,[74,75,77] this most recent study suggests that at least one epitope on the carboxy terminus of type VII collagen is in fact present, although in somewhat reduced amounts, in skin from patients with recessive dystrophic EB. Therefore, it is likely that there may be in recessive dystrophic EB skin an incomplete synthesis of type VII collagen and/or abnormal assembly into intact anchoring fibrils, rather than a total absence of the molecule within skin basement membrane zone. Alternatively, it is possible that these data may indicate degradation of all but small portions of the type VII collagen molecule by the elevated collagenase levels previously demonstrated in skin from such patients.

Two additional epitopes identified by polyclonal or monoclonal antibodies that are of interest in inherited EB are AA3 and GB3 (BM600).[80–82] Both are present as early as 7 to 8 gestational weeks in normal human fetal skin,[83] and have been localized ultrastructurally to the level of the lamina lucida. When EB skin has been examined with each antibody, AA3 showed reduced or absent staining only in junctional EB skin[84]; unfortunately, due to the limited nature of the source of this particular polyclonal antibody (i.e., rabbit), the supply of AA3 is now completely exhausted, thereby preventing its use in any future diagnostic studies. As originally reported in a rather limited series of patients, no binding of GB3 monoclonal antibody was noted in specimens from patients with junctional EB.[85] A subsequent multicenter study confirmed the complete or virtual absence of GB3 staining in Herlitz variant junctional EB specimens; however, normal staining was noted in about half of all non-Herlitz junctional EB patients, suggesting the limitation of GB3 as a reliable diagnostic probe for all forms of junctional disease.[86,87]

It has also been demonstrated that human skin basement membrane zone (to include DEJ, vasculature, and adnexae) contains two distinct groups of proteoglycans—heparan sulfate proteoglycan and chondroitin-6-sulfate proteoglycan.[61,88,89] Whereas the heparan sulfate proteoglycan is expressed in all forms of inherited EB, it has been found that chondroitin-6-sulfate proteoglycan is undetectable in recessive dystrophic EB and reduced in intensity or undetectable in dominant dystrophic EB skin specimens.[61,63] Interestingly, the aberrant expression of chondroitin-6-sulfate proteoglycan is noted solely within the DEJ; that is, vascular and adnexal basement membranes are still recognized by the monoclonal antibody (3B3) specific for this particular proteoglycan even though the DEJ shows no evidence of binding. Multiple interpretations exist to explain the latter findings, since the monoclonal antibody recognizing chondroitin-6-sulfate proteoglycan actually identifies a specific epitope on the carbohydrate side chain rather than the core protein of the proteoglycan. It is possible that basement membranes within human skin contain multiple core proteins bearing chondroitin-6-sulfate, and that only one specific core protein is aberrantly expressed within the DEJ in recessive and dominant dystrophic EB. Alternatively, it is possible that there may be either specific degradation of that carbohydrate side chain in the DEJ from such patients, or that the assembly of that particular proteoglycan is abnormal only within selective skin sites in these two forms of inherited EB.

Most recently, a monoclonal antibody referred to as 19-DEJ-1 has been produced by immunization with intact viable human keratinocytes.[90] Its corresponding antigen is present along the DEJ and in the basement membrane of arrector pili muscles of human skin, as well as in other selected human organs (including cornea). Ultrastructurally, 19-DEJ-1 has been localized to the mid–lamina lucida and is present only underneath hemidesmosomes. This antigen is not expressed until approximately 81 gestational days, closely coinciding with the time of expression of bullous pemphigoid antigen[66] and hemidesmosomes.[91] More recent studies using immunogold technique suggest that this antigen likely resides within the anchoring filament, although further confirmatory studies are still needed. Other data have shown that 19-DEJ-1 is normally expressed in both simplex and dominant dystrophic EB skin.[92,93] In contrast, 19-DEJ-1 is undetectable along the DEJ in all specimens from patients with junctional EB, correlating well with the absence or reduction of hemidesmosomes and/or anchoring filaments in this form of EB. Interestingly, approximately 25% of patients with recessive dystrophic EB also lack expression of this particular antigen,[75] further suggesting the probability that this monoclonal antibody may recognize a filamentous structure, such as the anchoring filament, capable of spanning more than a single ultrastructural region of human skin basement membrane zone. For example, possibly its lack of expression in some recessive dystrophic EB patients relates to abnormal insertion of anchoring filaments.

Finally, it has been shown that both bullous pemphigoid and cicatricial pemphigoid antigens appear to be reduced or absent along the DEJ of skin from some patients with various forms of EB, most notably EB simplex.[94] Since the level of skin cleavage in EB simplex is well above the level of the hemidesmosome and the lamina lucida, the sites of localization for these two antigens, it is unlikely that these findings represent primary structural defects. Instead, such findings presumably are a secondary effect of functionally abnormal basal keratinocytes.

What do these particular findings with monoclonal and polyclonal antibodies suggest, and how can they be used practically for diagnostic purposes? First, it should be emphasized that only selected antigens or antigenic epitopes are abnormally expressed in inherited EB skin, and that the site of ultrastructural localization for each of these antigens in normal skin correlates closely with the level shown to be mechanically fragile in those subsets of inherited EB having abnormal expression of that particular antigen. As such, it is likely that the reduction or absence of at least some of these antigenic epitopes may directly contribute to altered integrity of the DEJ, thereby facilitating blister formation following mechanical trauma. Unfortunately, only some of these particular antigens have been even partially characterized biochemically, thereby making it difficult to ascertain whether we are dealing with multiple distinct antigenic defects or alternatively, abnormal composition of a smaller number of macromolecules containing many of these particular antigenic epitopes. In addition, it is still possible that some or all of the undetectable antigens may be present in reduced amounts in human skin but cannot be recognized by routine immunohistochemical techniques due to either limitations in technique (i.e., indirect immunofluorescence) or an alteration in organization of these macromolecules in EB skin basement membrane zone such that antigenic masking occurs.

Regarding practical application of this information, at least two possibilities exist. First, each of these polyclonal or monoclonal antibodies has been employed as a means of further subclassifying patients with various subsets of inherited EB. Of most importance, the use of immunofluorescence mapping in combination with LH 7:2 or AF1 or AF2 has permitted identification of neonates with dominant dystrophic EB in the absence of positive family pedigree. Similarly, most types of recessive dystrophic EB may be diagnosed shortly after birth, before the development of more characteristic phenotypic features. In addition, at least some of these monoclonal antibodies have now been used for successful prenatal diagnosis or exclusion of junctional and dystrophic forms of EB.[83,95-97] Finally, one or more of these monoclonal antibodies may eventually be used to develop specific probes to permit examination of EB patients by molecular biologic approaches, thereby providing an opportunity to identify structural or regulatory defects at the level of the gene.

Alterations in Fibroblast Contractility

Erlich et al.[98] examined the interaction of human fibroblasts with artificial collagen matrices in vitro.[98] They reported that fibroblasts derived from patients with recessive dystrophic EB were less able to contract collagen matrices than normal human fibroblasts that were placed within an identical microenvironment. However, fibroblast attachment appeared to be normal. Subsequently, these investigators demonstrated that supernatants from biomatrices impregnated with recessive dystrophic EB fibroblasts contained excessive amounts of prostaglandin E2 and cyclic adenosine monophosphate, and that reduction of prostaglandin synthesis with indomethacin resulted in normalization of matrix contraction.[99,100] Unfortunately, more recent work by Eisen et al. suggests that there is a wide range of contractility exhibited by recessive dystrophic EB fibroblasts in vitro; in particular, some showed completely normal activity in tissue culture conditions that were identical to that previously described.[101] As such, these more recent data place into considerable doubt the functional significance and clinical relevance of these previously described findings.

Keratinocyte Lectin Binding Studies

Lectins recognize specific carbohydrate sequences in biologic tissues. Using such immunoreagents, many studies have now been performed addressing various aspects of glycosylation in a variety of cell membranes. Recently a study was reported in which eight affinity-purified fluorescein-conjugated lectins were used as probes for cell surface and basement membrane zone staining of skin specimens from patients with each of the subsets of inherited EB.[102] Whereas normal binding was noted with seven of the lectins, markedly irregular granular binding was noted by peanut agglutinin to epidermal cell membranes in skin specimens only from patients with EB simplex. These findings were noted in patients with both localized and generalized forms of EB simplex, including the Dowling-Meara variant. As such, these findings suggest the possibility of abnormal glycosylation of one or more cell membrane components (glycoproteins, glycolipids) in EB simplex, which could potentially lead to abnormal cell-to-cell interaction within such epidermis, thereby enhancing mechanical fragility and the occurrence of intraepidermal blister formation.

Recombinant Graft Experiments

Many years ago Briggaman and Wheeler described an elegant set of experiments that addressed the origin of anchoring fibrils in normal and EB skin.[103] Epidermis and dermis were separated from specimens from both normal individuals and patients with recessive dystrophic EB. Subsequently the isolated dermis was inverted, placed on a chick chorioallantoic membrane, and then epidermis recombined. All possible combinations were made between normal and abnormal epidermal sheets and dermis. In so doing, it was possible to examine temporally for new basement membrane development, including anchoring fibrils. Whereas the hybrid combination of recessive dystrophic EB epidermis and normal human dermis led to development of anchoring fibrils, anchoring fibrils were absent in all recombinants containing dermis from recessive dystrophic EB skin, regardless of the source of epidermis. These findings clearly demonstrated that anchoring fibrils were a product of dermal fibroblasts, and that they could not be produced or at least visualized in recombinants containing recessive dystrophic EB dermal elements.

Keratin-related Studies

For some time it has been postulated that cytolysis and intraepidermal blister formation in EB simplex may result from a defect in the structure or organization of one or more keratins. Heightened interest in this hypothesis has been spurred by the observation of clumped tonofilaments within keratinocytes in the Dowling-Meara variant of this disease. Earliest attempts at immunohistochemically demonstrating such a defect were unsuccessful.[102,104] However, at that time only a limited number of monoclonal antibodies (i.e., AE1, AE2, and AE3) recognizing major groups of keratins were available for study. Despite this, one group of investigators subsequently reported that keratin intermediate filaments within cultured EB simplex keratinocytes appeared somewhat abnormal in their organization,[105] again raising the possibility of the existence of keratin abnormalities in this major EB group. Recently, Vassar et al. produced transgenic mice that expressed a truncated form of keratin K14. This keratin molecule differed from its normal counterpart by the absence of 135 amino acid residues from its carboxy terminus. Mice expressing this keratin had mechanically fragile skin, developed spontaneous blisters, and died shortly after birth. Ultrastructurally, cytolysis and keratin aggregation were noted within basilar keratinocytes, reminiscent of findings observed in EB simplex skin. In attempting to demonstrate a further correlation with human disease, these investigators then demonstrated that antibodies specific for keratins K14 and K5 bound to those aggregated keratins present within a skin sample from a patient with EB simplex. In further support of the concept of abnormal keratin structure in EB simplex, Bonifas et al.[107] have recently demonstrated in two EB simplex kindreds the linkage of disease to probes in the region of keratin gene clusters located at chromosomes 12q and 17q.

Other Laboratory Studies

Increased amounts of chondroitin sulfate have been noted within skin and urine from a patient with the Pasini variant of dominant dystrophic EB.[108] Fibroblasts from the same EB subtype were shown in tissue culture to contain excessive amounts of sulfated glycosaminoglycans.[109] However, others have been unable to confirm this latter finding.[110]

In one kindred of patients with the generalized (Köbner) variant of EB simplex, a deficiency was reported in the expression of galactosylhydroxylysyl glucosyltransferase, an enzyme involved in the glycosylation of collagen.[111] However, these findings were not present in all of the affected members of this kindred, and abnormal findings were noted in some unaffected members, making the significance of these findings rather unclear. However, taken together with previously described work with specific lectins, this may be yet further evidence of abnormal glycosylation as one possible mechanistic defect in simplex forms of inherited EB.

Using hemagglutination technique, it has been reported that some patients with EB simplex have circulating antibodies to a portion of type IV collagen (collagen C chain).[112] Subsequently, it has been demonstrated that patients with all forms of inherited and acquired EB have an increased frequency of autoantibodies to several extracellular matrix components (collagenous and noncollagenous), whereas no similar findings were noted in patients with two other autoimmune bullous diseases (i.e., bullous pemphigoid, pemphigus vulgaris), normal individuals, or patients being treated for extensive second and third degree thermal injuries.[113] Although it is unlikely that these autoantibodies play a primary role, since only one form of inherited EB (i.e., dystrophic EB) is associated with structural abnormalities in direct apposition to extracellular matrix of the dermis, it is possible that these findings reflect continued and/or excessive secondary injury to connective tissue components, leading to their recognition as foreign proteins and the subsequent generation of autoantibodies.

In one study, α-fetoprotein levels were reported to be elevated in amniotic fluid in patients with EB simplex.[114] Others have reported a similar alteration in amniotic fluid levels of acetylcholinesterase in association with dystrophic EB.[115] Although amniocentesis is not routinely performed in pregnancies at risk for EB simplex, such fluid is available for study in pregnancies at risk for junctional EB. Using samples from 10 of the latter at-risk pregnancies, it has been recently shown that both proteins are present in normal amounts, regardless of the status (i.e., affected vs. unaffected) of the fetus.[116] As such, these latter data argue against the routine performance of amniocentesis for the determination of such levels as a means of prenatal screening of inherited EB.

Mechanical fragility has been assessed in patients with various forms of EB by the induction of mechanical suction blisters.[117] Using this technique, it has been shown that patients with the severest forms of EB (i.e., recessive dystrophic and junctional EB) have reduced blister times, correlating clinically with their marked mechanical fragility. In contrast, no significant difference was noted between control individuals and patients with EB simplex and dominant dystrophic EB. Interestingly, it has been recently shown that some patients with recessive dystrophic EB develop skin cleavage at the level of the lamina lucida following mechanical suction blister induction, rather than at the level of the sublamina densa, the site of spontaneous blister formation in this disease.[118] This suggests the possibility of abnormal mechanical fragility in more than a single ultrastructural level in a subset of patients with recessive dystrophic EB. Whether the latter correlates with the findings seen in some patients with recessive dystrophic EB using 19-DEJ-1 monoclonal antibody[75] will await further comparative studies.

Epidermal cell cultures have been grown from some EB patients.[119] In some, spontaneous bleb formation was noted. Of particular interest, reduced numbers of hemidesmosomelike structures were noted in cultured junctional EB keratinocytes.[120] Although these studies have been performed in the absence of an underlying collagenous substratum, similar studies using more physiologic biomatrices may shed additional light on the specificity of these reported findings as well as provide possibly excellent in vitro models for one or more of the subsets of inherited EB.

Recent work has been performed in an attempt to address the issue of possible nutritional deficiencies in patients with various forms of inherited EB.[121,122] In general, no significant abnormalities have been noted other than those expected on the basis of a generalized debilitating disorder (i.e., low serum zinc and/or iron levels). These essentially negative findings are important, however, in that one theoretical possibility for enhanced collagenolysis in some subsets of dystrophic EB relates not merely to elevated collagenase levels but also to abnormally produced collagen, as a result of altered vitamin C levels. Similar abnormalities in macromolecule production might have also resulted from the presence of aberrant copper levels, although this possibility was not borne out by recent comprehensive studies.

Over the past several years occasional animals have been reported that have phenotypic and ultrastructural features reminiscent of specific subtypes of inherited EB.[123-126] The most promising one, which appears to represent a condition analogous to recessive dystrophic EB, occurs in a particular breed of sheep.[127] Of interest, type VII collagen cannot be detected in such skin using two known immunohistochemical probes to the molecule, consistent with published data on some patients with severe generalized recessive dystrophic EB.

Possible Mechanisms for Pathogenesis in Inherited EB

EB Simplex

To date, little is known about the pathophysiology of EB simplex. Considering the number of distinctive phenotypes in this as well as other forms of EB, it is certainly possible that multiple mechanisms may apply, depending on specific subtype or even specific affected family. For example, a precedent for the latter is data recently accumulated on osteogenesis imperfecta.[128] Despite this, it appears clear that, in general, basement membrane and dermal elements play little if any direct role in the mechanical fragility observed in EB simplex. Very recent studies, both in humans and transgenic mice, strongly suggest that the most likely cause for cytolysis in EB simplex is the presence of a mutation within keratin molecules.[106,107] Whether identical point mutations on a single keratin protein will be eventually demonstrated in all of the subsets of this disease awaits further studies. In addition, other immunohistochemical work with lectins suggests the possibility that abnormal glycosylation of keratinocyte cell membranes may also play some contributory role in the mechanical fragility observed in this disease.[102] In contrast, studies examining other keratinocyte components, including involucrum, have not resulted in identification of other cytoplasmic defects as possible sources for abnormal keratinocyte functioning in this disease. There are also some published data to suggest that neutral proteases may play a direct role in blister formation in all forms of inherited EB.[49-53] However, these findings do not appear to be specific ones, when more critically reevaluated,[55] suggesting that they at most may be contributory to intraepidermal cleavage only after preceding injury has befallen EB simplex keratinocytes.

Junctional EB

The uniform development of intralamina lucida cleavage in all patients with junctional EB suggests the likely importance of one or more structural defects within this particular ultrastructural region. This has been borne out by the finding of absence or marked reduction of hemidesmosomes and subbasal dense plates in skin from patients with the most severe form of junctional EB, the Herlitz variant.[34] However, the presence of apparent normal numbers of hemidesmosomes in noninherited forms of junctional EB suggest that hemidesmosomal abnormalities may facilitate but are not necessary for skin cleavage at the level of the lamina lucida. As a correlate of the latter, it is interesting to note that bullous pemphigoid antigen, a hemidesmosome-associated antigen, is normally expressed in virtually all patients with junctional EB even in the absence of detectable hemidesmosomes.[129] In contrast, the lack of expression of three other intralamina lucida antigens (AA3, GB3, 19-DEJ-1) correlates well with the development of intralamina lucida cleavage in junctional EB, suggesting a possibly direct role, via their absence, in the presence of marked mechanical fragility and the occurrence of intralamina lucida blister formation in junctional EB skin.[84,85,93]

With regard to the role of proteases in junctional EB, data have been reported that suggest that blister fluid from patients with junctional EB contain proteases with degradative specificity for the lamina lucida. However, as previously discussed, these findings have not been reproduced by other investigators, thereby making their role less certain in the overall pathogenesis of this disease. It should be furthermore noted that the addition of most enzymes (i.e., trypsin) to normal human skin results in cleavage at the level of the lamina lucida.[56] Therefore, it would be expected that the presence of such proteases would have a permissive effect on intralamina lucida cleavage in such patients.

Finally, it should be noted that some patients with junctional EB have been reported to have elevated levels of fibroblast-derived collagenase.[42,43] Similarly, some patients with junctional EB may clinically benefit by treatment with phenytoin, a drug known to have an inhibitory effect on collagenase synthesis.[130,131] It is as yet unknown how collagenase might lead to blister formation in junctional EB skin. For example, the two major types of basement membrane collagen, types IV and VII, are ultrastructurally localized within the lamina densa and within anchoring fibrils, respectively. Furthermore, whereas recently published work suggests the presence of type V collagen at the level of the lamina lucida,[64,132] no abnormalities have been noted immunohistochemically in the expression of type V collagen in EB skin.

Dystrophic EB

There is overwhelming evidence to suggest that elevated levels of a biochemically abnormal tissue collagenase contribute to blister formation in recessive dystrophic EB[35-41]; such findings are discussed in detail elsewhere within this volume (Chapter 4). However, there is also now increasing data to suggest the absence of several noncollagenous antigenic epitopes at the level of the lamina densa in skin from patients with dominant and/or recessive dystrophic EB.[63,68,69,75] It does not appear that these latter findings can be simply attributed to concurrent elevated levels of tissue collagenase. For example, no normalization in the expression of any of these antigens has been reported in patients successfully treated with phenytoin. Recent evidence with LH 7:2 monoclonal antibody, which recognizes an epitope of type VII collagen, suggests that the absence of this epitope correlates with the well-known absence or marked diminution of anchoring fibrils in skin from patients with severe generalized recessive dystrophic EB.[75] On the other hand, recent work with L3d monoclonal antibody, which recognizes yet another epitope on the carboxy terminus of type VII collagen, suggests that some portions of type VII collagen still exist in recessive dystrophic EB skin even in the absence of visible anchoring fibrils.[79]

Finally, even though multiple basement membrane antigenic defects have now been described in dominant and/or recessive dystrophic EB skin, these findings do not by themselves lead to the conclusion that such antigens or antigenic epitopes are truly lacking in such skin. For example, it is possible that these antigens are normally produced by keratinocytes and/or fibroblasts, but are undetectable due to "masking" as a result of abnormal assembly of such basement membrane. Similarly, there may be other as yet undefined degradative enzymes that may lead to destruction of such antigens or portions thereof, so as to make selected epitopes inapparent when examined with monoclonal and polyclonal antibody probes. Furthermore, it is possible that the macromolecules containing such antigenic epitopes may be produced, but that point mutations in other portions of such molecules lead to conformational changes, thereby altering the binding site for such monoclonal antibodies. Finally, it is possible that these antigens are normally synthesized by the appropriate cell type (i.e, keratinocyte and/or fibroblast) but that functional abnormalities of such cells may lead to abnormal sequestration of such macromolecules into intracellular pools, thereby preventing their ready detection within the basement membrane zone by conventional immunohistochemical techniques. As a precedent for the latter, it has been shown that both intracellular and extracellular pools of bullous pemphigoid antigen exist, and that specific chemical pretreatments may be necessary to "unmask" the former, similarly, an intracytoplasmic pool of type VII collagen has been noted in one subset of dominant dystrophic EB (transient bullous dermolysis of the newborn).[133]

Future Directions for Research into Pathogenesis of Inherited EB

There are now a number of antigenic defects that have been described by immunohistochemical techniques in skin from patients with junctional and dystrophic forms of EB; similar findings have been noted with at least one specific lectin in EB simplex. Further definition of these defects awaits biochemical isolation and identification of the specific proteins, glycoproteins, or glycolipids defined by these probes, as extractable from normal human skin. Subsequently, identical studies need to be pursued in tissue extracts from various forms of EB, so as to permit determination of the true presence or absence of such molecules in various types of EB tissue. Subsequent studies should then be forthcoming that will allow investigations into the synthesis and degradation of each of these extracellular matrix and cell membrane components in both normal and diseased states. Furthermore, the use of one or more of these immunohistochemical probes should allow for screening of complementary DNA libraries from human keratinocytes, thereby possibly allowing for the eventual definition of one or more of the genetic defects present in patients with various subsets of inherited EB.

Further studies should be pursued using more refined artificial biomatrices, so as to develop a rather physiologic tissue culture model for each of the subsets of EB. Using the latter, it should then be possible to assess more critically the role of keratinocytes, basement membrane zone, extracellular matrix, and fibroblasts in the development of ultrastructural and functional defects attributable to the pathogenesis of mechanical fragility and skin cleavage in these diseases.

Additional animal models for each of the major types of inherited EB should be developed, since these afford not only the opportunity to study multiple affected organs in vivo, but also a means whereby novel therapies can be explored before initiation of clinical trials in affected patients.

Finally, additional studies employing linkage analysis, similar to those recently performed in EB simplex, should be pursued in genetically well-defined subsets of inherited EB.

Acknowledgements. Supported in part by NIH (NIAMS) grant RO1 AR34861 and contract NO1 AR62271.

References

1. Gedde-Dahl T Jr. *Epidermolysis Bullosa. A clinical, Genetic and Epidemiologic Study.* Baltimore: The Johns Hopkins Press; 1971.
2. Gedde-Dahl T Jr. Sixteen types of epidermolysis. On the clinical discrimination, therapy, and prenatal diagnosis. *Acta Derm (Stockh).* 1981; suppl 95:74–87.

3. Pearson RW. Clinicopathologic types of epidermolysis bullosa and their non-dermatological complications. *Arch Dermatol.* 1988; 124: 718–725.
4. Fine J-D. Epidermolysis Bullosa. In: Demis DJ, ed. *Clinical Dermatology*. Philadelphia: Harper & Row Publishers; 1991: 1–31.
5. Fine JD, Bauer EA, Briggaman RA, et al. Revised clinical and laboratory criteria for subtypes of inherited epidermolysis bullosa: a consensus report by the Subcommittee on Diagnosis and Classification of the National Epidermolysis Bullosa Registry. *J Am Acad Dermatol.* 1991; 24: 119–135.
6. Pearson RW. Studies on the pathogenesis of epidermolysis bullosa. *J Invest Dermatol.* 1962; 39: 551–575.
7. Pearson RW. Histopathologic and ultrastructural findings in certain genodermatoses. *Clin Dermatol.* 1985; 3: 143–174.
8. Haneke E, Anton-Lamprecht I. Ultrastructure of blister formation in epidermolysis bullosa hereditaria: V. Epidermolysis bullosa simplex localisata type Weber-Cockayne. *J Invest Dermatol.* 1982; 78: 219–223.
9. Anton-Lamprecht I, Schnyder UW. Epidermolysis bullosa herpetiformis Dowling-Meara: a report of a case and pathomorphogenesis. *Dermatologica.* 1982; 164: 221–235.
10. Buchbinder LH, Lucky AW, Ballard E, et al. Severe infantile epidermolysis bullosa simplex: Dowling-Meara type. *Arch Dermatol.* 1986; 122: 190–198.
11. Pearson RW, Potter B, Strauss F. Epidermolysis bullosa hereditaria letalis: clinical and histological manifestations and course of the disease. *Arch Dermatol.* 1974; 109: 349–355.
12. Hashimoto I, Schnyder UW, Anton-Lamprecht I. Epidermolysis bullosa hereditaria with junctional blistering in an adult. *Dermatologica.* 1976; 152: 72–86.
13. Anton-Lamprecht I, Schnyder UW. Zur ultrastruktur der epidermolysen mit junktionaler blasenbildung. *Dermatologica.* 1979; 159: 377–382.
14. Schachner L, Lazarus GS, Dembitzer H. Epidermolysis bullosa hereditaria letalis: pathology, natural history, and therapy. *Br J Dermatol.* 1977; 96: 51–58.
15. Paller AS, Fine J-D, Kaplan S, Pearson RW. The generalized atrophic benign form of junctional epidermolysis bullosa: experience with four patients in the United States. *Arch Dermatol.* 1986; 122: 704–710.
16. Hashimoto I, Gedde-Dahl T Jr., Schnyder UW, Anton-Lamprecht I. Ultrastructural studies in epidermolysis bullosa hereditaria. IV. Recessive dystrophic types with junctional blistering (infantile or Herlitz-Pearson type and adult type). *Arch Dermatol Res.* 1976; 257: 17–32.
17. Hashimoto I, Anton-Lamprecht I, Gedde-Dahl T Jr, Schnyder UW. Ultrastructural studies in epidermolysis bullosa hereditaria I: Dominant dystronhic type of Pasini. *Arch Dermatol Res.* 1975; 252: 167–178.
18. Hashimoto I, Gedde-Dahl T Jr, Schnyder UW, Anton-Lamprecht I. Ultrastructural studies in epidermolysis bullosa: II. Dominant dystrophic type of Cockayne and Touraine. *Arch Dermatol Res.* 1976; 255: 285–295.
19. Hashimoto I, Schnyder UW, Anton-Lamprecht I, Gedde-Dahl T Jr, Ward S. Ultrastructural studies in epidermolysis bullosa hereditaria: III. Recessive dystrophic types with dermolytic blistering (Hallopeau-Siemens types and inverse type). *Arch Dermatol Res.* 1976; 256: 137–150.
20. Tidman MJ, Eady RAJ. Dystrophic epidermolysis bullosa: ultrastructural morphometry of the dermo-epidermal junction. *J Invest Dermatol.* 1983; 80: 342.

21. Tidman MJ, Eady RAJ. Evaluation of anchoring fibrils and other components of the dermal–epidermal junction in dystrophic epidermolysis by a quantitative ultrastructural technique. *J Invest Dermatol.* 1985;84:374–377.

22. Hashimoto K, Matsumoto M, Iacobelli D. Transient bullous dermolysis of the newborn. *Arch Dermatol.* 1985;121:1429–1438.

23. Hashimoto K, Burk JD, Bale GF, et al. Transient bullous dermolysis of the newborn: two additional cases. *J Am Acad Dermatol.* 1989;21:708–713.

24. Fine JD. Epidermolysis bullosa: clinical aspects, pathology, and recent advances in research. *Int J Dermatol.* 1986;25:143–157.

25. Hintner H, Stingl G, Schuler G, et al. Immunofluoresence mapping of antigenic determinants within the dermal-epidermal junction in mechanobullous diseases. *J Invest Dermatol.* 1981;76:113–118.

26. Mutasim DF, Takahashi Y, Labib RS, Anhalt GJ, Patel HP, Diaz LA. A pool of bullous pemphigoid antigen(s) is intracellular and associated with basal cell cytoskeleton-hemidesmosome complex. *J Invest Dermatol.* 1985;84:47–53.

27. Westgate GE, Weaver AC, Couchman JR. Bullous pemphigoid antigen localization suggests an intracellular association with hemidesmosomes. *J Invest Dermatol.* 1985;84:218–224.

28. Foidart J-M, Bere EW, Yaar M, et al. Distribution and immunoelectron microscopic localization of laminin, a non-collagenous basement membrane glycoprotein. *Lab Invest.* 1980;42:336–342.

29. Laurie GW, Leblond CP, Martin GR. Localization of type IV collagen, laminin, heparan sulfate proteoglycan and fibronectin to the basal lamina of the basement membranes. *J Cell Biol.* 1982;95:340–344.

30. Fleischmajer R, Timpl R, Dziadek M, Lebwohl M. Basement membrane proteins, interstitial collagens, and fibronectin in neurofibroma. *J Invest Dermatol.* 1985;85:54–59.

31. Horiguchi Y, Abrahamson D, Fine J-D. Epitope mapping of the laminin molecule in murine skin basement membrane zone: demonstration of spatial differences in ultrastructural localization. *J Invest Dermatol.* 1991;96:309–313.

32. Yaoita H, Foidart J-M, Katz S. Localization of the collagenous component in skin basement membrane. *J Invest Dermatol.* 1978;70:191–193.

33. Tidman MJ, Eady RAJ. Ultrastructural morphometry of normal human dermal-epidermal junction: the influence of age, sex, and body region on laminar and nonlaminar components. *J Invest Dermatol.* 1984;83:448–453.

34. Tidman MJ, Eady RAJ. Hemidesmosomes herterogeneity in junctional epidermolysis bullosa revealed by morphometric analysis. *J Invest Dermatol.* 1986;86:51–56.

35. Eisen AZ. Human skin collagenase: relationship to the pathogenesis of epidermolysis bullosa dystrophica. *J Invest Dermatol.* 1969;52:449–453.

36. Lazarus GS. Collagenase and connective tissue metabolism in epidermolysis bullosa. *J Invest Dermatol.* 1972;58:242–248.

37. Bauer EA, Gedde-Dahl T Jr, Eisen AZ. The role of human skin collagenase in epidermolysis bullosa. *J Invest Dermatol.* 1977;68:119–124.

38. Bauer EA, Eisen AZ. Recessive dystrophic epidermolysis bullosa: evidence for increased collagenase as a genetic characteristic in cell culture. *J Exp Med.* 1978;148:1378–1387.

39. Valle K-J, Bauer EA. Enhanced biosynthesis of human skin collagenase in fibro-

blast cultures from recessive dystrophic epidermolysis bullosa. *J Clin Invest.* 1980;66:176–187.

40. Stricklin GP, Welgus HG, Bauer EA. Human skin collagenase in recessive dystrophic epidermolysis bullosa: purification of a mutant enzyme from fibroblast cultures. *J Clin Invest.* 1982;69:1373–1383.
41. Bauer EA. Abnormalities in collagenase expression as in vitro markers for recessive dystrophic epidermolysis bullosa. *J Invest Dermatol.* 1982;79:105s–108s.
42. Kero M. Epidermolysis bullosa in Finland: clinical features, morphology and relation to collagen metabolism. *Acta Derm Venereol (Stockh).* 1984; suppl 110: 1–51.
43. Kero M, Palotie A, Peltonen L. Collagen metabolism in two rare forms of epidermolysis bullosa. *Br J Dermatol.* 1984;110:177–184.
44. Bauer EA, Cooper TW, Tucker DR, Esterly NB. Phenytoin therapy of recessive dystrophic epidermolysis bullosa. Clinical trial and proposed mechanism of action on collagenase. *N Engl J Med.* 1980;303:776–781.
45. Lin AN, Stern RS, Caldwell-Brown D, Carter DM, and collaborators. Phenytoin for recessive dystrophic epidermolysis bullosa. *J Invest Dermatol.* 1989;92:472.
46. Sakai LY, Keene DR, Morris NP, Burgeson RE. Type VII collagen is a major structural component of anchoring fibrils. *J Cell Biol.* 1986;103:1577–1586.
47. Sanchez G, Seltzer JL, Eisen AZ, Stapler P, Bauer EA. Generalized dominant epidemlolysis bullosa simplex. Decreased activity of a gelatinolytic protease in cultured fibroblasts as a phenotypic marker. *J Invest Dermatol.* 1983;81:576–579.
48. Winberg J-O, Gedde-Dahl T Jr. Gelatinase expression in generalized epidermolysis bullosa simplex fibroblasts. *J Invest Dermatol.* 1986;87:326–329.
49. Takamori K, Naito K, Ogawa H. Epidermolysis bullosa simplex blister fluid induces an intra-epidermal blister in cultured normal skin. *Br J Dermatol.* 1983; 109:643–646.
50. Manabe M, Naito K, Ikeda S, Takamori K, Ogawa H. Production of blister in normal human skin in vitro by blister fluids from epidermolysis bullosa. *J Invest Dermatol.* 1984;82:283–286.
51. Matsumoto M, Hashimoto K. Blister fluid from epidermolysis bullosa letalis induces dermal–epidermal separation at lamina lucida. *J Invest Dermatol.* 1984; 82:392–393.
52. Matsumoto M, Hashimoto K, Ohkawara A. The role of lysosomal protease in junctional blister formation in epidermolysis bullosa letalis. *J Invest Dermatol.* 1985;84:354.
53. Takamori K, Ikeda S, Naito K, Ogawa H. Proteases are responsible for blister formation in recessive dystrophic epidermolysis bullosa and epidermolysis bullosa simplex. *Br J Dermatol.* 1985;112:533.
54. Takamori K, Naito K, Taneda A, Ogawa H. Increased neutral protease and collagenase activity in recessive dystrophic epidermolysis bullosa. *Br J Dermatol.* 1983;108:687–694.
55. Fine JD, Stewart B, Austin R. Epidermolysis bullosa blister fluid and human skin organ culture: an unreliable in vitro model for the disease. *J Invest Dermatol.* 1986;37:139.
56. Fine JD. The skin basement membrane zone. In: Callen J, ed. *Advances in Dermatology.* Chicago: Year Book Publishers; 1986:283–303.

57. Fine JD. Antigenic features and structural correlates of basement membranes: relationship to epidermolysis bullosa. *Arch Dermatol.* 1988;124:713–717.

58. Fine J-D. Structure and antigenicity of the skin basement membrane zone. *J Cutan Pathol.* 1991;18:401–409.

59. Fine JD. Altered skin basement membrane antigenicity in epidermolysis bullosa. In: Wuepper KD, Gedde-Dahl T Jr, ed. *Biology of Heritable Skin Diseases.* Basel: Karger; 1987:111–126.

60. Eady RAJ, Tidman MJ, Heagerty AHM, Kennedy AR. Approaches to the study of epidermolysis bullosa. *Curr Probl Dermatol.* 1987;17:127–141.

61. Caughman SW, Krieg T, Timpl R, Hintner H, Katz SI. Nidogen and heparan sulfate proteoglycan: detection of newly isolated basement membrane components in normal and epidermolysis bullosa skin. *J Invest Dermatol.* 1987;89:547–550.

62. Fine JD, Gay S. LDA-1 monoclonal antibody: an excellent reagent for immunofluorescence mapping studies in patients with epidermolysis bullosa. *Arch Dermatol.* 1986;122:48–51.

63. Fine JD, Couchman JR. Chondroitin 6-sulfate proteoglycan but not heparan sulfate proteoglycan is abnormally expressed in skin basement membrane from patients with dominant and recessive dystrophic epidermolysis bullosa. *J Invest Dermatol.* 1989;92:611–616.

64. Fine JD, Horiguchi Y, Madri JA. Ultrastructural localization of AB2 type V collagen in human skin basement membrane and its expression in epidermolysis bullosa. *Clin Res.* 1989;37:358A.

65. Breathnach SM, Fox PA, Neises GR, Stanley JR, Katz SI. A unique squamous epithelial basement membrane antigen defined by a monoclonal antibody (KF-1). *J Invest Dermatol.* 1983;80:392–395.

66. Fine JD, Smith LT, Holbrook KA, Katz SI. The appearance of four basement membrane zone antigens in developing human fetal skin. *J Invest Dermatol.* 1984;83:66–69.

67. Bernard BA. Biochemical characterization of the epithelial membrane antigen defined by the monoclonal antibody KF-1. *J Invest Dermatol.* 1986;87:86–88.

68. Fine JD, Breathnach SM, Hintner H, Katz SI. KF-1 monoclonal antibody defines a specific basement membrane antigenic defect in dystrophic forms of epidermolysis bullosa. *J Invest Dermatol.* 1984;82:35–38.

69. Goldsmith LA, Briggaman RA. Monoclonal antibodies to anchoring fibrils for the diagnosis of epidermolysis bullosa. *J Invest Dermatol.* 1983;81:464–466.

70. Lane AT, Helm KF, Goldsmith LA. Identification of bullous pemphigoid, pemphigus, laminin, and anchoring fibril antigens in human fetal skin. *J Invest Dermatol.* 1985;84:27–30.

71. Leigh IM, Purkis PE. LH 7:2: a new monoclonal antibody to a lamina densa protein. *J Invest Dermatol.* 1985;84:448.

72. Heagerty AHM, Kennedy AR, Leigh IM, Purkis P, Eady RAJ. Identification of an epidermal basement membrane defect in recessive forms of dystrophic epidermolysis bullosa by LH 7:2 monoclonal antibody: use in diagnosis. *Br J Dermatol.* 1986;115:125–131.

73. Leigh IM, Purkis P, Bruckner-Tuderman L. LH 7:2 monoclonal antibody detects type VII collagen in the basement membrane of ectodermally derived epithelia including skin. *Epithelia.* 1987;1:17–29.

74. Leigh IM, Eady RAJ, Heagerty AHM, Purkis P, Whitehead PA, Burgeson RA. Type VII collagen is a normal component of epidermal basement membrane which shows altered expression in recessive dystrophic epidermolysis bullosa. *J Invest Dermatol.* 1988;90:639–642.
75. Fine JD, Johnson LB, Wright T. Type VII collagen and 19-DEJ-1 antigen: comparison of expression in inversa and generalized variants of recessive dystrophic epidermolysis bullosa. *Arch Dermatol.* 1990;126:1587–1593.
76. Bruckner-Tuderman L, Ruegger S, Odermatt B, Mitsuhashi Y, Schnyder UW. Lack of type VII collagen is unaffected skin of patients with severe recessive dystrophic epidermolysis bullosa. *Dermatologica.* 1988;176:57–64.
77. Bruckner-Tuderman L, Mitsuhasshi Y, Schnyder UW, Bruckner P. Anchoring fibrils and type VII collagen are absent from skin in severe recessive dystrophic epidermolysis bullosa. *J Invest Dermatol.* 1989;93:3–9.
78. Bruckner-Tuderman L, Niemi KM, Kero M, Schnyder UW, Reunala T. Type-VII collagen is expressed but anchoring fibrils are defective in dystrophic epidermolysis bullosa inversa. *Br J Dermatol.* 1990;122:383–390.
79. Rusenko KW, Gammon WR, Fine JD, Briggaman RA. The carboxyl-terminal domain of type VII collagen is present at the basement membrane in recessive dystrophic epidermolysis bullosa. *J Invest Dermatol.* 1989;92:623–627.
80. Verrando P, Ortonne J-P, Pautrat G, Hsi B-L, Yeh C-J. Identification of a 37 kilodalton protein at the epidermal basement membrane by anti-serum to human amnion. *J Invest Dermatol.* 1986;86:190–196.
81. Verrando P, Hsi B-L, Yeh C-J, Pisano A, Serleys N, Ortonne J-P. Monoclonal antibody GB3, a new probe for the study of human basement membranes and hemidesmosomes. *Exp Cell Res.* 1987;170:116–128.
82. Verrando P, Pisani A, Ortonne J-P. The new basement membrane antigen recognized by the monoclonal antibody GB3 is a large size glycoprotein: modulation of its expression by retinoic acid. *Biochim Biophys Acta.* 1988;942:45–56.
83. Heagerty AHM, Kennedy AR, Gunner DB, Eady RAJ. Rapid prenatal diagnosis and exclusion of epidermolysis bullosa using novel antibody probes. *J Invest Dermatol.* 1986;86:603–605.
84. Kennedy AR, Heagerty AHM, Ortonne J-P, Hsi B-L, Yeh C-JG, Eady RAJ. Abnormal binding of an anti-amnion antibody to epidermal basement membrane provides a novel diagnostic probe for junctional epidermolysis bullosa. *Br J Dermatol.* 1985;113:651–659.
85. Heagerty AHM, Kennedy AR, Eady RAJ, et al. GB3 monoclonal antibody for diagnosis of junctional epidermolysis bullosa. *Lancet.* 1986;1:860.
86. Fine JD. GB3 antigen is an accurate marker of only the Herlitz subset of junctional epidermolysis bullosa. *Clin Res.* 1990;38:72A.
87. Schofield OMV, Fine JD, Pisani A, Heagerty AHM, Ortonne JP, Eady RAJ. GB3 monoclonal antibody for the diagnosis of junctional epidermolysis bullosa: results of a multicentre study. *J Am Acad Dermatol.* 1990;23:1078–1083.
88. Horiguchi Y, Couchman JR, Ljubimov AV, Vasiliev JM, Yamasaki H, Fine JD. Organ specificity, ontogeny, and ultrastructural localization of the core protein of heparan sulfate proteoglycan, a new component of human skin basement membrane zone. *J Histochem Cytochem.* 1989;37:961–970.
89. Fine JD, Couchman JR. Chondroitin-6-sulfate-containing proteoglycan: a new component of human skin dermoepidermal junction. *J Invest Dermatol.* 1988;90:283–288.

90. Fine JD, Horiguchi Y, Jester J, Couchman J. Detection and partial characterization of a mid-lamina lucida—hemidesmosome—associated antigen (19-DEJ-1) present within human skin. *J Invest Dermatol.* 1989;92:825–830.

91. Holbrook KA, Smith LT. Ultrastructural aspects of human skin during embryonic, fetal, neonatal and adult periods of life. In: Blandau RJ, ed. *Morphogenesis and Malformations of the Skin.* New York: Alan R Liss; 1981:9–38.

92. Fine JD, Horiguchi Y, Couchman JR. 19-DEJ-1, a hemidesmosome-anchoring filament complex-associated monoclonal antibody. Definition of a new skin basement membrane antigenic defect in junctional and dystrophic epidermolysis bullosa. *Arch Dermatol.* 1989;125:520–523.

93. Fine JD. 19-DEJ-1, a monoclonal antibody to the hemidesmosome-anchoring filament complex, is the only reliable immunohistochemical probe for all major forms of junctional epidermolysis bullosa. *Arch Dermatol.* 1990;126:1187–1190.

94. Fine JD. Epidermolysis bullosa: variability of expression of cicatricial pemphigoid, bullous pemphigoid, and epidermolysis bullosa acquisita antigens. *J Invest Dermatol.* 1985;85:47–49.

95. Heagerty AHM, Eady RAJ, Kennedy AR, et al. Rapid prenatal diagnosis of epidermolysis bullosa letalis using GB3 monoclonal antibody. *Br J Dermatol.* 1987;17:271–275.

96. Fine JD, Eady RAJ, Levy ML, et al. Prenatal diagnosis of dominant and recessive dystrophic epidermolysis bullosa: application and limitations in the use of KF-1 and LH 7:2 monoclonal antibodies and immunofluorescence mapping. *J Invest Dermatol.* 1988;91:465–471.

97. Fine JD, Holbrook KA, Elias S, Anton-Lamprecht I, Rauskolb R. Applicability of 19-DEJ-1 monoclonal antibody for the prenatal diagnosis or exclusion of junctional epidermolysis bullosa. *Prenatal Diagn.* 1990;10:219–229.

98. Erhlich HP, Buttle D, Trelstad R, Hayashi K. Epidermolysis bullosa dystrophica recessive fibroblasts altered behavior within a collagen matrix. *J Invest Dermatol.* 1983;80:56–60.

99. Erhlich HP, White M. Effects of increased concentrations of prostaglandin E levels with epidermolysis bullosa dystrophica recessive fibroblasts within a populated collagen lattice. *J Invest Dermatol.* 1983;81:572–575.

100. Erhlich HP, Griswold TR. Epidermolysis bullosa dystrophica recessive fibroblasts produce increased concentrations of cAMP within collagen matrix. *J Invest Dermatol.* 1984;83:230–233.

101. Eisen AZ, Pentland AP, Bauer EA, Goldberg GI. The behavior of epidermolysis bullosa fibroblasts in a hydrated collagen lattice. *J Invest Dermatol.* 1986;87:138.

102. Fine JD, Griffith RD. A specific defect in glycosylation of epidermal cell membranes. Definition in skin from patients with epidermolysis bullosa simplex. *Arch Dermatol.* 1985;121:1292–1296.

103. Briggaman RA, Wheeler CE Jr. Epidermolysis bullosa dystrophica-recessive: a possible role of anchoring fibrils in the pathogenesis. *J Invest Dermatol.* 1975;65:203–211.

104. Tidman MJ, Eady RA, Leigh IM, MacDonald DM. Keratin expression in epidermolysis bullosa simplex (Dowling-Meara). *Acta Derm Venereol.* 1988;68:15–20.

105. Kitajima Y, Inoue S, Yaoita H. Abnormal organization of keratin intermediate filaments in cultured keratinocytes of epidermolysis bullosa simplex. *Arch Dermatol Res.* 1989;281:5–10.

106. Vassar R, Coulombe PA, Degenstein L, Albers K, Fuchs E. Mutant keratin expression in transgenic mice causes marked abnormalities resembling a human genetic skin disease. *Cell.* 1991;64:365–380.
107. Bonifas JM, Rothman AL, Epstein E. Linkage of epidermolysis bullosa simplex to probes in the region of keratin gene clusters on chromosomes 12q and 17q. *J Invest Dermatol.* 1991;39(2):503A.
108. Endo M, Yamamoto R, Yosizawa Z, Sasai Y, Saito N. Urinary chondroitin of epidermolysis bullosa dystrophica et albo-papuloidea (Pasini). *Clin Chim Acta.* 1974;57:249–253.
109. Bauer EA, Fiehler WK, Esterly NB. Increased glycosaminoglycan accumulation as a gene ic characteristic in cell cultures of one variety of dominant dystrophic epidennolysis bullosa. *J Clin Invest.* 1979;64:32–39.
110. Priestley GC. Glycosaminoglycans production by cultured skin fibroblasts from the Pasini and Cockayne-Touraine forms of dominant dystrophic epidermolysis bullosa. *J Invest Dermatol.* 1991;96:168–171.
111. Savolainen E-R, Kero M, Pihlajaniemi T, Kivirikko KI. Deficiency of galacto-sylhydroxylysyl glucosyltransferase, an enzyme of collagen synthesis, in a family with dominant epidermolysis bullosa simplex. *N Engl J Med.* 1981;304:197–204.
112. Gay S, Ward WQ, Gay R, Miller EJ. Autoantibodies to basement membrane collagen: epidermolysis bullosa simplex versus bullous pemphigoid. *J Cutan Pathol.* 1980;7:315–317.
113. Gay S, Fine JD, Storer JS. Autoantibodies to extracellular collagen matrix components in epidermolysis bullosa and other bullous diseases. *Arch Dermatol. Res* 1988;280:333–337.
114. Yacoub T, Campbell CA, Gordon YB, Kirby JD, Kitau MJ. Maternal serum and amniotic fluid concentrations of alphafetoprotein in epidermolysis bullosa simplex. *Br Med J.* 1979;1:307.
115. Bick DP, Balkite EA, Baumgarten A, Hobbins JC, Mahoney MJ. The association of congenital skin disorders with acetylcholinesterase in amniotic fluid. *Prenatal Diagn.* 1987;7:543–549.
116. Shulman LP, Elias S, Andersen RN, et al. Alpha-fetoprotein and acetylcholine-sterase are not predictive of fetal junctional epidermolysis bullosa, Herlitz variant. *Prenatal Diagn.* 1991;11:813–818.
117. Briggaman RA, Meador P, Wheeler CE Jr. Suction blister studies in epidermolysis bullosa. *J Invest Dermatol.* 1977;68:231.
118. Tidman MJ, Eady RAJ. Evidence for a functional defect of the lamina lucida in recessive dystrophic epidermolysis bullosa demonstrated by suction blisters. *Br J Dermatol.* 1984;111:379–387.
119. Leigh [M, Tidman MJ. Eady RAJ. Epidermolysis bullosa preliminary observations of blister formation in keratinocyte cultures. *Br J Dermatol.* 1984;111:527–532.
120. Chapman SJ, Leigh IM, Tidman MJ, Eady RAJ. Abnormal expression of hemidesmosome-like structures by junctional epidermolysis bullosa keratinocytes in vitro. *Br J Dermatol.* 1990;123:137–144.
121. Cunnane SC, Kent ET, McAdoo KR, Caldwell D, Lin AN, Carter DM. Abnormalities of plasma and erythrocyte essential fatty acid composition in epidermolysis bullosa: influence of treatment with diphenylhydantoin. *J Invest Dermatol.* 1987;89:395–399.

122. Fine JD, Tamura T, Johnson L. Blood vitamin and trace metal levels in epidermolysis bullosa. *Arch Dermatol.* 1989;125:374–379.
123. Alley MR, O'Hara PJ, Middelberg A. An epidermolysis bullosa of sheep. *N Z Vet J.* 1974;22:55–59.
124. Bassett E. Bovine epidermolysis: an inherited skin disease in cattle. Dublin: 1986:75–80. In: Proceedings of the 14th World Congress on disease of cattle, Dublin, Ireland. 1986, 75–80.
125. Dunstan RW, Sills RC, Wilkinson JE, Paller AS, Hashimoto KH. A disease resembling junctional epidermolysis bullosa in a toy poodle. *Am J Dermatopathol.* 1988;10:442–447.
126. Thompson KG, Crandell RA, Rugeley WW, Sutherland RJ. A mechanobullous disease with sub-basilar separation in Brangus calves. *Vet Pathol.* 1985;22:283–285.
127. Bruckner-Tuderman L, Guscetti F, Ehrensperger F. Animal model for dermolytic mechanobullous disease: sheep with recessive dystrophic epidermolysis bullosa lack collagen VII. *J Invest Dermatol.* 1991;96:452–458.
128. Byers PH, Wenstrup RJ, Bonadio JF, et al. Molecular basis of inherited disorders of collagen biosynthesis: implications for prenatal diagnosis. *Curr Probl Dermatol.* 1987;16:158–174.
129. Fine JD. Cicatricial pemphigoid, bullous pemphigoid, and epidermolysis bullosa acquisita antigens: differences in organ and species specificities and localization in chemically-separated human skin of three basement membrane antigens. *Coll Rel Res.* 1985;5:369–377.
130. Rogers RB, Yancey KB, Allen BS, Guill MF. Phenytoin therapy for junctional epidermolysis bullosa. *Arch Dermatol.* 1983;119:925–926.
131. Fine JD, Johnson L. Efficacy of systemic phenytoin in the treatment of junctional epidennolysis bullosa. *Arch Dermatol.* 1988;124:1402–1406.
132. Woodley DT, Scheidt VJ, Reese MJ, et al. Localization of the alpha 3 (V) chain of type V collagen in human skin. *J Invest Dermatol.* 1987;88:246–252.
133. Fine JD, Horiguchi Y, Stein DH, Esterly NB, Leigh IM. Intraepidermal type VII collagen. Evidence for abnormal intracytoplasmic processing of a major basement protein in rare patients with dominant and possibly localized recessive forms of dystrophic epidermolysis bullosa. *J Am Acad Dermatol.* 1990;22:188–195.

4
Collagenase and Connective Tissue Remodeling in Recessive Dystrophic Epidermolysis Bullosa

ELKE VOGES, ANNEMARIE KRONBERGER, ROSALIND A. GRYMES, and EUGENE A. BAUER,

The basement membrane zone (BMZ) of the skin is defined as the ultra-structurally identifiable region that includes the basal keratinocytes, the lamina lucida, the lamina densa, and the uppermost papillary dermis. The lower dermal "boundary" of the BMZ is unclear but must extend at least to the depth of the anchoring fibrils where they insert into anchoring plaques.[1]

The mechanisms involved in remodeling of the BMZ are proteolytic in nature and involve two major cell types: keratinocytes and fibroblasts.[2-4] Both keratinocytes and fibroblasts display many proteases that may participate in this process.[5] Fibroblasts and keratinocytes also synthesize an inhibitor of metalloproteases, the tissue inhibitor of metalloproteases (TIMP), which functions locally to regulate proteolytic activity.[6] Last, keratinocytes elaborate epidermal cell–derived thymocyte activating factor,[7] a cytokine identical to interleukin-1 (IL-1), and thus capable of affecting stromal cells' expression of metalloproteases and TIMP.[8]

These three observations—protease expression, TIMP expression, and cytokine expression by cells found in the BMZ—lead to the conclusion that at least three means exist for controlling BMZ remodeling. These include (a) direct expression of proteases by cells of the epidermis and/or dermis, (b) alteration of normal tissue-level regulatory controls (e.g., inadequate levels or functionally impaired protease inhibitors), and (c) induction or repression of protease expression through the effects of cytokines.

Tissue Remodeling as Part of Pathogenesis

The interactions of the entire repertoire of structural proteins of the BMZ. provide stability and resiliency to this critical region of the skin.[1] Thus, as stated earlier,[9] "any concept of BMZ remodeling, irrespective of whether it is physiologically or pathologically driven, must accommodate the possibility that proteolytic degradation of one of these major structural proteins may lead to a secondary effect on one or more proteins or cells with which it interacts with resultant profound effects on the stability of the BMZ."

At present, no conclusions can be made about the genetic defect(s) in recessive dystrophic epidermolysis bullosa (EB). Nevertheless, it is likely, from both clinical and experimental evidence, that decreased numbers and/or function of anchoring fibrils are an important component of the pathology of recessive dystrophic EB.[10,11] Whether this is due to diminished synthesis or abnormal structure of the constituent type VII collagen,[1] to increased expression of human skin collagenase,[12] or to both is under investigation. Alternatively, it is possible that neither diminished synthesis of anchoring fibrils nor increased collagenase production represents the genetic defect. For example, the observations of Smith and Sybert[13] suggest failure of type VII collagen secretion that might be secondary to defective posttranslational modification of the protein. Thus, it must be remembered that in any given disease process there is often a profound difference between the precise genetic abnormality and the overall pathogenesis of the disease.[14]

To understand the defective wound healing that occurs in recessive dystrophic EB, we must first look more closely at normal wound healing events. By probing events of wound healing, we reveal the complexity of control mechanisms and the redundancies that exist in the response of the organism to a cutaneous wound. A crucial part of normal wound healing is remodeling of the newly synthesized and deposited collagen. To accomplish this task, human skin collagenase is synthesized by one or more cell types and can be shown to follow a pattern of expression that parallels ultrastructually observable reorganization (see below). In contrast, in recessive dystrophic EB, the repeated trauma inflicted on the skin and mucous membranes never allows the healing wound to mature properly. Thus, there is chronic "up-regulation" of proteases—both collagenase and noncollagenolytic enzymes[12,15-19]—and the circumstance is one in which the wound healing response has gone awry.

Tissue Sources of Collagenase

Under normal circumstances, the major source of collagenase in human skin is the dermis. The original investigations of Eisen[20] and Lazarus and Fullmer[21] in organ explant cultures showed that almost all of the collagenase activity was located in the dermis. This conclusion was supported by later immunohistochemical observations of normal human skin in which the papillary dermis was the site of collagenase localization.[2] Similarly, cultured skin fibroblasts were found to be a major source of the enzyme.[2]

There is abundant evidence that more than one protease is critical to the remodeling of connective tissue matrix during wound healing.[5] Especially important is the family of zinc metalloproteases,[22] of which interstitial collagenase is the prototype. The cells of origin of these proteases vary somewhat; however, the cell types involved in this aspect of the wound healing response at least include keratinocytes, fibroblasts, and macrophages, any one of which could be directly expressing collagenase and/or TIMP and/or producing cytokines capable of inducing synthesis of collagenase and/or TIMP in a secondary target cell.

As noted above, the first investigations of wound healing involved organ cultures of experimentally wounded guinea pig[23] and human[20] skin. In these systems, the data suggested both dermal and epidermal origins of interstitial collagenase. In an intriguing model developed several years later, Woodley et al.[24] observed thinning of connective tissue subjacent to migrating keratinocytes, suggesting elaboration of collagenase by the keratinocytes as might occur during debridement of a wound. Such findings were in contrast to immunohistochemical observations with nonwounded skin and with fibroblasts in monolayer culture.[2] Here, the major, if not the total, elaboration of collagenase was attributable to the dermis and, more specifically, to the dermal fibroblasts.[25]

The role of keratinocytes in collagenase expression, despile the early organ culture data,[20,23] remained in question until techniques for culturing keratinocytes in monolayer culture were developed. When keratinocytes are cultured under conditions that permit growth of the cells, that is, under subconfluent growth conditions, they synthesize interstitial collagenase that is identical to the collagenase produced by the fibroblasts.[3,6] The synthesis of collagenase by keratinocytes is significantly attenuated when they reach confluence and are contact inhibited.[6] The addition of phorbol esters to the culture medium induces the expression of the enzyme[3] even in confluent cultures. Similar events seem to dictate expression of TIMP by the keratinocytes, although TIMP is present only transiently and in much lower concentrations than found in fibroblast cultures.[6]

Indirect Mechanisms Affecting Collagenase Expression

In addition to the direct elaboration of collagenase and TIMP by keratinocytes, indirect mechanisms can be seen to occur (i.e., cytokine-mediated induction of collagenase occurs in fibroblasts). Following wounding there is activation of clotting mechanisms. The degranulation of platelets[26] results in a series of wound repair events. Especially important is the release of platelet-derived growth factor (PDGF), a peptide of ~28.5 kDa that is chemoattractant and mitogenic for fibroblasts.[27] Fibroblast migration and activation are accompanied by synthesis and deposition of interstitial collagen.[28,29] As initial scar formation occurs, morphologic analysis reveals connective tissue reorganization, presumably enzymatically mediated,[9] which results in the evolution of a mature scar.

Epithelial–stromal interactions, particularly as mediated by cytokines such as IL-1, are also involved in the wound healing response. Proliferative cultured keratinocytes release a cytokine, or cytokines, capable of inducing collagenase in normal human fetal skin fibroblasts.[4] Like both collagenase and TIMP synthesis, the expression of this cytokine is attenuated once the cultured keratinocytes reach confluence. The principal cytokine elaborated by the keratinocytes and thus far isolated that shows the collagenase-stimulatory function is IL-1.[4,6,8]

Local Control of Collagen Degradation

Control mechanisms also exist to exert control over collagenase activity at a local level. The tissue inhibitor of metalloproteases (TIMP) appears to be critical. TIMP has a molecular mass of ~28.5 kDa and acts to control the activities of the matrix metalloproteases family of enzymes within tissues locally.[30,31] TIMP is present in normal concentrations in the serum of patients with recessive dystrophic EB.[32] It is preferentially concentrated in the blister fluids from patients with a wide variety of diseases, including all forms of EB, where it is believed to be controlling excessive connective tissue matrix destruction in the wounded skin.[32] In contrast, alpha-2-macroglobulin, an antiprotease of molecular mass ~780 kDa, exerts its antiprotease activity within vascular spaces.[33]

BMZ Structure and Function in Recessive Dystrophic EB

The protein–protein interactions that stabilize the BMZ are highly complex. Burgeson et al.[1,34,35] have shown that anchoring fibrils—made largely of type VII collagen—stream from the basal lamina to "insert" into so-called anchoring plaques containing type IV collagen. This creates a series of loop-like structures that embrace the interstitial collagens (types I and III) of this region. This picture can then be joined to, or superimposed on, another that includes, for example, fibronectin with its collagen and cell-binding domains. The resultant hierarchy of interactions makes it clear that disruption of the expression of one of the collagenous components—whether due to defective synthesis or secretion or to enhanced proteolysis—could destabilize the BMZ.

Several hypotheses can be offered to account for the BMZ fragility in recessive dystrophic EB. In one version, the synthesis of the interstitial collagens (types I and III) and type VII collagen comprising the anchoring fibrils is normal, but there is overexpression of collagenase[12] resulting in degradation of the interstitial collagens to which the BMZ has been attached by loops of anchoring fibrils. Degradation of the interstitial collagens liberates the anchoring fibrils and destabilizes the BMZ. The anchoring fibrils might then be degraded, by collagenase or other proteases,[36] accounting for the inability to demonstrate these structures.[10,11] That this might in fact occur is supported by the recent observation that human skin collagenase, both from normal and recessive dystrophic EB fibroblasts, can degrade type VII collagen.[36] In a second hypothetical model, reduced anchoring fibrils result from an abnormality in the synthesis of type VII collagen. Type VII collagen might be absent, reduced, or defective and result in a structurally abnormal collagen molecule. Any of these possibilities almost certainly would lead to defective formation of the anchoring fibrils, disrupting critical interactions among structural macromolecules. Once such interactions are lost, it is likely signals are transmitted[14] to fibroblasts in the papillary dermis to adopt a wound-healing phenotype, one component of which is induction of the expression of proteases such as collagenase. The existence of a partial cDNA clone for type VII collagen[37] should now permit these two possibilities to be addressed.

Even if none of the hypotheses is correct, an alteration in one of the BMZ structures will almost certainly compromise the functional integrity of all. Thus, not only interstitial collagenase but also other proteases expressed in the skin should be examined. The members of the family of matrix metallo-proteases, including interstitial collagenase, stromelysin, 72-kDa type IV collagenase, and 92-kDa type V collagenase, are closely related structurally and probably arose by gene duplication.[22] They also share substrate specificities, at least to some extent. Interstitial collagenase preferentially degrades types I and III collagens but can also attack denatured collagen (gelatin) and types IV, V, and VII collagens. Stromelysin preferentially degrades proteoglycans and one form of type IV collagen but also acts on gelatin, fibronectin, laminin, and type VII collagen. The 72-kDa type IV collagenase degrades gelatin preferentially but also degrades types IV, V, and VII collagens.[22,36,38,39]

Mechanisms that regulate the expression of this entire family of enzymes may be critical to understanding pathophysiology and therapy in EB. Coordinated regulation of these proteases may occur following certain stimuli,[38,39] but will not be uniform. Indeed, particularly in the use of pharmacologic agents,[40] capacity to modulate differentially the expression of the structural proteins of the BMZ and the enzymes that degrade these structures probably represents a key to therapeutic success in recessive dystrophic EB.

Acknowledgments. This work was supported in part by USPHS grants 5R37 AR 19537, T32 AR 07422, and N01 AR 6-2273 from the National Institute of Arthritis and Musculoskeletal and Skin Diseases and by grant NCA2-483 from NASA.

References

1. Burgeson RE, Morris NP, Murray LW, Duncan KG, Keene DR, Sakai LY. The structure of type VII collagen. *Ann NY Acad Sci.* 1985;460:47–57.
2. Reddick ME, Bauer EA, Eisen AZ. Immunocytochemical localization of collagenase in humanskin and fibroblasts in monolayer culture. *J Invest Dermatol.* 1974;62:361–366.
3. Petersen MJ, Woodley DT, Stricklin GP, O'Keefe EJ. Production of procollagenase by cultured human keratinocytes. *J Biol Chem.* 1987;262:835–840.

4. Bauer EA, Pentland AP, Kronberger A, Wilhelm SW, Goldberg GI, Welgus HG, Eisen AZ. Keratinocyte- and tumor-derived inducers of collagenase. *Ann NY Acad Sci.* 1988;548:174–179.

5. He C, Wilhelm SM, Pentland AP, Marmer BL, Grant GA, Eisen AZ, Goldberg GI. Tissue cooperation in a proteolytic cascade activating human interstitial collagenase. *Proc Natl Acad Sci.* 1989;86:2632–2636.

6. Pentland AP, Kronberger A, Wilhelm SW, et al. Epidermal modulation of dermal collagen metabolism: Evidence for direct participation of keratinocyte collagenase and for indirect modulation by cytokines. 1991. In preparation.

7. Sauder DN. Interleukins. *Prog Dermatol.* 1988;22:1–8.

8. Postlethwaite AE, Lachman LB, Mainardi C, Kang AH. Interleukin 1 stimulation of collagenase production by cultured fibroblasts. *J Exp Med.* 1983;157:801–806.

9. Bauer EA. The role of proteinases in epidermolysis bullosa. General principles of basement membrane zone remodelling in relationship to the pathogenesis of epidermolysis bullosa. In: Priestly GC, Tidman MJ, Weiss JB, Eady RAJ, eds. *Epidermolysis Bullosa: A Comprehensive Review of Classification, Management and Laboratory Studies.* Crowthorne: DEBRA, 1990:141–151.

10. Goldsmith LA, Briggaman RA. Monoclonal antibodies to anchoring fibrils for the diagnosis of epidermolysis bullosa. *J Invest Dermatol.* 1983; 81:464–466.

11. Fine J-D, Breathnach SM, Hintner H, Katz SI. KF-1 monoclonal antibody defines a specific basement membrane antigen defect in dystrophic forms of epidemolysis bullosa. *J Invest Dermatol.* 1984;82:35–38.

12. Bauer EA. Collagenase in recessive dystrophic epidermolysis bullosa. *Ann NY Acad Sci.* 1986;460:311–320

13. Smith LT, Sybert VP. Intra-epidermal retention of type VII collagen in a patient with recessive dystrophic epidermolysis bullosa. *J Invest Dermatol.* 1990;94:261–264.

14. Trelstad RL. The extracellular matrix is a soluble and solid-phase agonist and receptor. *Arch Dermatol.* 1988;124:706–708.

15. Takamori K, Naito K, TAneda A, Ogawa H. Increased neutral protease and collagenase activity in recessive dystrophic epidermolysis bullosa. *Br J Dermatol.* 1983;108:687–694.

16. Ikeda S, Naito K, Imai R, Manabe M, Takamori K, Ogawa H. Origin and properties of the blister formation factor in blister fluids from recessive dystrophic epidermolysis bullosa. *Br J Dermatol.* 1985;113:661–667.

17. Takamori K, Shigaku I, Naito K, Manabe M, Ogawa H. Blister formation mechanisms of epidermolysis bullosa simplex and recessive dystrophic epidermolysis bullosa. In: Urabe H, Kimura M, Yamamoto K, Ogawa H, eds. *Proceedings of the IVth International Congress of Pediatric Dermatology.* Tokyo: University of Tokyo Press, 1987:143–151.

18. Takamori K, Yoshiike T, Morioka S, Ogawa H. The role of proteases in the pathogenesis of bullous dermatoses. *Int J Dermatol.* 1988;27:533–539.

19. Sawamura D, Sugawara T, Hashimoto I, et al. Increased gene expression of matrix metalloproteinase-3 (stromelysin) in skin fibroblasts from patients with severe recessive dystrophic epidermolysis bullosa. *Biochem Biophys Res Commun.* 1991;174:1003–1008.

20. Eisen AZ. Human skin collagenase: localization and distribution in normal human skin. *J Invest Dermatol.* 1969;52:442–448.

21. Lazarus GS, Fullmer HM. Collagenase production by human dermis in vitro. *J Invest Dermatol.* 1969;52:545–547.

22. Collier IE, Smith J, Kronberger A, et al. The structure of the human skin fibroblast collagenase gene. *J Biol Chem.* 1988;263:10711–10713.
23. Donoff RB, McLennan JE, Grillo HC. Preparation and properties of collagenases from epithelium and mesenchyme of healing mammalian wounds. *Biochim Biophys Acta.* 1971;227:639–653.
24. Woodley DT, Kelebec T, Banes AJ, Link W, Prunieras M, Liotta LA. Adult human keratinocytes migrating over nonviable dermal collagen produce collagenolytic enzymes that degrade type I and type IV collagen. *J Invest Dermatol.* 1986; 86:418–423.
25. Valle K-J, Bauer EA. Biosynthesis of collagenase by human skin fibroblasts in monolayer culture. *J Biol Chem.* 1979;254:10115–10122.
26. Ross R, Vogel A. The platelet-derived growth factor. *Cell.* 1978;14:203–210.
27. Deuel TF, Huang JS. Platelet-derived growth factor. Structure, function, and roles in normal and transformed cells. *J Clin Invest.* 1984;74:669–676.
28. Odland G, Ross R. Human wound repair. I. Epidermal regeneration. *J Cell Biol.* 1968;39:135–151.
29. Ross R, Odland G. Human wound repair. II. Inflammatory cells, epithelial-mesenchymal interrelations, and fibrogenesis. *J Cell Biol.* 1968;39:152–168.
30. Stricklin GP, Welgus HG. Human skin fibroblast collagenase inhibitor: purification and biochemical characterization. *J Biol Chem.* 1983;258:12252–12258.
31. Welgus HG, Stricklin GP. Human skin fibroblast collagenase inhibitor: comparative studies in human connective tissues, serum and amniotic fluid. *J Biol Chem.* 1983;258:12259–12264.
32. Welgus HG, Bauer EA, Stricklin GP. Elevated levels of human collagenase inhibitor in blister fluids of diverse etiology. *J Invest Dermatol.* 1986;87:592–596.
33. Werb Z, Burleigh MC, Barrett AJ, Starkey PM. The interaction of alpha-2-macroglobulin with proteinases. Binding and inhibition of mammalian collagenases and other metal proteinases. *Biochem J.* 1974;139:359–368.
34. Sakai LY, Keene DR, Morris NP, Burgeson RE. Type VII collagen is a major structural component of anchoring fibrils. *J Cell Biol.* 1986;103:1577–1586.
35. Keene DR, Sakai LY, Lunstrum GP, Morris NP, Burgeson RE. Type VII collagen forms an extended network of anchoring fibrils. *J Cell Biol.* 1987;104: 611–621.
36. Seltzer JL, Eisen AZ, Bauer EA, Morris NP, Glanville RW, Burgeson RE. Cleavage of type VII collagen by interstitial collagenase and type IV collagenase (gelatinase) derived from human skin. *J Biol Chem.* 1989;264:3822–3826.
37. Parente MG, Chung LC, Ryynänen J et al. Human type VII collagen: cDNA cloning and chromosomal mapping of the gene. *Proc Natl Acad Sci.* 1991;88: 6931–6935.
38. Goldberg GI, Wilhelm SW, Kronberger A, Bauer EA, Grant GA, Eisen AZ. Human fibroblast collagenase. Complete primary structure and homology to an oncogene transformation-induced rat protein. *J Biol Chem.* 1986;261:6600–6605.
39. Wilhelm SM, Collier IE, Kronberger A, et al. Human skin fibroblast stromelysin: structure, glycosylation, substrate specificity, and differential expression in normal and tumorigenic cells. *Proc Natl Acad Sci.* 1987;84:6725–6729.
40. Clark SD, Kobayashi DK, Welgus HG. Regulation of the expression of tissue inhibitor of metalloproteinases and collagenase by retinoids and glucocorticoids in human fibroblasts. *J Clin Invest.* 1987;80:1280–1288.

5
Linkage Studies in
Epidermolysis Bullosa

Ervin H. Epstein, Jr.

The search for the fundamental defect in the various forms of epidermolysis bullosa (EB) has relied on careful clinical, histologic, and biochemical analysis of the skin of patients. Although many detailed analyses have been performed, thus far they have not demonstrated convincingly what primary genetic abnormality underlies the skin disease. Despite remarkable insights into a few diseases (e.g., mutant hemoglobins in sickle cell disease, decreased enzyme activity in some porphyrias, etc.) this situation in EB has been similar to the status of investigation of most other hereditary disorders, both cutaneous and extracutaneous.

More recently, however, the study of extracutaneous hereditary disorders has been revolutionized by shifting the primary investigative focus from enzyme activity and protein abundance to the DNA itself to the inherited sequences whose mutations are the actual stuff of heredity. Study of DNA instead of protein offers several advantages: one need not collect large amounts of affected skin—extracutaneous DNA (e.g., from peripheral blood leukocytes) is identical to that of skin; cloning or polymerase chain reaction (PCR) amplification allows one to replicate the DNA and hence to produce many identical molecules for analysis; cutting and separating fragments and determining the sequence of the monomers (bases) making up the polymer (DNA) is much easier; and genes are linked together physically—they are arranged in a specific order along 1 of the 22 autosomal or the X or Y chromosomes. It is this physical linkage that permits linkage analysis.

Linkage analysis allows one to answer the question "What is the physical location of the gene whose mutation(s) underlie an inherited disease?"; that is, on which part of which chromosome is the "disease gene" located? For such a study, one gathers specimens from affected and unaffected members of a kindred in which the disease of interest is inherited and compares the inheritance of the disease with the inheritance of each chromosomal region. For example, for an autosomal dominant disease in a three-generation kindred one expects that all affected grandchildren will inherit the mutant allele from the affected grandparent and that all unaffected grandchildren will inherit the normal allele from the unaffected grandparent. If there is no correlation between the inheritance of the disease versus normal status on the one hand and the inheritance of one or the other copy of the region of a chromosome that is tested, then the disease gene must not be on the chromosomal region that has been tested. One may as well abandon the tested region and go on to another chromosomal site.

Changing from study of protein polymorphisms to study of DNA polymorphisms has produced an explosion of interest in linkage analysis for two reasons: it has allowed the development of many more tools for identifying which chromosomal region came, in the above example, from the grandmother and which from the grandfather. Literally thousands of probes are now available to analyze the inheritance of each part of each chromosome, so the major hurdle to linkage analysis is the gathering of DNA from carefully studied, large kindreds.

Second, once the location of the disease gene has been found, other molecular biological techniques allow, currently with great effort, the identification of the actual disease gene and its mutation, so the genetic basis of disease can be uncovered even if one has no clue as to the deranged biochemical function that causes the phenotype. The pursuit of this strategy has produced the recent increasingly rapid and well publicized elucidation of the primary gene defects in cystic fibrosis, neurofibromatosis, Marfan's syndrome, and several hereditary cancers. Very recently, the pursuit of this strategy has produced strong evidence that defects in keratins and in type VII collagen genes underlie EB simplex and dominant dystrophic EB, respectively.

EB Simplex

Several years ago we developed the hypothesis that disorders of keratin genes—of genes coding for the major proteins of the keratinocyte "cytoskeleton"—might be responsible for the cellular fragility in EBS. Since it would be difficult to obtain large amounts of patient epidermis from which keratins could be extracted and since the defect potentially could be so subtle as to defy identification even if purified proteins were available, we chose instead to test the hypothesis by linkage analysis in families with EBS. We began by gathering DNA from leukocytes from members of large kindreds with EBS as well as collecting probes that identify polymorphisms at DNA loci near the keratin genes—the type I keratin gene cluster on chromosome 17q and the type II keratin gene cluster on chromosome 12q. Such probes enabled us to compare the inheritance, for example, of 12q with that of EBS. Thus, the question we asked was whether within a single family the inheritance of the paternal 12q was associated with EBS and of the maternal 12q with normal skin or whether the inheritance of the paternal and maternal 12q was independent of the ineritance of EBS. To our great satisfaction, we found that in the first family we studied, the inheritance of EBS was linked tightly to that of 12q (i.e., the EBS gene in this family is on 12q and lies very close to/within the cluster of type II keratin genes) and in a second family EBS was linked tightly to 17q (i.e., the EBS gene in this family lies very close to/within the cluster of type I keratin genes). Furthermore, in the second family we identified a single base pair substitution within keratin 14 (the type I keratin of basal keratinocytes) DNA that causes substitution of a proline for a leucine in the protein, a change expected to disrupt an α-helix and thereby to weaken the keratin filaments.[1] Others too have identified families with EBS in which the inheritance of the disease is linked strongly to 12q or 17q,[2] and it seems likely that in most (all?) patients with EBS, the fragility of the basal keratinocyte is caused by defects in its cytoskeleton.

Simultaneously, Fuchs and colleagues reached the same conclusion from a quite different approach.[3,4] They found that introduction into mice of a mutated gene producing abnormal keratins caused these transgenic mice to have basal keratinocyte fragility and blistering highly reminiscent of human EBS. Their work thus offers a second proof of the relationship between keratins and EBS.

This recent flurry was not the first attempt at linkage analysis in EBS. Olaissen and Gedde-Dahl[5,6] two decades ago analyzed protein polymorphisms and found very strong evidence localizing the gene for the Ogna subtype of EBS to a region quite close to the gene coding for the enzyme glutamic-pyruvic transminase (GPT). This gene is now believed to be on chromosome 8, and so it must be a gene quite separate from the keratin genes whose mutations underlie the thus-far studied cases of Köbner and Weber-Cockayne forms of EBS.

Dystrophic EB

As discussed elsewhere in this book, many years of elegant histological and biochemical effort have produced two prime suspects for the fundamental defect in dystrophic EB—primary defective anchoring fibrils versus a primary abnormal collagenase causing secondary destruction of anchoring fibrils. Linkage analysis from two groups now indicates the former is correct.

First, Uitto and colleagues[7] found the gene-encoding type VII collagen, the major constituent of the anchoring fibrils. Next, they identified a DNA polymorphism within the type VII collagen gene, and they used this polymorphism to determine that the gene for dominant dystrophic EB is very close/identical to the VII collagen gene.[8] Such data are now available for three families, and hence it seems extremely likely that mutations in this gene underlie disease in most (all?) kindreds with dominant dystrophic EB.

Simultaneously, Hovnanian and colleagues[9] identified polymorphisms in the collagenase gene and showed that, at least in some families, the gene causing recessive dystrophic EB is not linked to the collagenase gene. Hence in those families the increased collagenase enzyme activity must be secondary to some other fundamental defect. These successes can be contrasted with earlier efforts at linkage analysis of dystrophic EB using protein polymorphisms.[10,11] The comparison illustrates not only the increased power of studying DNA instead of proteins but also, of course, the greater power of testing a correct hypothesis (e.g., type VII collagen mutations underlie dystrophic EB) versus the more difficult effort to hunt for a disease gene at random sites.

Conclusions

The identification of gene abnormalities in these diseases by different groups nearly simultaneously indicates the immense increase in analytic power wrought by the new concentration on DNA and, especially, by linkage analysis rather than study of proteins. The finding of the type VII collagen gene as the defect in dominant dystrophic EB rather quickly should allow prenatal diagnosis to be DNA-based, thus obviating the current need for the technically more difficult biopsy of fetal skin. Last, identification of these primary defects may permit us finally to start devising therapies that might truly correct the skin abnormalities.

References

1. Bonifas JM, Rothman AL, Epstein EH Jr. Epidermolysis bullosa simplex: evidence in two families for keratin gene abnormalities. *Science*. 1991;254:1202–1205.
2. Ryynanen M, Knowlton RG, Uitto J. Mapping of epidermolysis bullosa simplex mutation to chromosome 12, *Am J Hum Genet*. 1991;49:978–984.
3. Coulombe PA, Hutton ME, Letai A, Hebert A, Paller AS, Fuchs E. Point mutations in human keratin 14 genes of epidermolysis bullosa simplex patients: genetic and functional analysis. *Cell*. 1991;66:1301–1311.
4. Vassar R, Coulombe PA, Degenstein L, Albers K, Fuchs E. Mutant keratin expression in transgenic mice causes marked abnormalities resembling a human genetic skin disease. *Cell*. 1991;64:365–380.
5. Olaisen B, Gedde-Dahl T Jr. GPT—epidermolysis bullosa simplex (EBS Ogna) linkage in man. *Hum Hered*. 1973;23:189–196.
6. Olaisen B, Gedde-Dahl T Jr. Gpt-EBS linkage group. *Hum Hered*. 1974;24:178–185.
7. Parente MG, Chung LC, Ryynanen J, et al. Human type VII colagen: cDNA cloning and chromosomal mapping of the gene. *Proc Natl Acad Sci*. 1991;88:6931–6935.
8. Ryynanen M, Knowlton RG, Parente MG, Clung LC, Chu M-1, Uitto J. Human type VII collagen: genetic linkage of the gene (COL7A1) on chromosome 3 to dominant dystrophic epidermolysis bullosa. *Am J Hum Genet*. 1991;49:797–803.
9. Hovnanian A, Duquesnoy P, Amselem S, et al. Exclusion of linkage between the collagenase gene and generalized recessive dystropic epidermolysis bullosa phenotype. *J Clin Invest*. 1991;88:1716–1721.

10. Joensen HD, Hansen HE, Henningsen K,Svejgaard A, Anderson I. A study of the linkage relations of epidermolysis bullosa dystrophica. *Hum Hered.* 1979;29: 221–225.
11. Mulley JC, Turner T, Nicholls C, Propert D, Sutherland GR. Genetic linkage analysis of epidermolysis bullosa dystrophica, Cockayne-Touraine type. *Clin Genet.* 1985;28:31–35.

6
Epidermolysis Bullosa Acquisita

DAVID T. WOODLEY, W. RAY GAMMON, and ROBERT A. BRIGGAMAN

History and Nosology

Acquired forms of epidermolysis bullosa have been recognized since 1895.[1] Although epidermolysis bullosa acquisita (EBA) is an acquired disease, it was given the name "epidermolysis bullosa" because the clinical features of the disease were reminiscent of hereditary dystrophic epidermolysis bullosa. The early published cases[1-4] were diagnosed by the clinical appearance of the disease, and it is likely that at least some of these cases were not bonafide cases of EBA. Since these early cases of EBA were reported before the advent of porphyrin biochemistry, immunofluorescent staining, and electron microscopy, it is possible that early reported cases of EBA may have included cases of porphyria cutanea tarda, pseudo-porphyria cutanea tarda, cicatricial pemphigoid, bullous vasculitis, or bullous pemphigoid.

In 1972, Roenigk and colleagues[5] reviewed the world literature on EBA and identified three new cases. These investigators recognized that EBA was a poorly defined entity and established the first firm criteria for the diagnosis. These criteria included that the patient have an acquired blistering disease in the absence of a family history of such a disorder in addition to skin fragility and a blister distribution in trauma-prone sites akin to the clinical features of hereditary epidermolysis bullosa. The final criterion was that all other blistering disorders be excluded.

It was thought at that time that direct immunofluorescent staining for immunoglobulin G (IgG) and complement at the cutaneous basement membrane zone was specific for the pemphigoid group of disorders. However, as the use of immunofluorescent methods became more widespread as an aid to the diagnosis of cutaneous diseases, it was soon recognized by Kushniruk[6] and later by Gibbs and Minus[7] that EBA, like bullous pemphigoid, could have IgG deposits and complement at the dermal–epidermal junction (DEJ).

Since both bullous pemphigoid and EBA were chronic, disabling, subepidermal blistering disorders with IgG deposits at the DEJ, could EBA be nothing more than a clinical variant of bullous pemphigoid? This question was put to rest by Nieboer and colleagues[8] and Yaoita and colleagues[9] who extended the immunofluorescent findings of Kushniruk[6] and Gibbs and Minus[7] by performing immunoelectron microscopy on perilesional skin of EBA patients and demonstrating that the precise localization of the immune complexes within the DEJ was different from bullous pemphigoid complexes. In EBA, the complexes were found to be within and below the lamina densa zone of the junction whereas the complexes in bullous pemphigoid were above the lamina densa in the lamina lucida space apposed to hemidesmosomes.[10-13]

Although perhaps not widely recognized at the time, the implications of the immunofluorescence and ultrastructural studies was that EBA and bullous pemphigoid could not be distinguished by immunofluorescence methods and that immunoelectron microscopy would be required to distinguish these two diseases. However, one reason that this notion was probably not popularized was because most dermatologists felt that they could easily distinguish these two diseases by the clinical features of the diseases. EBA was supposed to be a noninflammatory mechanobullous disease whereas bullous pemphigoid was supposed to be an inflammatory vesiculobullous disorder without skin fragility. Nevertheless, there were many patients with chronic blistering disorders who did not fall comfortably into these two clinical constellations, and many investigators reported series of "outlier" cases of EBA with a variety of clinical features.[14-20]

Gammon, Briggaman, and colleagues[14,15] used the most up-to-date methods of immunofluorescent and immunoelectron microscopy along with biochemical methods to document firmly that EBA could indeed present clinically as an inflammatory vesiculobullous disease with features identical to those of bullous pemphigoid. Using a novel method of immunofluorescent microscopy, they showed that between 8% and 14% of cases that had been diagnosed as bullous pemphigoid by two academic, immunodermatology units were, in fact, EBA cases that had been misdiagnosed.[21] These findings were later confirmed by others (personal communication, Jean-Claude Bystryn, New York, NY). The point of these studies is that EBA documented by immunological, ultrastructural, and biochemical parameters can present clinically as an inflammatory vesiculobullous disorder reminiscent of bullous pemphigoid or cicatricial pemphigoid. In addition, we have seen one patient witn a noninflammatory mechanobullous disease akin to the clinical features of "classical" EBA who by immunoelectron microscopy and biochemical methods (immunoprecipitation and Western blotting of specific antigen) was shown to have bullous pemphigoid.[22]

Since it is apparent that patients with EBA can present with clinical features of bullous pemphigoid and patients with bullous pemphigoid can present with a clinical appearance of a noninflammatory mechanobullous disease, the "bottom line" message is that special immunological tests (indirect immunofluorescence on salt split skin, immunoelectron microscopy, immunoprecipitation, and/or Western immune blotting against specific antigen) are methods that must be invoked to confirm the diagnosis of these disorders.

What is Known About EBA

EBA is a chronic, debilitating, blistering disease of the skin in which the full spectrum of clinical presentation is not fully established. There is good evidence to suggest that EBA may present clinically as a noninflammatory mechanobullous disorder with skin fragility, milia, and scarring, the so-called classical presentation that is reminiscent of hereditary dystrophic EB or porphyria cutanea tarda. However, the same disease (as strictly defined with histological, immunological, ultrastructural, and biochemical parameters) can also present as an inflammatory vesiculobullous disease akin to bullous pemphigoid or with prominent mucosal scarring reminiscent of cicatricial pemphigoid.[14-20] It is also possible that other new clinical presentations of EBA will be defined in the future.

Since the studies of Yaoita et al., positive direct immunofluorescent staining for IgG deposits in the DEJ of perilesional skin has been added as a diagnostic criterion. In addition, the localization of these IgG deposits within the DEJ by direct immunoelectron microscopy should be below the lamina densa zone, and no immune deposits should be found within the lamina lucida space (where the immune deposits are found in bullous pemphigoid).

In addition to immune deposits within the DEJ, about 50% of patients with EBA have autoimmune, anti–basement membrane zone antibodies circulating in their plasma. These can be detected by indirect immunofluorescence on normal human skin substrate. Alternatively, normal human skin can be incubated in cold 1 M salt for 72 to 96 hours, at which time the DEJ can be separated through the lamina lucida space.[23] This salt-separated skin can be used as substrate for indirect immunofluorescent testing and has the advantage of placing the bullous pemphigoid antigen on the epidermal roof of the separation and the EBA antigen on the dermal floor of the separation.[21,23] Gammon and colleagues[21,24] have shown that indirect immunofluorescent staining of salt-separated skin substrate with patient sera can be used to distinguish whether the serum antibodies are to the bullous pemphigoid antigen (epidermal roof staining) or to the EBA antigen (dermal floor staining). This immunofluorescent test is a rapid screening procedure that is useful when a patient with an unknown blistering disorder has a serum antibody to the basement membrane zone detected by routine indirect immunofluorescence. By simply repeating the test with salt-split skin substrate, it can be determined if the target for the antibody is the bullous pemphigoid antigen or the EBA antigen.

Recently, it has been shown that the target for EBA antibodies is type VII collagen.[25] This type of collagen is specifically localized to anchoring fibrils within the DEJ.[26] Anchoring fibrils are wheat-stack–shaped structures aligned perpendicular to the lamina densa zone of the junction.[27] Anchoring fibrils are decreased in lesional skin of EBA patients.[7,20,28-30] In situations in which there are few anchoring fibrils, epidermal–dermal adherence appears to be compromised.[31] Although not directly proven, there is the notion that anchoring fibrils serve to "anchor" the epidermis to dermal connective tissue. It has been shown that the EBA antigen/type VII collagen has specific affinity for fibronectin, a major dermal glycoprotein.[32] This interaction may play a role in the maintenance of normal epidermal–dermal adherence. The EBA antigen/type VII collagen in vitro can be immunoprecipitated from both human keratinocyte cultures and human dermal fibroblast cultures suggesting that both cell types can contribute to the formation of anchoring fibrils.[33–35] It is unclear which cell type in vivo contributes to anchoring fibril formation, and it is conceivable that under different situations (gestation, wound healing, etc.) one or both cell types may be invoked to make anchoring fibril collagen.

The structure of the EBA antigen/type VII collagen is not fully known. It is known that the molecule has a large noncollagen, carboxyl domain of approximately 145 to 150 kDa. The other half of the molecule consists of a typical helical collagen domain that ends with the amino terminus.[36,37] The noncollagen, carboxyl domain is globular and the helical collagen domain is rodlike. Therefore, the entire molecule (or chain) is shaped something like a baton with a soft ball attached to one end. Each chain has the approximate size of near 290 to 300 kDa and is related to two other chains in a triple helix. So, one would predict that native type VII collagen in vivo would have a molecular size near 900 kDa. These triple helical macromolecules are attached at the globular, carboxyl terminus to the lamina densa. The helical chain then "hangs" perpendicularly from the lamina densa into the papillary dermis where its amino terminus is attached to a second macromolecule by its amino terminus (i.e., like-end to like-end). These two type VII macromolecules aligned like-end to like-end by their amino termini then laterally aggregate with other identically aligned duets of type VII collagen macromolecules to form wheat-stack–shaped anchoring fibrils.[36,37] Both bacterial collagenase[38,39] and human skin collagenase call cleave type VII collagen.[40,41]

How is EBA Related to Hereditary Dystrophic EB?

An important question, at least with regard to this volume on hereditary EB, is how acquired EB is related to the hereditary forms of EB. Although EBA has a variety of clinical presentations as outlined above, certainly a predominant presentation is that of a noninflammatory mechanobullous disease characterized by skin fragility and healing with milia and scar formation (Figs. 6.1, 6.2, 6.3), a presentation reminiscent of hereditary dystrophic EB. We do not know the etiology of EBA or of any of the forms of hereditary EB. Therefore, to say how these entities are related is completely speculative at this point. However, it is fair to say that the initiating events in EBA and hereditary dystrophic EBs must be very different. EBA is an autoimmune blistering disorder, and although there is no proof to date that the auto-

(text continued on page 82)

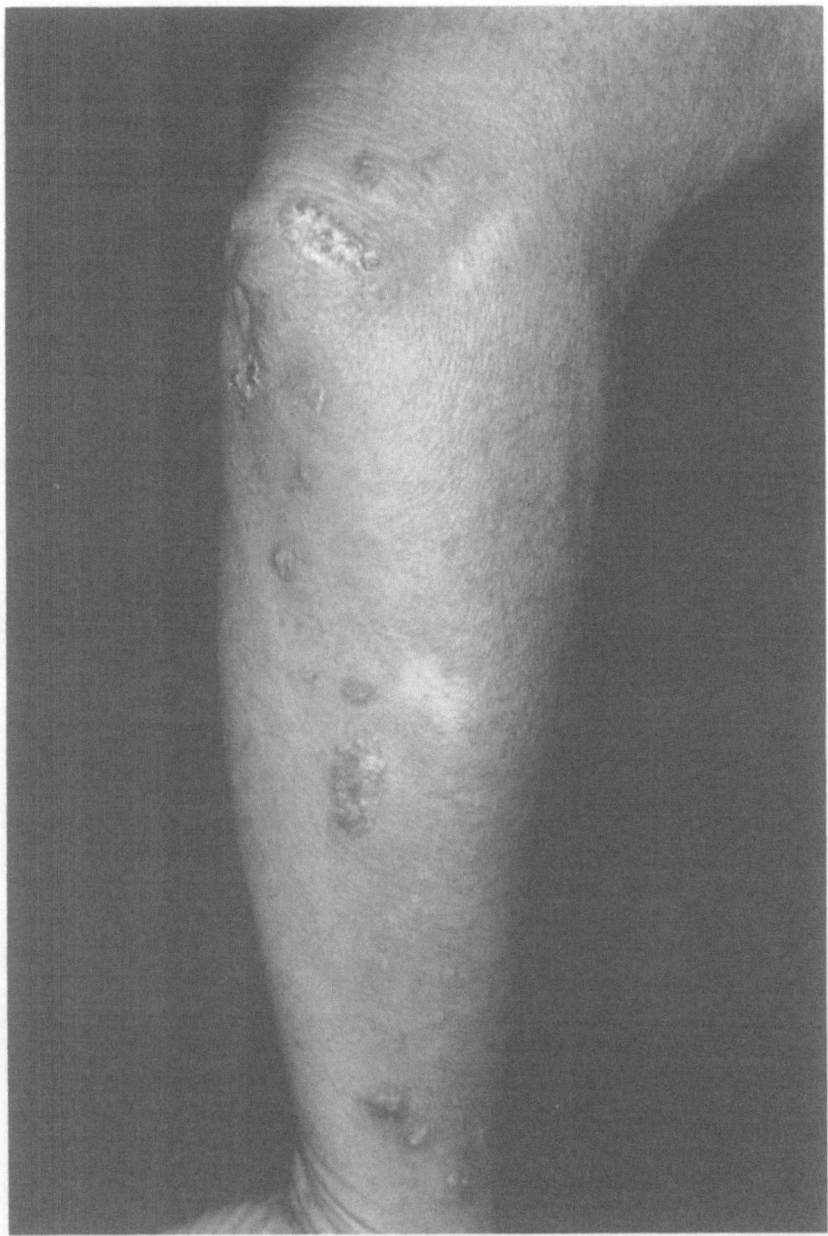

FIGURE 6.1. Erosions and scars with milia formation on the elbow and forearm of a patient with EBA.

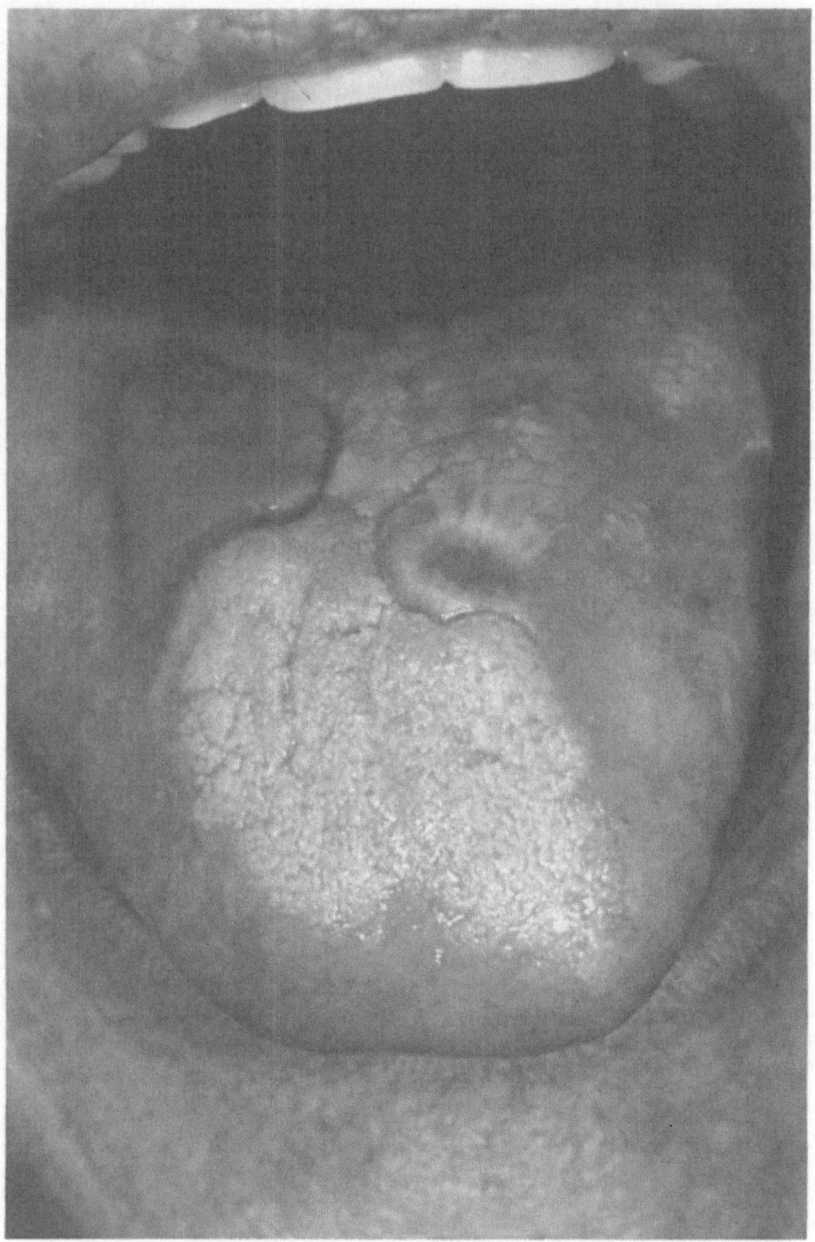

FIGURE 6.2. Severe oral mucosal involvement in a patient with EBA.

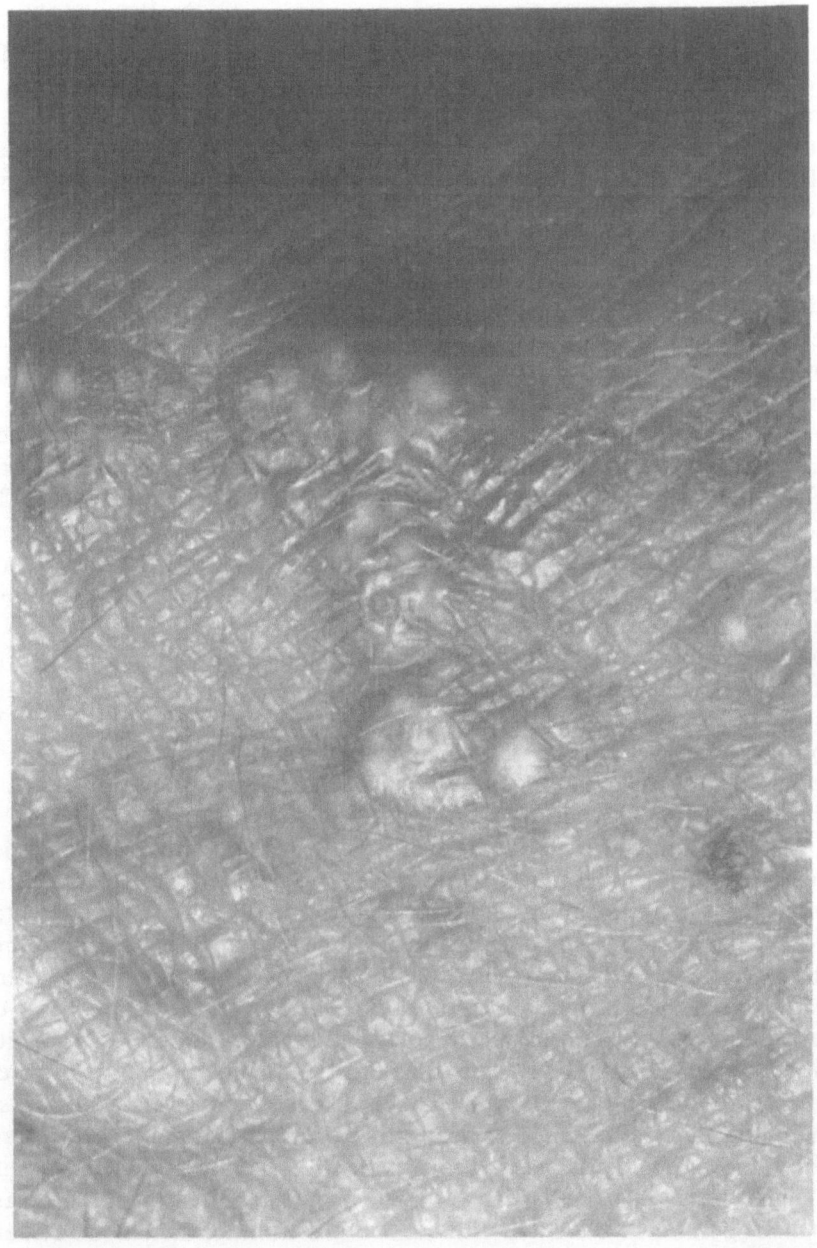

FIGURE 6.3. Multiple milia cysts within a scarred area of an extensor surface of a patient with EBA.

antibodies to type VII collagen in a patient's skin and plasma are pathogenic, there is evidence to suggest that these antibodies do play a role in EBA. Gammon and colleagues[42] have shown that in organ culture immune deposits within the DEJ of EBA skin will fix complement and induce human leukocytes to migrate to the junction, a situation analogous in many ways to EBA in humans. In another set of experiments, normal human skin was incubated in culture with EBA antibodies, complement, and neutrophils. The EBA antibodies were capable of binding to the EBA antigen within the DEJ of the normal skin and fix complement. Neutrophils migrated and adhered to the junction and induced a separation of the epidermis from the dermis.[42] Although this is not classical in vivo passive transfer of the disease, this is the in vitro equivalent and strongly suggests a pathogenic role for EBA antibodies.

EBA patients have a very high incidence of the HLA-DR2 phenotype,[43] which strongly suggests that there is a genetic predisposition to the disease. HLA-D antigens are thought to be linked to human immune functions. The fact that HLA-DR2 is also highly represented in bullous lupus erythematosus patients[43] who often have autoantibodies to type VII collagen[44] would suggest that this HLA phenotype may be broadly implicated in hyperimmune states in which autoantibodies to type VII collagen are a feature. So, in common with hereditary dystrophic EB, one could argue that EBA is sort of a genetic disease in which there is an HLA phenotype clustering that is associated with a predisposition to autoimmunity and antibodies to type VII collagen. However, to our knowledge, patients with recessive dystrophic EB do not have a particular clustering of HLA antigens, hyperimmunity, or a propensity for making autoantibodies.

EBA patients and recessive dystrophic EB patients both have decreased anchoring fibrils,[28,30,45-47] scarring, and skin fragility. However, the reason for the paucity of anchoring fibrils in the two diseases appears different: in those with recessive dystrophic EB, anchoring fibrils are thought to be diminished due to an overabundance of skin collagenase produced by EB fibroblasts within the dermis.[45,46] It is known that human skin collagenase can degrade type VII (anchoring fibril) collagen[40,41] in addition to dermal interstitial collagens I and III. Despite the paucity of anchoring fibrils in hereditary dystrophic EB patients, Rusenko et al.[48] have shown that remnants of anchoring fibril collagen, specifically the carboxyl domain, is still present within the lamina densa. This is consistent with the notion that this domain is highly resistant to collagenase digestion.[38,39] The reason for decreased anchoring fibrils in EBA is not understood. Currently, there is no evidence that EBA patients have increased levels of collagenase in their skin or that their fibroblasts synthesize increased levels of the enzyme. It is more likely that the anchoring fibril degradation (and type VII collagen degradation) is due to an inflammatory process that is initiated by some immune event such as immune complexes of IgG and complement being bound to type VII collagen molecules in the DEJ. It is also likely that decreased anchoring fibrils correlate with poor DEJ adherence and blister formation,[31] but this point has not been proven.

In addition to blister formation and decreased anchoring fibrils, the other common features of both EBA and hereditary dystrophic EB include a healing pattern characterized by scar formation and milia. This healing response is not specific for EB since it is a common feature of porphyria cutanea tarda and may be seen, although rarely, in bullous pemphigoid.[22] Despite the different initiating events in EBA and recessive dystrophic EB, it is hard to imagine that there are not "final pathway" events that are held in common in these two diseases that lead to the characteristic scarring and milia formation seen in healed lesions of both entities. Said another way, there may be pathomechanisms of these two diseases that are similar, and understanding the mechanisms of one disease will probably provide clues that lead to the understanding of pathomechanisms involved in the other.

EBA has been reported to occur in association with various systemic diseases, many of which are autoimmune in nature. The association with inflammatory bowel diseases (Crohn's disease and ulcerative colitis) is likely to be significant,[49] as is the association with systemic lupus erythematosis.[50] Association with other diseases is based mainly on isolated case reports, and the significance of such associations remains unclear. Examples include[5,51] rheumatoid arthritis, amyloidosis, diabetes mellitus, autoimmune thyroiditis, hypothyroidism, multiple endocrinopathy syndrome, and a lymphomalike illness. It is interesting that a number of the associated disorders are thought to have an autoimmune pathogenesis. Most patients respond poorly to various topical and systemic medications. Favorable response to oral cyclosporine A has been reported,[52,53] but the potential for irreversible renal toxicity requires extreme care in the use of this agent, and only as a last resort.[54]

Acknowledgments. Supported by grants AM33625, AR30475, AR10546, and AR30475 from the National Institutes of Health.

References

1. Elliott GT. Two cases of epidermolysis bullosa. *J Cutan Genitourin Dis.* 1895;13: 10–18.
2. Wise F, Lautman MF. Epidermolysis bullosa beginning in adult life. The acquired form of the disease, with the report of a case and review of the literature. *J Cutan Dis.* 1915;33:44–52.
3. Kablitz R. Ein Reitrag Zur Frage der Epidermolysis bullosa (hereditaria et acquisita) Rostock, 1904:Dissertation.
4. Hundley JL, Smith DC. Epidermolysis bullosa acquisita. *South Med J.* 1941;34: 364–367.
5. Roenigk HH, Ryan JG, Bergfeld WF. Epidermolysis bullosa acquisita: report of three cases and review of all published cases. *Arch Dematol.*1971;103:1–10.

6. Kushniruk W. The immunopathology of epidermolysis bullosa acquisita. *Can Med Assoc J*. 1973;108:1143–1146.
7. Gibbs RB, Minus HR. Epidermolysis bullosa acquisita with electron microscopical studies. *Arch Dermatol*. 1975;111:215–220.
8. Nieboer C, Boorsma DM, Woerdeman MJ, Kalsbeck GL. Epidermolysis bullosa acquisita: immunofluorescence, electron microscopic and immunoelectron microscopic studies in four patients. *Br J Dermatol*. 1980;102:383–392.
9. Yaoita H, Briggaman RA, Lawley TJ, Provost TT, Katz SI. Epidermolysis bullosa acquisita: ultastructural and immunological studies. *J Invest Dermatol*. 1981; 76:288–292.
10. Schaumberg-Lever G, Rule RA, Schmidt-Ullrich B, Lever WF. Ultrastructural localization of in vivo bound immunoglobulins in bullous pemphigoid: a preliminary report. *J Invest Dermatol*. 1975;64:47–49.
11. Holubar K, Wolff K, Konrad K, Beutner EH. Ultrastructural localization of immunoglobulins in bullous pemphigoid skin. *J Invest Dermatol*. 1975;64:220–227.
12. Mutasim DF, Takahashi Y, Ramzy LS, Anhalt GJ, Patel HP, Diaz LA. A pool of bullous pemphigoid antigen(s) is intracellular and associated with the basal cell cytoskeleton-hemidesmosome complex. *J Invest Dermatol*. 1986;84:47–53.
13. Regnier M, Vaigot P, Michel S, Prunieras M. Localization of bullous pemphigoid antigen in isolated human keratinocytes. *J Invest Dermatol*. 1985;85:187–190.
14. Gammon WR, Briggaman RA, Wheeler CE Jr. Epidermolysis bullosa acquisita presenting as an inflammatory bullous disease. *J Am Acad Dermatol*. 1982;7: 382–387.
15. Gammon WR, Briggaman RA, Woodley DT, Heald PW, Wheeler CE Jr. Epidermolysis bullosa acquisita—a pemphigoid-like disease. *J Am Acad Dermatol*. 1984;11:820–832.
16. Dahl MGC. Epidermolysis bullosa acquisita—a sign of cicatricial pemphigoid? *Br J Dermatol*. 1979;101:475–483.
17. Richter BJ, McNutt NS. The spectrum of epidermolysis bullosa acquisita. *Arch Dermatol*. 1979;115:1325–1328.
18. Provost TT, Maize JC, Amed AR. Unusual subepidermal bullous diseases presenting as an inflammatory bullous disease. *Arch Dermatol*. 1979; 115:156–160.
19. Palestine RF, Kossard S, Dicken CH. Epidermolysis bullosa acquisita: a heterogeneous disease. *J Am Acad Dermatol*. 1981;5:43–53.
20. Wilson BD, Brinkrant AF, Beutner EH, Maize JC. Epidermolysis bullosa acquisita: a clinical disorder of varied etiologies: two cases and a review of immunologic and other reported findings. *J Am Acad Dermatol*. 1980;3:280–291.
21. Gammon WR, Briggaman RA, Inman AO, Queen LL, Wheeler CE Jr. Differentiating anti-lamina lucida and anti-sublamina densa anti-BMZ antibodies by direct immunofluorescence on 1.0 M sodium chloride-separated skin. *J Invest Dermatol*. 1984;82:139–144.
22. Mutasim D, Anhalt G, Woodley DT, Briggaman RA, Diaz LA, Patel HP. Immunological and ultrastructural characterization of a subepidermal bullous disease with features of bullous pemphigoid and epidermolysis bullosa acquisita. *Clin Res*. 1986;34:77A.
23. Woodley DT, Sauder D, Talley MJ, Silver M, Grotendorst G, Qwarnstrom E. Localization of basement membrane components after dermal–epidermal junction separation. *J Invest Dermatol*. 1983;81:149–153.

24. Woodley DT, Briggaman RA, O'Keefe EJ, Inman AO, Queen LL, Gammon WR. Identification of the skin basement membrane autoantigen in epidermolysis bullosa acquisita. *N Engl J Med.* 1984;310:1007–1013.
25. Woodley DT, Burgeson RE, Lunstrum GP, Reese MJ, Bruckner-Tuderman L, Briggaman RA. The epidermolysis bullosa acquisita antigen is the globular carboxyl terminus of type VII procollagen. *J Clin Invest.* 1988;81:683–687.
26. Sakai LY, Keene DR, Morris NP, Burgeson RE. Type VII collagen is a major structural component of anchoring fibrils. *J Cell Biol.* 1986;103:1577–1586.
27. Briggaman RA, Wheeler CE Jr. The epidermal-dermal junction. *J Invest Dermatol.* 1975;65:71–84.
28. Woerdeman MJ. Epidermolysis bullosa dystrophica acquisita. *Dermatologica.* 1974;149:184–186.
29. Ray TL, Levine JB, Weiss W, Ward PA. Epidermolysis bullosa acquisita and inflammatory bowel disease. *J Am Acad Dermatol.* 1982;6:242–252.
30. Benedetto AV, Bergfeld WF, Taylor JS, Osborne DG. Epidermolysis bullosa acquisita Diagnosis by electron microscopy. *Cleve Clin Q.* 1976;43:283–293.
31. Woodley DT, Peterson HD, Herzog SR, et al. Burn wounds resurfaced by cultured epidermal autografts show abnormal reconstitution of anchoring fibrils. *J Am Acad Dermatol.* 1988;259:2566–2571.
32. Woodley DT, O'Keefe EJ, McDonald JA, Reese MJ, Briggaman RA, Gammon WR. Specific affinity between fibronectin and the epidermolysis bullosa acquisita antigen. *J Clin Invest.* 1987;179:1826–1830.
33. Woodley DT, Briggaman RA, Gammon WR, O'Keefe EJ. Epidermolysis bullosa acquisita antigen is synthesized by human keratinocytes cultured in serum-free medium. *Biochem Biophys Res Commun.* 1985;130:1267–1272.
34. Woodley DT, Briggaman RA, Gammon WR, et al. Epidermolysis bullosa acquisita antigen, a major cutaneous basement membrane component is synthesized by human dermal fibroblasts and other cutaneous tissues. *J Invest Dermatol.* 1986;87:227–231.
35. Stanley JR, Rubinstein N. Klaus-Kovtun V. Epidermolysis bullosa acquisita antigen is synthesized by both human keratinocyte and human dermal fibroblasts. *J Invest Dermatol.* 1985;85:542–545.
36. Keene DR, Sakai LY, Lunstrum GP, Morris NP, Burgeson RE. Type VII collagen forms an extended network of anchoring fibrils. *J Cell Biol.* 1987;104:611–622.
37. Lundstrum GP, Kuo H-J, Rosenbaum LM, et al. Anchoring fibrils contain the carboxyl-terminal globular domain of type VII procollagen, but lack the amino-terminal globular domain. *J Biol Chem.* 1987;262:13, 706–13, 712.
38. Yoshiike T, Woodley DT, Briggaman RA. Epidermolysis bullosa acquisita: relationship between the collagenase-sensitive and -insensitive domains. *J Invest Dermatol.* 1988;90:127–133.
39. Woodley DT, O'Keefe EJ, Reese MJ, Mechanic GL, Briggaman RA, Gammon WR. Epidermolysis bullosa acquisita antigen, a new major component of cutaneous basement membrane, is a glycoprotein with collagenous domains. *J Invest Dermatol.* 1986;86:668–672.
40. Seltzer JI, Eisen AZ, Bauer EA, Morris NP, Glanville RW, Burgeson RE. Cleavage of type VII collagen by interstitial collagenase and type IV collagenase (gelatinase) derived from human skin. *J Cell Biol.* 1989;264:3822–3826.
41. Woodley DT, Petersen MJ, Wynn KC, Briggaman RA O'Keefe EJ. Human skin

collagenase degrades epidermolysis bullosa acquisita antigen (EBA-Ag) type VII (anchoring fibril) collagen. *J Invest Dermatol.* 1989;92:543.

42. Gammon WR, Inman AO, Wheeler CE Jr. Differences in complement-dependent chemotactic activity generated by bullous pemphigoid and epidermolysis bullosa acquisita immune complexes: demonstration by leukocyte attachment and organ culture methods. *J Invest Dermatol.* 1984;83:57–61.

43. Gammon WR, Heise ER, Burke WA, Dole KC, Woodley DT, Briggaman RA. Production of epidermolysis bullosa acquisita autoantibodies is associated with the HLA-DR2 phenotype. *J Invest Dermatol.* 1986;86:476.

44. Gammon WR, Woodley DT, Dole KC, Briggaman RA. Evidence that antibasement membrane zone antibodies in bullous eruption of systemic lupus erythematosus recognize epidermolysis bullosa acquisita autoantigens. *J Invest Dermatol.* 1985;84:472–476.

45. Bauer EA, Eisen AZ. Recessive dystrophic epidermolysis bullosa: evidence for increased collagenase as a genetic characteristic in cell culture. *J Exp Med.* 1978; 148:1378–1387.

46. Bauer EA, Gedde-Dahl T, Eizen AZ. The role of human skin collagenase in epidermolysis bullosa. *J Invest Dermatol.* 1977;68:119–124.

47. Briggaman RA. Hereditary epidermolysis bullosa with special emphasis on newly reorganized syndromes and complications. *Dermatol Clin.* 1983;1:263–280.

48. Rusenko KW, Gammon WR, Fine JD, Briggaman RA. The carboxyl-terminal domain of type VII collagen is present at the basement membrane in recessive dystrophic epidermolysis bullosa. *J Invest Dermatol.* 1989;92:623–627.

49. Raab B, Fretzin DF, Bronson DM, Scott MJ, Roenigk Jr HH, Medenica M. Epidermolysis bullosa acquisita and inflammatory bowel disease. *JAMA.* 1983; 250:1746–1748.

50. Boh E, Roberts LJ, Lieu T-S, Gammon WR, Sontheimer RD. Epidermolysis bullosa acquisita preceding the development of systemic lupus erythematosus. *J Am Acad Dermatol.* 1990;22:587–593.

51. Burke WA, Briggaman RA, Gammon WR. Epidermolysis bullosa acquisita in a patient with multiple endocrinopathies syndrome. *Arch Dermatol.* 1986;122:187–189.

52. Crow LL, Finkle JP, Woodley DT, Gammon WR. Clearing of epidermolysis bullosa acquisita on cyclosporine A. *J Am Acad Dermatol.* 1988;19:937–941.

53. Merle C, Blanc D, Zultak M, Van Landuyt, Drobacheff C, Laurent R. Intractable epidermolysis bullosa acquisita: efficacy of cyclosporine A. *Dermatologica.* 1990; 181:44–47.

54. Woodley DT, Crow L. Reply to letter by Layton and Cunliffe (letter). *J Am Acad Dermatol.* 1990;22:535–536.

III
Clinical Overview

7
Epidermolysis Bullosa Simplex: A Clinical Overview

ANDREW N. LIN and D. MARTIN CARTER

Epidermolysis bullosa simplex (EBS) is characterized by formation of intra-epidermal blisters. As a rule, the degree of clinical involvement is mild, blisters generally heal without scarring unless lesions become infected, and milia generally do not occur. Mucosal involvement is usually restricted to the mouth, and estimates of the incidence of oral blistering range from 2%[1] to 30%.[2] Nails and teeth are usually normal. Corneal involvement[3] has been reported but is very uncommon. There is one reported case of ear involvement causing stricture of the external auditory canal,[4] but EBS cannot be substantiated in that patient because the pedigree suggested an autosomal recessive trait and ultrastructural findings were not presented. Patients may experience only occasional cutaneous blistering that does not significantly affect their lifestyle. This mild degree of involvement is reflected in the old terminology, now no longer used, where EBS was called "benign EB," in contrast to"malignant EB," which referred to dystrophic forms.[5]

Light microscopic examination of a blister may show intraepidermal separation, usually at the level of the basal cells (Fig. 7.1). However, because separation occurs so low in the epidermis, light microscopy often cannot identify precisely the level of split, but shows instead the presence of a blister at the area of the basement membrane zone, often indistinguishable from a blister occurring in the lamina lucida (as in junctional EB) or even a blister below the lamina densa (as in dystrophic EB). Confirmation is therefore required, either by electron microscopy or immunofluorescence mapping. Electron microscopy shows breakdown of the basal cell (Fig. 7.2), usually at the region below the nucleus ("subnuclear cytolysis"). The lamina densa occurs at the base of the blister cavity, and hemidesmosomes and anchoring fibrils remain normal in appearance. Immunofluorescence mapping shows intraepidermal separation with bullous pemphigoid antigen, laminin, and type IV collagen all located on the blister floor (see also Chapter 3). To emphasize the intraepidermal location of the blister cavity, EBS is sometimes called "epidermolytic" EB.

The literature contains numerous reports in which affected individuals

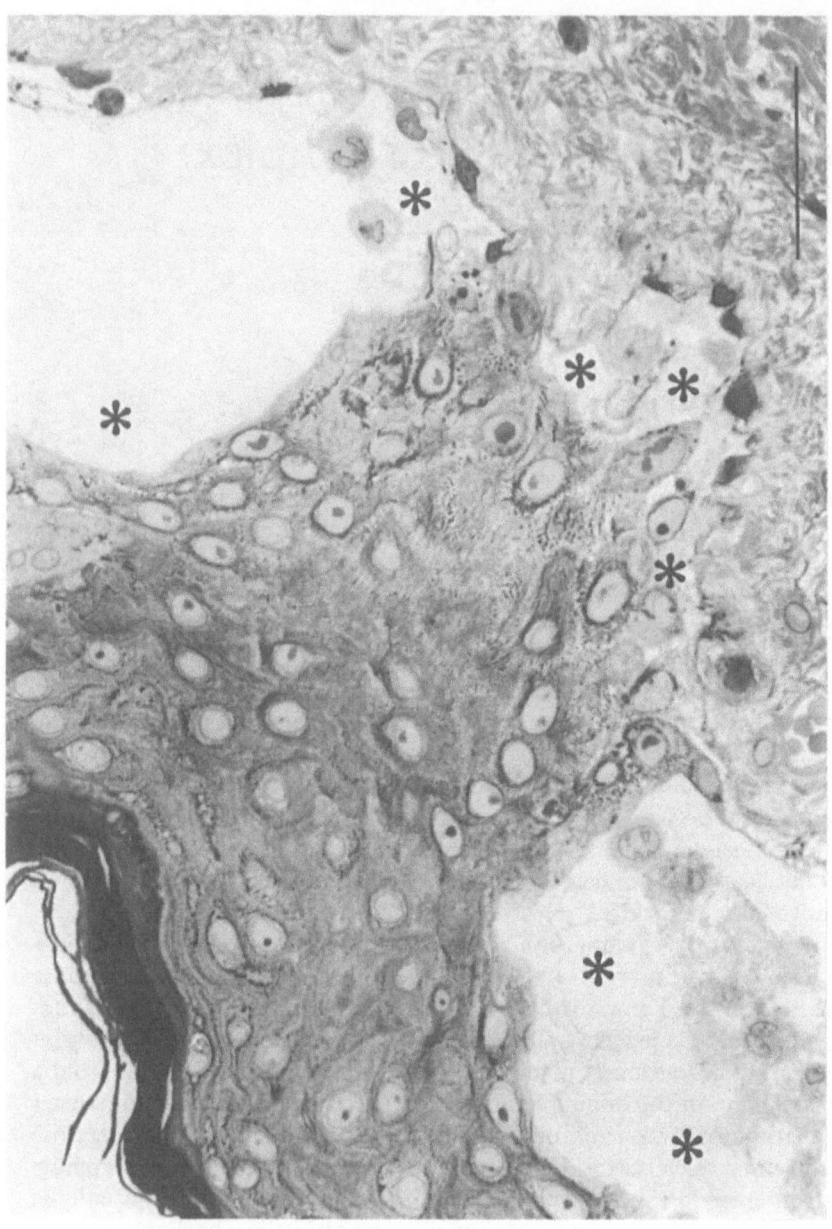

FIGURE. 7.1. Light micrograph of EBS. The blister cavity (*) is formed by lysis of basal keratinocytes. The basement membrane and remnants of the epidermis form the floor of the blister. Inflammatory cells are present within the cavity. (Bar = 50 μm, 522 ×). (Photomicrograph courtesy of Lynne T. Smith, Seattle, WA.)

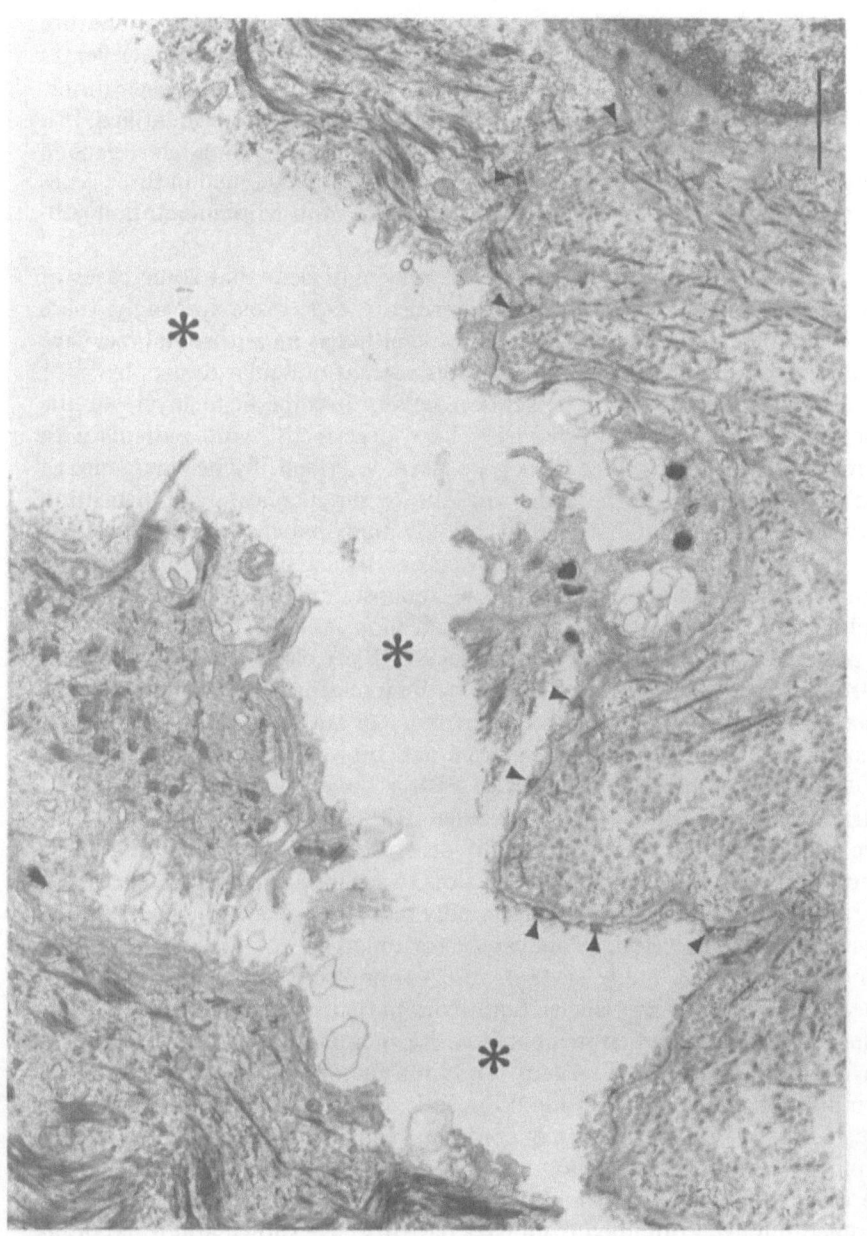

FIGURE. 7.2. Electron micrograph of EBS. The blister cavity (*) has formed within the basal keratinocytes. Remnants of the basal keratinocytes including intact hemidesmosomes (arrowheads) are attached along the dermal–epidermal junction. (Bar = 1 μm, 13,320×). (Electron micrograph courtesy of Lynne T. Smith, Seattle, WA.)

occur in consecutive generations, attesting to the autosomal dominant nature in which this disorder is inherited.[5-11] Spontaneous mutation, however, is common. In one kindred involving 83 affected individuals in six generations, three individuals with reduced expressivity of the gene were identified.[8] In one study of HLA antigens and EB, investigators reported that "close genetic linkage and, therefore, true association to HLA" was excluded in three types of EB simplex (the Ogna, Weber-Cockayne, and mottled pigmentation subtypes), and in five other types of EB.[12]

In the last few years it has become increasingly clear that some cases of EBS do not conform to the pattern described above. Most strikingly, there have been kindreds in which EBS was transmitted as an autosomal recessive trait and associated with systemic disorders such as muscular dystrophy.[13-16] In addition, cases in which separation occurs in superficial layers of the epidermis, above the basal cells, have been described,[17] and patients with severe skin involvement since birth have been described.[18] The emergence of these "atypical" cases of EBS may be due to the increasing sophistication with which EB is subclassified. Until recently many patients were classified as EBS solely on the basis of clinical features, which usually consist of the absence of scarring, of milia, and of mucosal involvement. Diagnostic histologic criteria were not established and biopsies were rarely performed. It is possible that as more and more cases of EB are classified on the basis of electron microscopic examination, and with increasing use of immunofluorescence mapping using an increasing repertory of antibodies directed against basement membrane constituents, more and more "atypical" cases will be uncovered. The complete spectrum of EBS is therefore more complex than the traditional concept of mild involvement with autosomal dominant inheritance and probably remains to be fully described[19] (Table 7.1). While these observations may initially lend confusion to existing schemes of classification, in the long run they will undoubtedly increase the accuracy with which prognosis and genetic counseling can be formulated.

Investigators have made several observations that may help to explain blister formation in EBS. Blister fluid from patients with EBS caused intraepidermal separation when incubated with organ cultures of normal human skin, suggesting that the fluid may contain a factor such as an enzyme that can induce blistering.[20-21] Using fluorescein-labeled affinity-purified lectins, a specific defect in glycosylation of epidermal cell membranes was seen in skin samples of EBS, but not junctional or dystrophic forms, suggesting there may be a selective defect in cell membrane glycoproteins or glycolipids.[22] Cultured keratinocytes obtained from EBS patients have shown abnormal organization of keratin intermediate filaments.[23] Elevated levels of alphafetoprotein have been noted in maternal serum and amniotic fluid obtained during delivery of an infant with EBS.[24] Sera from six patients in one family with EBS contained antibodies against the collagen C chain derived from basememnt membrane structures.[25] Because these studies have in-

TABLE 7.1. Clinical types of epidermolysis bullosa simplex (all autosomal dominant, except where noted).

Clinical type	Characteristic
Common types of EBS:	
EBS of Weber-Cockayne	Predominant involvement of hands and feet
Generalized EBS of Köbner	Generalized involvement of skin
EBS herpetiformis of	Grouped blisters
Dowling-Meara	Progressive hyperkeratosis of palms and soles
	Blistering can be severe at birth, but improvement may occur with age
	Clumping of tonofilament seen on electron microscopy
Uncommon types of EBS:	
EBS with mottled pigmentation	Mottled pigmentation of skin, especially on extremities and trunk
EBS Ogna	Tendency for cutaneous bruising
Autosomal recessive EBS with	Autosomal recessive inheritance
neuromuscular disease	Association with muscular dystrophy, myasthenia gravis
"Lethal autosomal recessive EBS	Early death (8 days to 20 months)
	Reported in only one kindred
Kallin's syndrome	Missing teeth, dystrophic nails, nonscarring alopecia
	Reported in only one kindred, pattern consistent with autosomal recessive
Autosomal recessive EBS of	Predominant involvement of hands and feet
Weber-Cockayne	Reported in only one kindred, pattern consistent with autosomal recessive
EBS superficialis	Subcorneal blistering
Conditions of uncertain nosology	
Mendes da Costa syndrome	X-linked recessive
	Blisters reported to occur spontaneously, not in response to mechanical friction
Bart's syndrome	Congenital absence of skin
	Skin and mucosal blistering that heals without scars
	Nail abnormalities

volved small numbers of patients, it is unclear how significant are the results in the pathogenesis of EBS.

An animal model of EBS has been described in the collie dog.[26] A radiation-induced autosomal recessive condition has been described in the rat; it is characterized by friction-induced blisters showing suprabasal, intraepidermal split, but it is unclear if there is a human analogue.[27] A familial blistering disorder in angus calves is characterized by acantholysis and resembles Hailey-Hailey disease rather than EBS.[28] A condition similar to EBS has been observed in transgenic mice expressing a mutant keratin in the basal layer of the stratified squamous epithelia.[29] These mice blister easily and often die prematurely. Light and electron microscopy showed basal cell cytolysis and keratin aggregates were seen in basal cells, but terminally differentiating cells in the suprabasal layers made keratin filaments and formed a stratum corneum.[29]

Weber-Cockayne EBS

This condition is the most common form of EBS[16,30] and is named after the physicians who characterized it.[31,32] Because of distinctive clinical features, it is one of the most readily recognizable forms of EB. Typically blistering is confined mainly to the hands and feet (Fig. 7.3), often after an identifiable physical activity such as gardening, ironing, or walking. Lesions may also occur on other sites, but these are usually not a prominent feature. Although onset is usually during infancy or early childhood,[31,33] some patients do not notice blistering until early adolescence.[34] The degree of blistering may be so mild that patients do not seek medical attention until the condition becomes bothersome because of a sudden increase in physical activity, such as enlisting in the army.[34-44] Oral mucosal involvement is either absent or mild. Nail involvement is not common, but pachyonychia has been reported.[45] Blistering tends to be worse during hot weather. Patients may also have hyperhidrosis of the palms and soles, which can severely worsen the blistering during summer months.[46,47] Treatment with 20% aluminum chloride hexahydrate has been found to decrease sweating and improve blistering,[48,49] whereas topical glutaraldehyde was useful but caused irritant and sensitizing effects.[50] Improvement with concomitant use of oral vitamin E and topical "hyperhidrosis powder" has been noted.[51] One patient noted marked reduction of blistering while taking oral isotretinoin.[52] A double-blind, controlled study involving nine patients with Weber-Cockayne EBS and one patient with the generalized type showed that topical bufexamac was ineffective.[53]

This condition is transmitted as an autosomal dominant trait.[35,38,54-60] Fine et al. described a kindred in which four patients presented with features consistent with Weber-Cockayne EBS, but analysis of pedigree suggested the trait was transmitted in autosomal recessive fashion.[16] The significance of this observation is unclear, but it might indicate a new subtype of EB simplex.

The ultrastructural defects of Weber-Cockayne EBS were studied by Haneke et al.[61,62] They induced fresh blisters by friction after patients took a hot bath. They found that blister formation started with dilution of organelles of the cells in the basal layer, followed by formation of cytoplasmic holes that merge to reuslt in blisters found between the dermal–epidermal junction and the nucleus. They did not observe structural abnormalities, and cell organelles remained intact. The occurrence of macular amyloidosis in a patient with Weber-Cockayne EBS has led to the speculation that both conditions may involve basal cell lysosomal activation.[63]

Generalized EBS of Köbner

The Köbner variant of generalized EBS differs from Weber-Cockayne EBS only in extent of cutaneous involvement. Instead of affecting mainly the hands and feet, the Köbner type of EBS can cause blister formation in the entire skin surface. Severe generalized involvement can occur at birth.[64] It is rarely associated with hyperkeratosis of the palms and soles.[65]

A recent study of an Irish kindred with Köbner EBS yielded evidence for linkage to genetic markers on the long arm of chromosome 1.[66] Further study of this kindred supported exclusion of the human nidogen gene (also mapped to long arm of chromosome 1) as a candidate gene for Köbner EBS.[67] Because of the similarity between the Köbner and Weber-Cockayne types of EBS, it has been suggested the two conditions represent different clinical diseases caused by allelic mutations of varying severity, and that the clinical heterogeneity within the two variants is mainly a quantitative kind.[68,69] Linkage analysis has supported the hypothesis that Köbner and Weber-Cockayne types of EBS may be determined by a single locus.[70] However, using linkage analysis to study a Northern Irish family with the Weber-Cockayne type of EBS, investigators showed that the causative gene in that family did not lie in the region on chromosome 1 to which the gene for Köbner EBS has been mapped.[71] By studying a Finnish kindred with Köbner EBS, investigators showed that mutations in genes coding for two bullous pemphigoid antigens (a 230-kDa antigen known as BPAG1, and a 180-kDa antigen known as BPAG2) are not the primary genetic defect in that kindred.[72] In two families with EBS, linkage of the disease has been demonstrated with keratin genes mapped on chromosomes 17q and 12q. These observations suggest that the blistering in EBS may be associated with abnormalities in cytoskeletal proteins leading to cellular fragility in response to trauma or to changes in temperature.[73] In a 1 month-old baby girl with Köbner EBS, ultrastructural examination of a skin biopsy specimen showed that cytoplasmic tonofilaments were lacking in the basal cells.[74] On immunohistochemical staining, a basal cell keratin was expressed in the suprabasal cell layers but not in the basal cell layer, suggesting that delayed keratin production by the epidermal cells may be the cause of cutaneous fragility.[74] A suspiciously high incidence of spontaneous abortions has been noted in a family with Köbner EBS, raising the question of an associated chromosomal abnormality.[75] A fragile site on chromosome 12 has been reported in one family with Köbner EBS.[76]

Various biochemical abnormalities have been described in patients with Köbner EBS. In 1981 Savolainen et al. measured the levels of galactosylhydroxylysyl glucosyltransferase (GGT) in one kindred with Köbner EBS.[77] This is a sugar transferase involved in collagen biosynthesis. They found that some, but not all, affected members showed decreased levels of this enzyme in serum, skin, and cultured skin fibroblasts. However, some unaffected

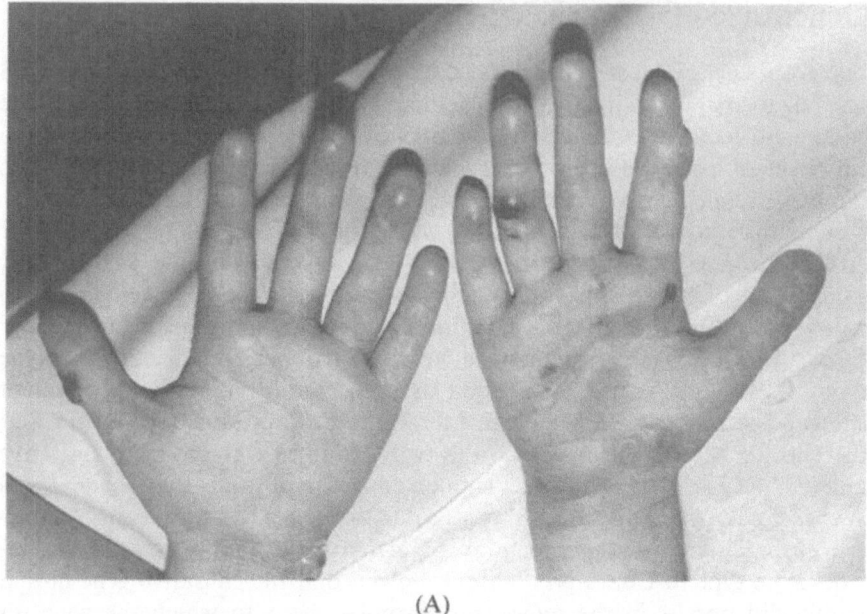

(A)

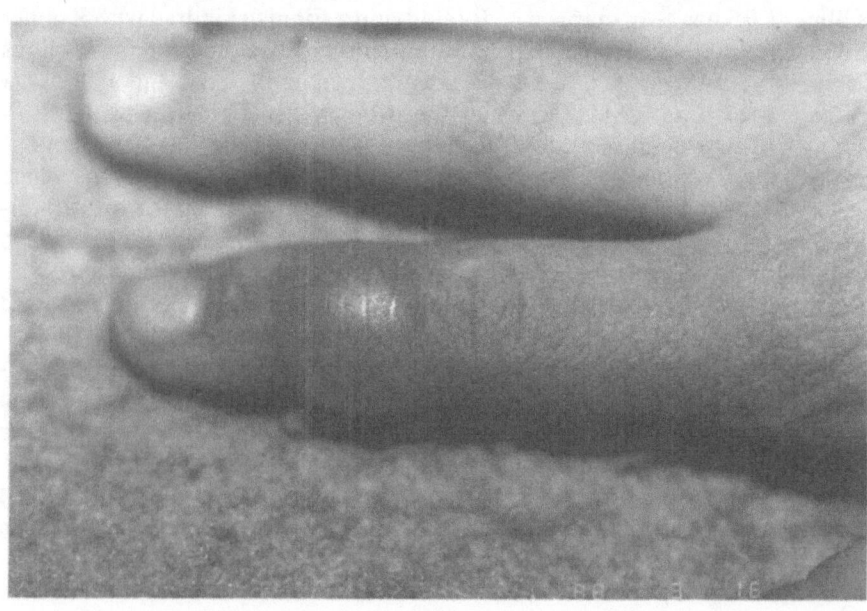

(B)

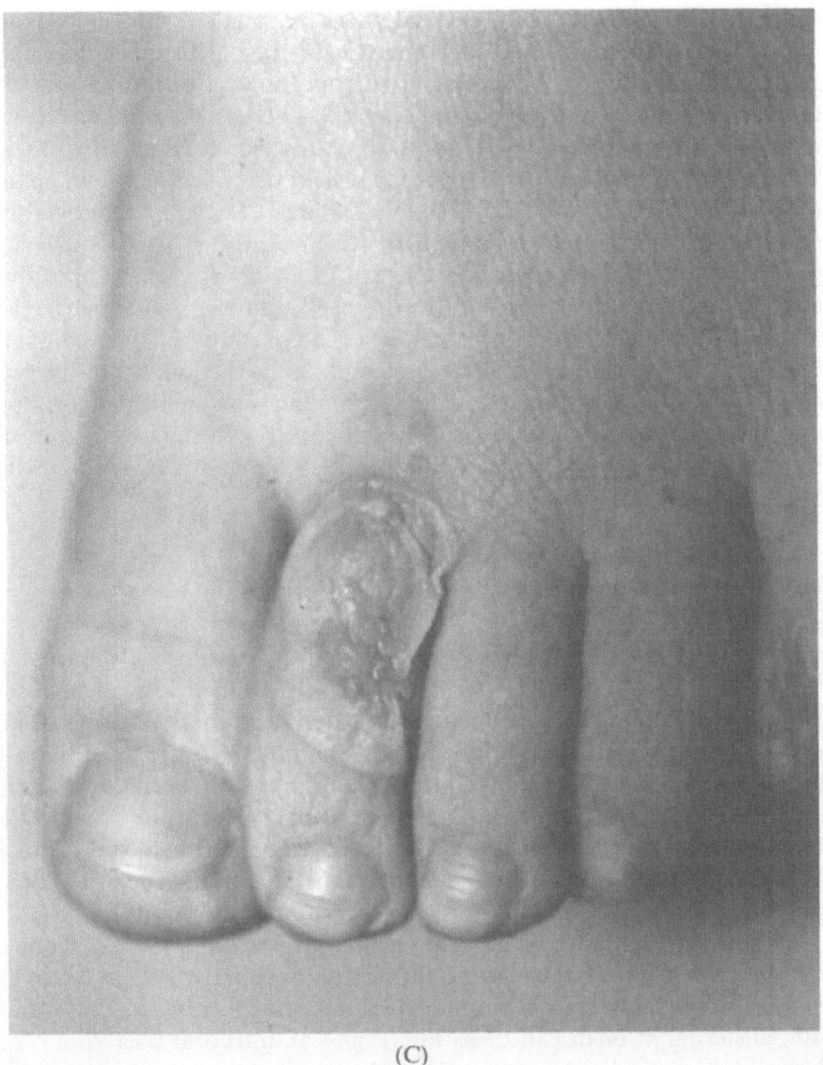

(C)

FIGURE. 7.3. Weber-Cockayne type of EBS, showing blisters on the hand (**A**, **B**, facing page) and foot (**C**).

members of the kindred also showed this abnormality, and in two other families with Köbner EBS no such abnormality was detectable. The significance of this finding is therefore unclear, and it was proposed that these observations may be due to the possibility that there is close linkage between the gene coding for the enzyme and that coding for Köbner EBS. In 1983 Sanchez et al. found decreased levels of a gelatinolytic protease in cultured fibroblasts obtained from patients with Köbner EBS from three kindreds, and suggested this may be a marker for Köbner EBS.[78] The significance of this observation, however, remains unclear, for Winberg et al. were unable to detect reduced gelatinase activity in dermal fibroblasts obtained from six Köbner EBS patients from three families.[79] Skin samples from six patients with Köbner EBS showed normal expression and distribution of "very late antigen (VLA) glycoproteins," a family of adhesion membrane receptors involved in cell–matrix and cell–cell interactions.[80] Normal results were also seen in one patient with Weber-Cockayne EBS, and another with Dowling-Meara type of EBS.[80]

EBS Herpetiformis of Dowling-Meara

In 1954 Dowling and Meara[81] described four unrelated children with trauma-induced skin blistering. The blisters showed a striking grouped configuration resembling those seen in juvenile dermatitis herpetiformis. Blisters healed without scarring, and three patients had hyperkeratosis of the palms and soles. This constellation of clinical findings has since been known as EBS herpetiformis of Dowling-Meara, and additional clinical and microscopic observations have since contributed to improved definition of this distinctive entity. It is felt to be probably the second most common type of EBS in the United Kingdom, second only to the Weber-Cockayne variety.[82]

Herpetiform grouping of blisters remains the cardinal clinical feature of this syndrome (Fig. 7.4). However, this feature is usually not present at birth and may not become apparent until childhood. In contrast to other forms of EBS, blistering at birth can be severe (Fig. 7.5), intraoral blistering is common, and even esophageal erosions have been noted; as a result, patients may initially be thought to have recessive dystrophic EB, and the correct diagnosis depends on electron microscopic examination of a blister.[18] However, extent of cutaneous blistering tends to improve as patients grow older. Another characteristic feature is progressive hyperkeratosis of palms and soles (Fig. 7.6), which has variably been described as "patchy,"[83] "diffuse,"[18,84] "irregular,"[85] and "punctate."[86] Palmar hyperkeratosis can be severe, causing flexion deformity of the hand,[87,88] but response to oral etretinate has been noted.[87] In one case blistering improved after administration of pipamperone, a neuroleptic agent belonging to the butyrophenone family used for treatment of psychological disturbance.[89] Blistering has been noted to improve during episodes of high fever (e.g., with measles),[86,90] but febrile episodes have also been known to exacerbate[83] or have no effect[87] on severity of blistering. Inheritance is autosomal dominant.[83]

The clinical impression of EBS herpetiformis of Dowling-Meara can be confirmed by electron microscopic examination of a biopsy specimen. This shows breakdown of the basal cells, and within these cells there is characteristic clumping of the tonofilaments[18,91] (Fig. 7.7), which has been noted to precede blister formation.[92] Tonofilament clumping has been observed in perilesional as well as nonlesional skin.[82,93,94,94a] Light microscopy is occasionally helpful, and may show hydropic and vacuolar degeneration of the basal cells.[18] Often, however, it shows only a subepidermal blister that is not helpful in establishing the diagnosis of EBS. Unusual histologic findings include abundant neutrophils and eosinophils in the dermis and the subepidermal blister,[89,95] and epidermolytic hyperkeratosis.[96]

It has been suggested that blister formation may be caused by an abnormality of the keratin cytoskeleton;[97,98] however Tidman et al. showed that the staining profile of antikeratin monoclonal antibodies was normal in perilesional skin, suggesting that tonofilament clumping may result from a postsynthetic modification of keratin molecules.[97,98] Ishida-Yamamoto et al.[94a] found tonofilament clumping in lesional skin of all 15 patients examined, and in non-lesional skin in six of nine patients examined. They also demonstrated abnormal round bodies, likely composed of keratin, in cultured keratinocytes obtained from perilesional skin, suggesting that tonofilament clumping is a primary phenomenon and not a consequence of blistering.[94a] Using immunoelectron microscopy, they also showed that clumped tonofilaments seen in patients' skin were labeled strongly with antibodies against the keratins K5 and K14 in basal and suprabasal layers, whereas suprabasal clumps were only slightly reactive with anti-K10 antibodies, suggesting that this type of EB is associated with an intrinsic abnormality of the keratin-filament network involving the K5 and K14 pair.[94a] Other investigators have recently shown that two patients with sporadic cases of EBS of Dowling-Meara have point mutations in the gene coding for the type I keratin K14, which is normally expressed in basal keratinocytes.[99] By engineering one of these point mutations in a cloned human K14 cDNA, they showed that a K14 with a mutation transforming an arginine residue to cysteine causes disruption of keratin network formation in transfected keratinocytes and perturbed filament assembly in vitro.[99] These observations will greatly enhance our understanding of molecular defects in EBS of Dowling-Meara.

EBS with Mottled Pigmentation

In 1979 Fischer and Gedde-Dahl[100] described a family in which blistering was associated with mottled pigmentation of the skin. In 11 individuals skin blistering was generalized and was thought to be consistent with Köbner type

(*text continued on page 105*)

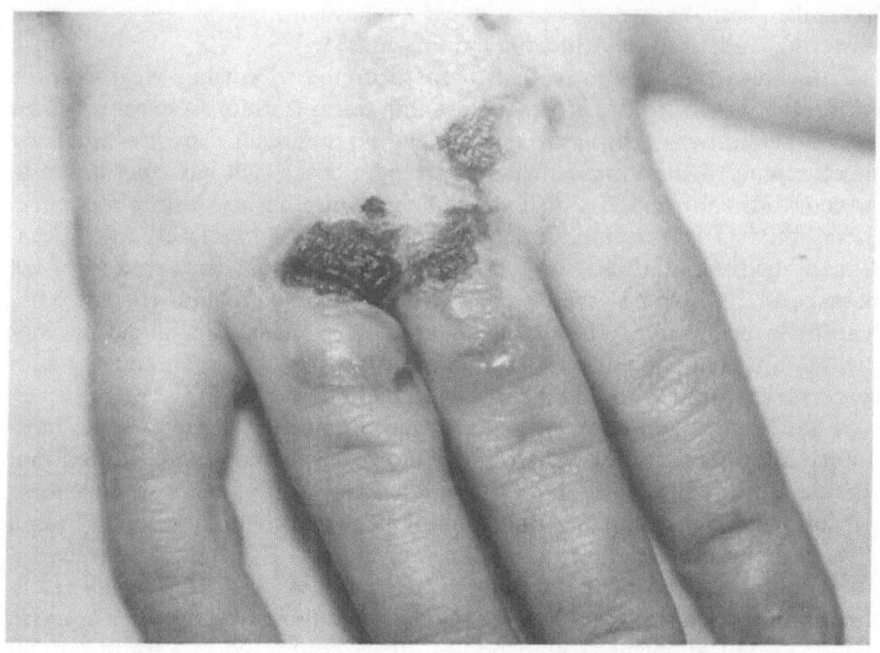

(A)

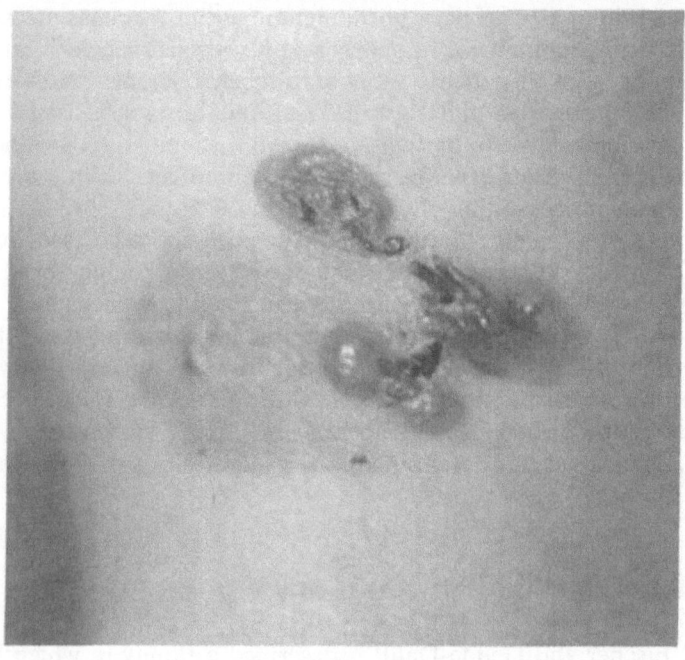

(B)

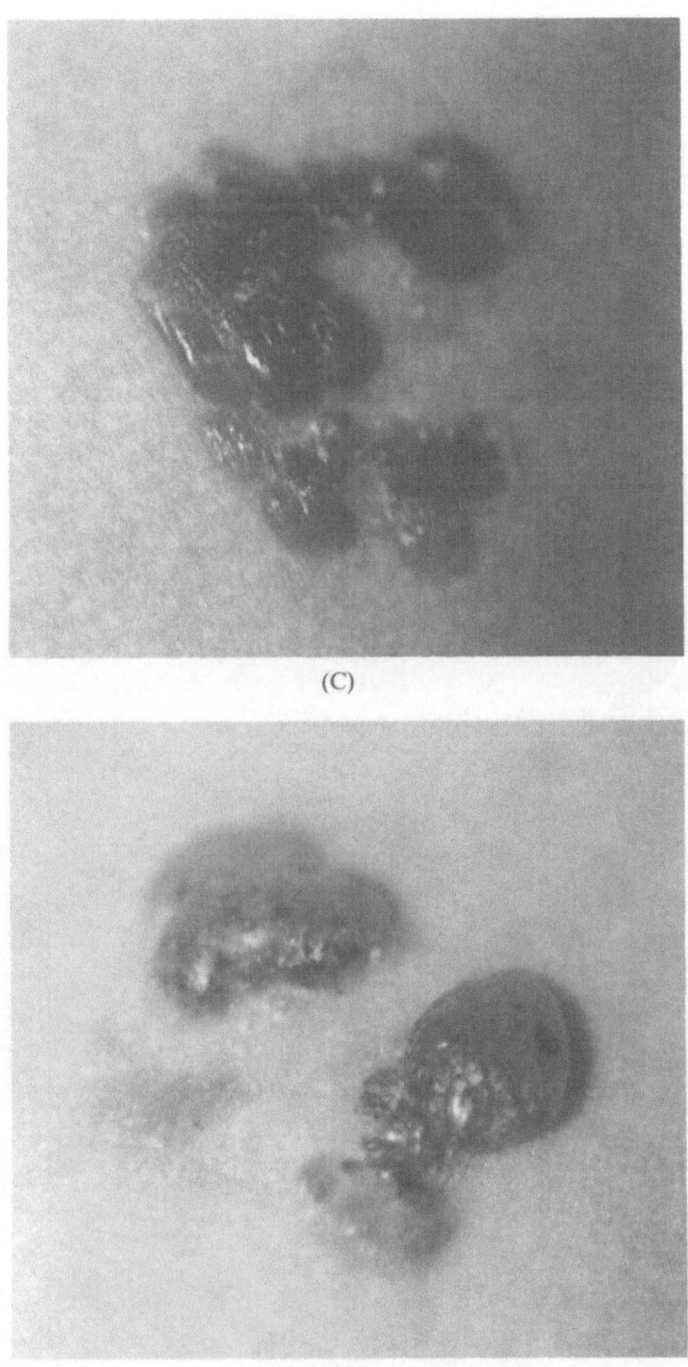

(C)

(D)

FIGURE. 7.4. Dowling-Meara type of EBS, showing herpetiform grouping of blisters (**A**, **B**, facing page; **C** and **D**).

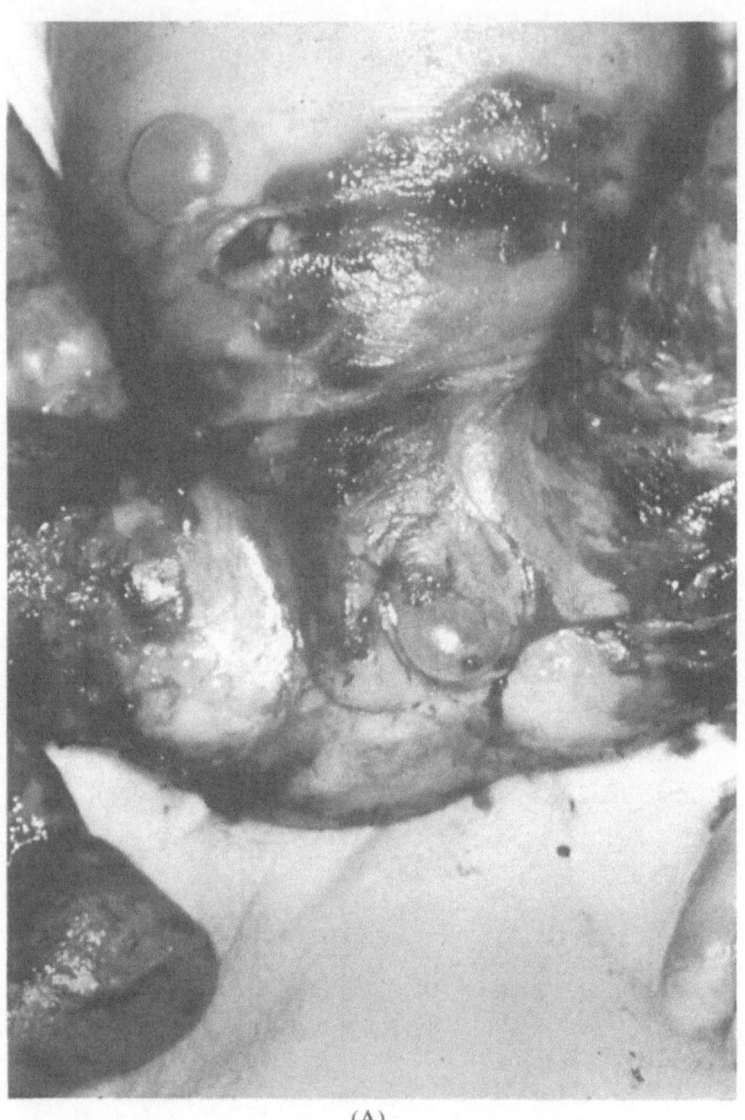

(A)

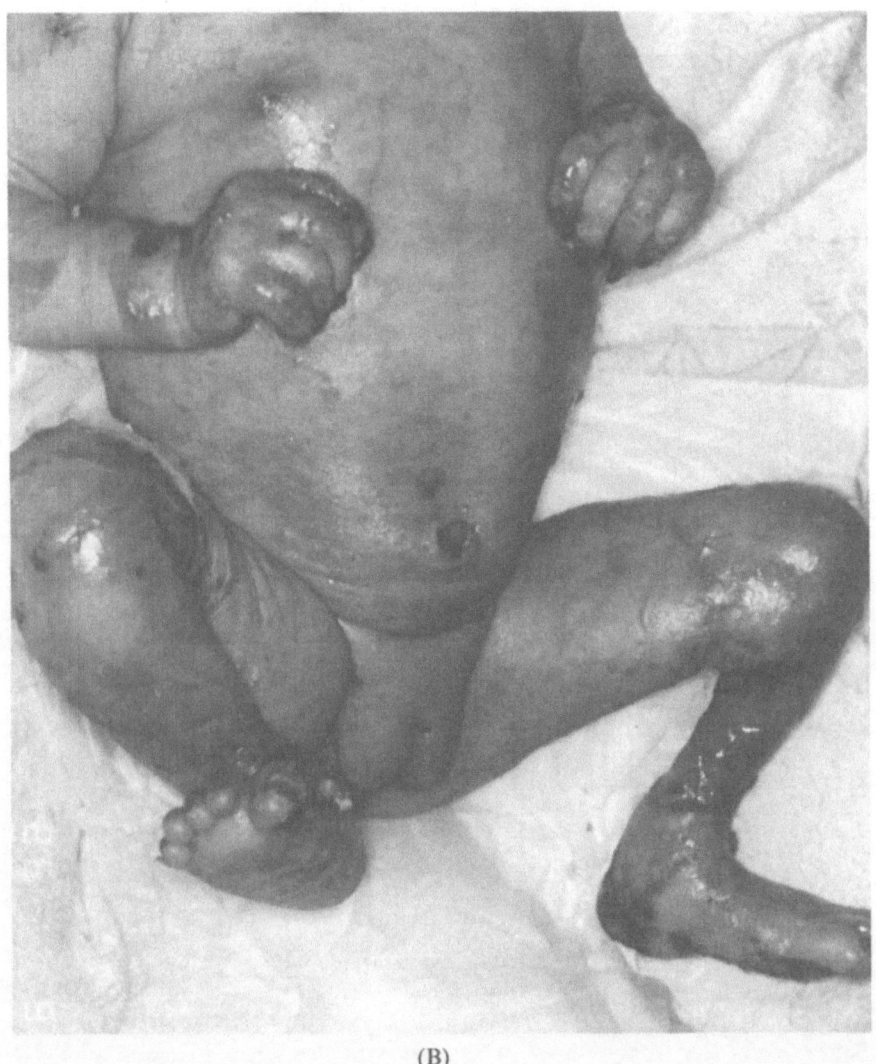

(B)

FIGURE. 7.5. Dowling-Meara type of EBS, showing extensive cutaneous blistering shortly after birth (**A**, facing page), followed by marked healing a few days later (**B**).

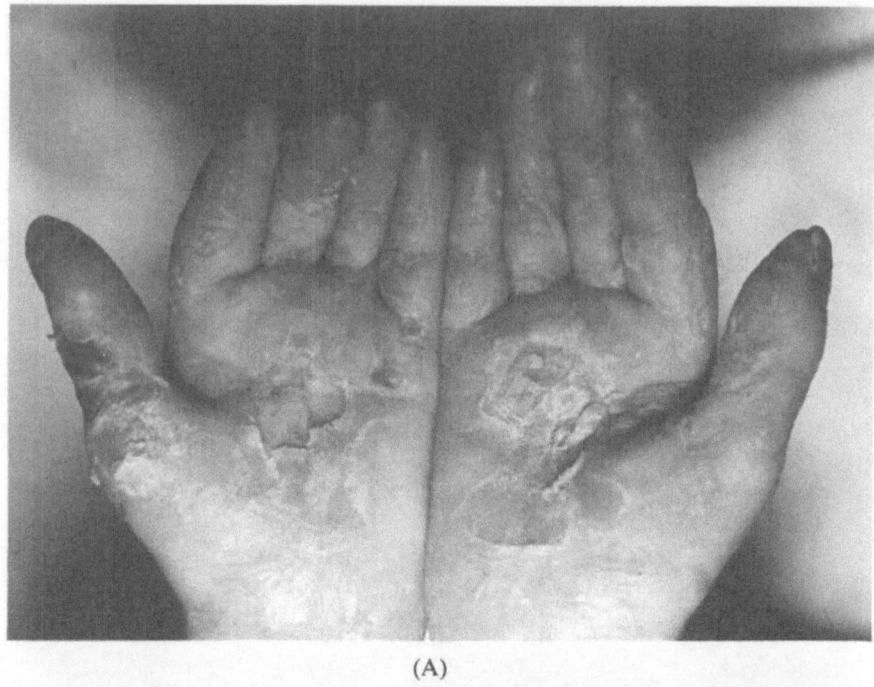

(A)

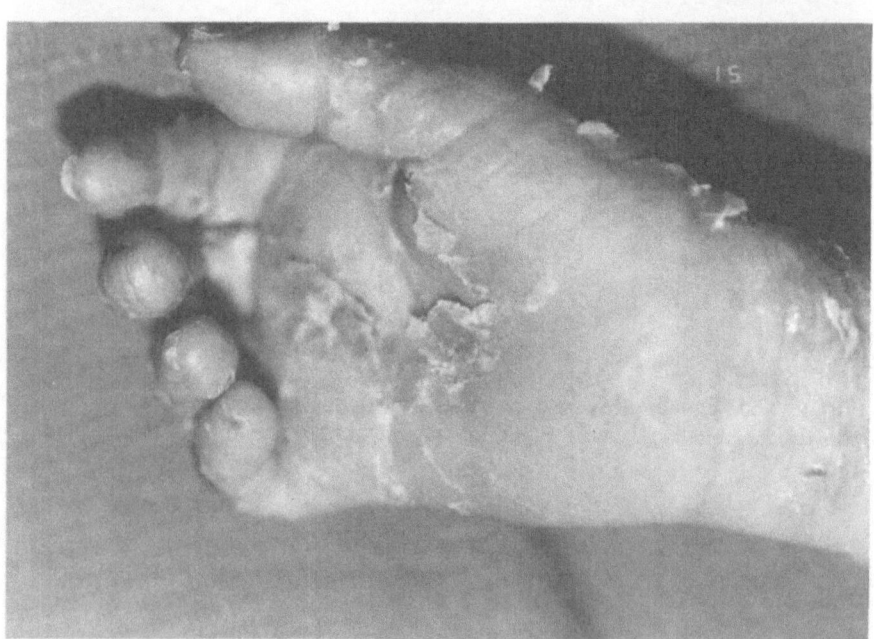

(B)

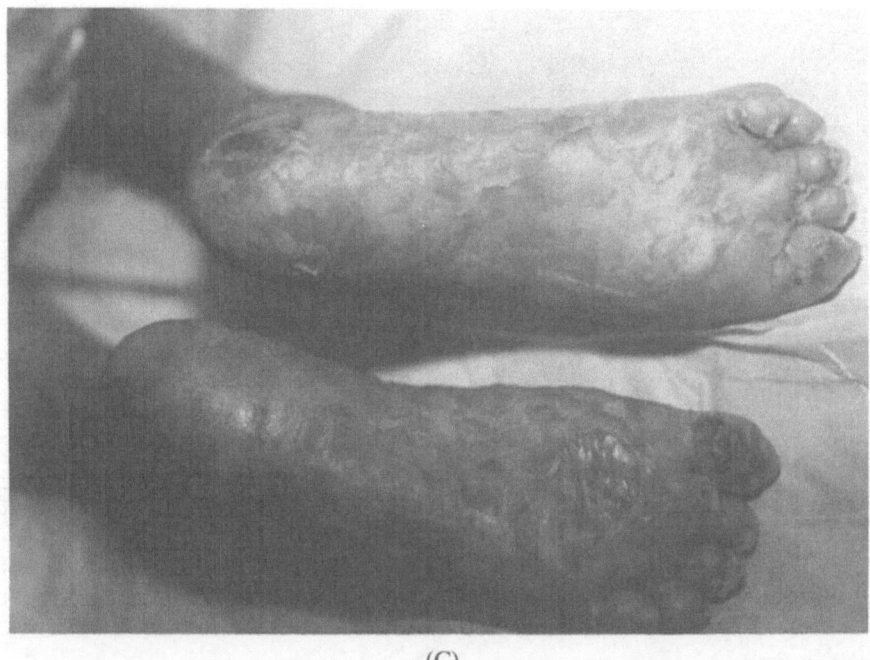

(C)

FIGURE. 7.6. Dowling-Meara type of EBS, featuring hyperkeratosis of the palms (**A–B** facing page) and soles (**C**).

of EBS. However, 10 of these individuals also had a striking pigment disorder in which 2 to 5 mm pigmented and depigmented spots formed a mosaic pattern mainly on the extremities and trunk, which tended to become blurred or even disappear with increasing age. The 11th individual had blistering without pigment disorder, suggesting the syndrome was due to genetic linkage of two independent genes instead of pleiotropic expression of a single mutant gene. Biopsy showed intraepidermal, suprabasal separation. When the authors first became aware of this family, it consisted of only nine affected individuals, all of whom were female, leading to the suspicion that the condition was transmitted as X-linked dominant and lethal for males. When the tenth affected individual was born and was a male, it was concluded that autosomal dominant transmission was more likely. The pigment disorder was thought to result from autosomal inactivation. Three individuals had occasional small oral blisters, and focal hyperkeratosis of palms and/or soles occurred in three patients. Ultrastructural analysis showed primary lipolytic changes in the basal cells.[101]

This syndrome is quite uncommon. In 1989 Bruckner-Tuderman et al.[102] described a patient with similar findings and extended the microscopic

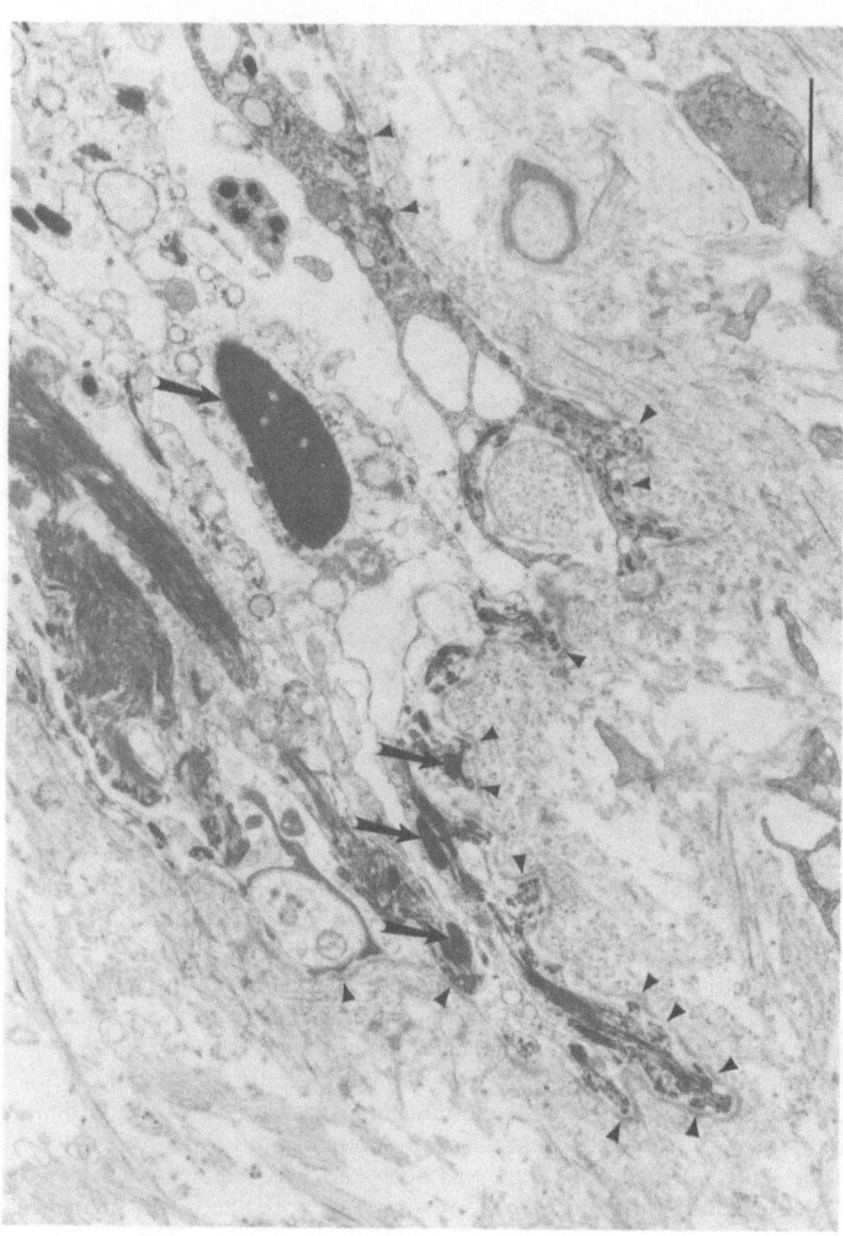

FIGURE. 7.7. Electron micrograph of Dowling-Meara EBS. A basal keratinocyte undergoing cytolysis has clumps (*arrows*) and dense whorls of keratin filaments. Along the dermal-epidermal junction are apparently normal hemidesmosomes (*arrowheads*), some of which have associated clumped keratin filaments. (Bar = 1 μm, 16,650 ×). (Electron micrograph courtesy of Lynne T. Smith, Seattle, WA.)

description, showing focal disruption of the basement membrane zone on immunofluorescence, and subnuclear splitting on electron microscopy. Another patient with EBS and mottled pigmentation was reported in 1986,[86] but this patient had herpetiform grouping of blisters and clumping of tonofilaments on electron microscopy, and is therefore best classified as EBS herpetiformis of Dowling-Meara. In 1981 Boss et al.[103] described two families with speckled hyperpigmentation, punctate keratoses of the palms and soles, and blistering predominantly of the hands and feet. The blistering, however, was mainly confined to infancy and in some patients was not clearly related to trauma. Although one of these families was intially thought to have EB,[104] it was subsequently thought this triad was a distinct entity.[103]

Bart's Syndrome

In 1966 Bart et al.[105,106] described a kindred of 103 in which 25 members had one or several of the following traits: (a) congenital absence of the skin, usually localized to the feet and medial sides of lower legs, (b) blistering of the skin or mucous membrane induced by slight friction, all healing with no scarring, (c) nail abnormalities such as congenital absence, deformity, and complete shedding. Inheritance was autosomal dominant with complete penetrance and variable expressivity. Although histologic analysis was not performed on this kindred, this condition has been variously classified as an epidermolytic form of EB,[90,107] dystrophic EB,[69,108,109] "uncertain EB,"[110] or a distinct type of "mildly scarring" EB.[111] Briggaman discusses Bart's syndrome and "congenital localized absence of skin" under the heading of "complications and special problems" of EB.[112] Sybert suggests Bart's syndrome should be considered a subtype of aplasia cutis congenita that sometimes occurs in association with EB.[113] Butler et al. presented evidence from ultrastructural and immunofluorescent mapping studies showing Bart's syndrome should be classed as a mild form of dominant dystrophic EB.[114,115] In one kindred with dominant dystrophic EB, certain affected individuals had congenital localized absence of skin, resembling Bart's syndrome.[116] "Congenital localized skin defect" has been reported in association with junctional EB.[117] Congenital absence of skin has also been reported in association with pyloric atresia, but the skin defect in such cases usually is not confined to the lower extremities but is quite extensive; ultrastructural studies usually show junctional EB,[118,119] although EBS has also been reported.[120] It is clear, therefore, that no consensus exists about the relation between Bart's syndrome and EB. Until this issue is clarified, Bart's syndrome should simply be reserved for the combination of findings set forth in Bart's original paper; it may not be a distinct genetic entity but may represent a combination of findings that may be seen in different types of EB.

EBS-Ogna

In his classical monograph on EB, Gedde-Dahl[121] described a large kindred from the Southwestern Norwegian community of Ogna afficted with a distinctive form of EB. He delineated three main clinical features: generalized bruising tendency of the skin, common occurrence of small hemorrhagic blebs, especially on the finger tips and palms, and serous blistering that mainly affects the hands and feet. The last feature resembled mild EBS of Weber-Cockayne.[90] A fourth inconstant feature was onychogryphosis of the big toe nails. Electron microscopy showed cytolysis of basal cells above the hemidesmosomes.[90] This disorder was established as a distinct genetic entity by demonstration of close linkage to the loci of erythrocyte-soluble glutamic pyruvic transaminase.[122,123] The gene for this condition is designated EBS1, and has been localized to chromosome 8.[124]

Autosomal Recessive EBS with Neuromuscular Diseases

Starting in 1988, several kindreds with a different type of EBS have been reported. In contrast to all other types of EBS, this type showed autosomal recessive inheritance, and was associated with severe extracutaneous involvement, most notably neuromuscular disorders such as muscular dystrophy[13-15] and myasthenia gravis.[14] The neuromuscular disorder often presents in infancy or childhood, sometimes at birth,[13] and tends to be progressive.[15] Other systemic manifestations include mental retardation,[15] anemia,[14] oral erosions,[14] and enamel defects of the teeth.[15] Cutaneous blistering is usually generalized, and scarring, milia, alopecia, and nail dystrophy have been noted.[14,15] Death has been reported.[13] This syndrome may represent a new, distinct, and uncommon autosomal recessive condition in which cutaneous blistering and muscular diseases are caused by pleiotropic effects of a single mutant gene. It is also possible that the skin and muscular disorders are caused by genes that are closely linked and are coinherited. It is unlikely to represent coincidental occurrence of two uncommon disorders. In contrast, the combination of EBS, mental retardation, and muscular hypertonicity in a patient described in 1965 probably occurred by chance, for this combination was seen in only 1 of 21 individuals affected with blistering in a kindred spanning four generations.[5]

Other Types of EBS

Lethal Autosomal Recessive EBS

In 1985 Salih et al.[125] reported a large Sudanese kindred in which 10 of 13 affected members died in early life (age at time of death ranged from 8 days to 20 months). Electron microscopic examination in two patients showed lysis of basal keratinocytes consistent with EBS. Cutaneous blistering was generalized and healed with no scarring, but a predilection for hands, feet, and elbows was noted. Mild oral erosions were common, but nails, hair, and teeth were not affected. Anemia was common. The causes of death were not readily apparent. Three died "without warning," four others died after febrile illness with "coughing and breathlessness," and the remaining four died after "pyrexia, diarrhea and vomiting." Asphyxiation due to laryngeal and esophageal involvement was considered a likely cause of death in some patients, but these were not documented.

Kallin's Syndrome

In 1985 Nielsen and Sjolund[126] reported two sisters with blistering affecting mainly the hands and feet, missing teeth, dystrophic nails, and nonscarring alopecia. Light microscopic examination of skin biopsy showed subcomeal cleavage in one patient, but cleavage in midepidermis was seen in the other. One of the affected patients had total loss of hearing in the left ear discovered at age 5 years. Although only one kindred with these findings was reported, it is noteworthy because it represents yet another example of epidermolytic EB in which transmission appears to be autosomal recessive. The name "Kallin's syndrome" was proposed, after the patients' surnames.

Autosomal Recessive EBS Weber-Cockayne

In 1989 Fine et al.[16] reported a kindred in which four patients had blisters affecting mainly the hands and feet with no extracutaneous involvement except oral erosions in one patient. Electron microscopy of a biopsy specimen showed separation at the level of the basal cells. Transmission was consistent with autosomal recessive.

EBS Superficialis

In 1989, Fine et al.[17] described seven patients in two kindreds showing blister formation just beneath the stratum corneum. Blistering was either generalized or affected predominantly the extremities. Transmission was autosomal dominant in the kindred, which contained six affected patients. Oral involvement was common, and abnormal nails, milia, atrophic scarring, and ocular involvement were noted. The condition was differentiated from peeling skin syndrome, in which there is continuous spontaneous peeling of the skin and which is usually transmitted as an autosomal recessive trait.

Mendes da Costa Syndrome

This refers to appearance of spontaneous blisters during the first three years of life, primarily on the extremities, as described in a Dutch kindred in

1957.[90,127] It is also called "dystrophia bullosa hereditaria, macular type of Mendes da Costa."[90] Associated findings are reticular erythema on the limbs, areas of hyperpigmentation and depigmentation, atrichia, microcephaly, dwarfism, and abnormalities of fingers and nails.[128] One patient showed syndactyly of second and third toes.[129] It is transmitted as an X-linked disorder.[124] Electron microscopy shows disruption of the cell membrane of basal cells with numerous anchoring fibrils.[128] Some consider it as a form of intraepidermal EB[90]; however, blisters appear spontaneously and cannot be induced by friction,[90,128] and for this reason this condition is best considered distinct from EB.[110,128]

Others

In 1983, a "new" histologic subgroup of EBS was reported in which two patients had blistering often occurring in groups. Light microscopy showed dyskeratotic keratinocytes and atypical mitoses, and electron microscopy showed tonofilament clumping.[130] Instead of creating another new subgroup, this condition fits into the Dowling-Meara type of EBS. Eisenberg et al.[131] reported a patient with blisters occurring mainly on the hands and feet, but ultrastructural analysis showed basal cell cytolysis and tonofilament clumping, combining the clinical features of the Weber-Cockayne and Dowling-Meara types of EBS. In 1987, a patient was reported to have the following at birth: skin fragility and extensive erosions, syndactyly of toes, dystrophic nails, and partial synechiae of eyelids.[132,133] Other abnormalities included cleft palate and low-set ears, and the patient died at age 3 days. Electron microscopy showed "splitting" of basal cells below the nucleus,[132] but the papillary dermis was edematous and anchoring fibrils were either absent or decreased.[133] These cases may represent rare, unusual forms of EBS, but the small number of reported cases does not allow precise classification.

Acknowledgments. Supported in part by a General Clinical Research Center grant (M01-RR00102) from the National Institutes of Health to The Rockefeller University Hospital; by a training grant (AR07525) from the National Institutes of Health to the Laboratory for Investigative Dermatology; by contracts AR62269 and AR62270 from the National Institutes of Health to the Laboratory for Investigative Dermatology; by a grant from the Dystrophic Epidermolysis Bullosa Research Association (D.E.B.R.A.) of America, Inc.; and with general support from the Pew Trusts.

References

1. Kahn S, Trieger N. Epidermolysis bullosa hereditaria letalis: a case report with special emphasis on oral manifestations. *J Oral Med.* 1976;31:32–35.

2. Wright TJ, Capps J, Johnson LB. Oral and ultrastructural dental manifestations of epidermolysis bullosa. *J Den Res.* 1988;67:249.
3. Granek H, Baden HP. Corneal involvement in epidermolysis bullosa simplex. *Arch Ophthalmol.* 1980;98:469–472.
4. Thawley SE, Black MJ, Dudek SE, Spector GJ. External auditory canal stricture secondary to epidermolysis bullosa. *Arch Otolaryngol.* 1977;103:55–57.
5. Passarge E. Epidermolysis bullosa hereditaria simplex, a kindred affected in four generations. *J Pediatr.* 1965;67:819–825.
6. Noojin RO, Reynolds JP, Croom WC. Genetic study of hereditary type of epidermolysis bullosa simplex. *Arch Dermatol Syphilol.* 1952;65:471–483.
7. Sehgal VN, Shamsuddin, Tyagi SP. Epidermolysis bullosa simplex in five consecutive generations. *Austr J Dermatol.* 1970;11:42–45.
8. Tilsley DA, Beard TC. Epidermolysis bullosa simplex in Tasmania. *The Lancet.* 1963;2:905–907.
9. Zimmerman MC. Epidermolysis bullosa simplex, hereditary dominant type. *Arch Dermatol.* 1966;94:809.
10. Norholm-Pedersen A, Nielsen NB. "Laeso disease"—epidermolysis bullosa simplex. *Acta Genet.* 1953;4:417–423.
11. Jain PK, Kaushik A. Epidermolysis bullosa simplex. *Indian Pediatr.* 1983;20:63–65.
12. Gedde-Dahl Jr T, Thorsby E. HLA and epidermolysis bullosa. *Arch Dermatol.* 1977;113:1722–1723.
13. Kletter G, Evans OB, Lee JA, Melvin B, Yates AB, Bock H-GO. Congenital muscular dystrophy and epidermolysis bullosa simplex. *J Pediatr.* 1989;114:104–107.
14. Fine J-D, Stenn J, Johnson L, Wright T, Bock H-GO, Horiguchi Y. Autosomal recessive epidermolysis bullosa simplex. Generalized phenotypic features suggestive of junctional or dystrophic epidermolysis bullosa, and association with neuromuscular diseases. *Arch Dermatol.* 1989;125:931–938.
15. Niemi K-M, Sommer H, Kero M, Kanerva L, Haltia M. Epidermolysis bullosa simplex associated with muscular dystrophy with recessive inheritance. *Arch Dermatol.* 1988;124:551–554.
16. Fine J-D, Johnson L, Wright T, Horiguchi Y. Epidermolysis bullosa simplex: identification of a kindred with autosomal recessive transmission of the Weber–Cockayne type. *Pediatr Dermatol.* 1989;6:1–5.
17. Fine J-D, Johnson L, Wright T. Epidermolysis simplex superficialis. A new variant of epidermolysis bullosa characterized by subcorneal skin cleavage mimicking peeling skin syndrome. *Arch Dermatol.* 1989;125:633–638.
18. Buchbinder L, Lucky AW, Ballard E, et al. Severe infantile epidermolysis bullosa simplex, Dowling-Meara type. *Arch Dermatol.* 1986;122:190–198.
19. Fine J-D. Changing clinical and laboratory concepts in inherited epidermolysis bullosa [editorial]. *Arch Dermatol.* 1988;124:523–526.
20. Takamori K, Naito K, Ogawa H. Epidermolysis bullosa simplex blister fluid induces an intra-epidermal blister in cultured normal skin. *Br J Dermatol.* 1983;109:643–646.
21. Manabe M, Naito K, Ikeda S, Takamori K, Ogawa H. Production of blister in normal human skin in vitro by blister fluids from epidermolysis bullosa. *J*
22. Fine J-D, Griffith RD. A specific defect in glycosylation of epidermal cell mem-

branes: definition in skin from patients with epidermolysis bullosa simplex. *Arch Dermatol.* 1985;121:1292–1296.

23. Kitajima Y, Inoue S, Yaoita J. Abnormal organization of keratin intermediate filaments in cultured keratinocytes of epidermolysis bullosa simplex. *Arch Dermatol Res.* 1989;281:5–10.

24. Yacoub T, Campbell CA, Gordon YB, Kirby JD, Kitau MJ. Maternal serum and amniotic fluid concentrations of alphafetoprotein in epidermolysis bullosa simplex. *Br Med J.* 1979;1:307.

25. Gay S, Ward WQ, Gay RE, Miller EJ. Autoantibodies to basement membrane collagen: epidermolysis bullosa simplex versus bullous pemphigoid. *J Cutan Pathol.* 1980;7:315–317.

26. Scott DW, Schultz RD. Epidermolysis bullosa simplex in the collie dog. *J A Vet Med Assoc.* 1977;171:721–727.

27. Lutzner MA, Hansen C. Skin blisters and hair loss in a rat mutant called vibrissaeless (vb). *J Invest Dermatol.* 1975;65:212–216.

28. Jolly RD, Alley MR, O'Hara PJ. Familial acantholysis of angus calves. *Vet Pathol.* 1973;10:473–483.

29. Vassar R, Coulombe PA, Degenstein L, Albers K, Fuchs E. Mutant keratin expression in transgenic mice causes marked abnormalities resembling a human genetic skin disease. *Cell.* 1991;64:365–380.

30. Fine J-D. Epidermolysis bullosa: clinical aspects, pathology, and recent advances in research. *Int J Dermatol.* 1986;25:143–157.

31. Weber FP. Recurrent bullous eruption of the feet in a child. *Proc Roy Soc Med.* 1926;19:72.

32. Cockayne EA. Recurrent bullous eruption of the feet. *Br J Dermatol.* 1938;55:358–367.

33. Jain SC, Sharma BK. Epidermolysis bullosa: a case report. *J Indian Med Assoc.* 1962;38:489–490.

34. Waisman M. Recurrent bullous eruption of the feet and hands (Weber-Cockayne). *J Am Med Assoc.* 1944;124:1247–1250.

35. Mansur HD. Hereditary epidermolysis bullosa. *J Am Med Assoc.* 1942;120:1122–1124.

36. Mooney JL. Epidermolysis bullosa. *Arch Dermatol.* 1944;50:167–169.

37. Leider M, Baer RL. Epidermolysis bullosa hereditaria, report of two cases with extensive family histories. *Arch Dermatol Syphilol.* 1942;46:419–424.

38. Haldane JBS, Poole R. A new pedigree of recurrent bullous eruption of the feet. *J Hered.* 1942;33:17–18.

39. Greenberg SI. Epidermolysis bullosa. *Arch Dermatol Syphilol.* 1944;49:333–334.

40. Franks AG, Davis MIJ. Epidermolysis bullosa. *Arch Dermatol Syphilol.* 1943;47:647–650.

41. Nippert PH, Fetter F. Epidermolysis bullosa: report of seven cases. *US Naval Med Bull.* 1945;44:154–158.

42. Catanzariti AR, Smith C, Shaps RS. Epidermolysis bullosa: a case presentation and review of the literature. *J Am Podiatr Assoc.* 1984;74:222–228.

43. Shelton JM. Epidermolysis bullosa: report of a case. *US Naval Med Bull.* 1944;42:424–427.

44. Franks AG, Davis MIJ, Dobes WL. Epidermolysis bullosa. *Urol Cutan Rev.* 1945;49:57–65.

45. May SB. Epidermolysis bullosa with pachyonychia in three generations. *Arch Dermatol.* 1962;185:662–662.
46. Thompson RG, Leedham CL, Hailey H. Epidermolysis bullosa hereditaria. *South Med J.* 1949;42:647–653.
47. Readett MD. Localized epidermolysis bullosa. *Br Med J.* 1961;1:1510–1511.
48. Tkach JR. Treatment of recurrent bullous eruption of the hands and feet (Weber-Cockayne Disease) with topical aluminum chloride (letter). *J Am Acad Dermatol.* 1982;6:1095–1096.
49. Jennings JL. Aluminum chloride hexahydrate treatment of localized epidermolyis bullosa. *Arch Dermatol.* 1984;120:1382.
50. DesGrosseilliers J-P, Brisson P. Localized epidermolysis bullosa: report of two cases and evaluation of therapy with glutaraldehyde. *Arch Dermatol.* 1974;109:70–72.
51. Ayres Jr S, Mihan R. Pseudoxanthoma elasticum and epidermolysis bullosa: response to vitamin E (tocopherol). *Cutis.* 1969;5:287–294.
52. Adreano JM, Tomecki KJ. Epidermolysis bullosa simplex responding to isotretinoin [letter]. *Arch Dermatol.* 1988;124:1445–1446.
53. Fine J-D, Johnson L. Evaluation of the efficacy of topical bufexamac in epidermolysis bullosa simplex: a double-blind placebo-controlled crossover study. *Arch Dermatol.* 1988;124:1669–1672.
54. Hall-Smith SP, Daunt FO'N. Recurrent bullous eruption of feet: report of a case. *Lancet.* 1948;I:66–67.
55. Cartledge JL, Myers VW. Inherited foot blistering in an American family. *J Hered.* 1943;34:24.
56. Anning ST. Recurrent bullous eruption of the feet. *Br J Dermatol.* 1951;63:104–110.
57. Johnson SAM, Test AR. Epidermolysis bullosa simplex of the hands and the feet: a genetic study of the hereditary type. *Arch Dermatol Syphilol.* 1946;53:610–619.
58. Cranko JAWM. Recurrent bullous eruption of the feet. *Central African J Med.* 1973;19:219–220.
59. Frank SB. An unusual variant of epidermolysis bullosa: recurrent bullous eruption of the feet. *Arch Dermatol Syphilol.* 1943;47:327–334.
60. Chowdhury SD, Ghosh S. Heredofamilial study of Weber-Cockayne disease. *Bull Calcutta School Trop Med.* 1968;XVI:12–14.
61. Haneke E, Anton-Lamprecht I. Ultrastructure of blister formation in epidermolysis bullosa hereditaria: V. Epidermlysis bullosa simplex localisata type Weber-Cockayne. *J Invest Dermatol.* 1982;78:219–223.
62. Haneke E, Anton-Lamprecht I. Blister formation in epidermolysis bullosa simplex Weber-Cockayne. *J Cutan Pathol.* 1980;7:171.
63. Kantor GR, Kasick JM, Bergfeld WF, McMahon JT, Krebs JA. Epidermolysis bullosa of the Weber-Cockayne type with macular amyloidosis. *Cleve Clin Q.* 1985;52:425–428.
64. Baker H. Epidermolysis bullosa simplex generalisata: importance of immunofluorescence studies in early diagnosis. *Arch Dermatol Res.* 1982;272:393–399.
65. Haber RM, Ramsay CA, Boxall LBH. Epidermolysis bullosa simplex with keratoderma of the palms and soles. *J Am Acad Dermatol.* 1985;12:1040–1044.
66. Humphries MM, Sheils D, Lawler M, et al. Epidermolysis bullosa: evidence for

linkage to genetic markers on chromosome 1 in a family with the autosomal dominant simplex form. *Genomics.* 1990;7:377–381.

67. Humphries M, Nagayoshi T, Sheils D, Hunphries P, Uitto J. Human nidogen gene: identification of multiple RFLP and exclusion as candidate gene in a family with epidermolysis bullosa (EBS2) with evidence for linkage to chromosome 1. *J Invest Dermatol.* 1990;95:568–570.

68. Gedde-Dahl Jr T. *Epidermolysis Bullosa: A Clinical, Genetic and Epidemiological Study.* Baltimore: The Johns Hopkins Press; 1971; 49–51.

69. Gedde-Dahl Jr T. Phenotype-genotype correlations in epidermolysis bullosa. *Birth Defects: Original Article Series.* 1971;7:107–111.

70. Mulley JC, Nicholls CM, Propert DN, Turner T, Sutherland GR. Genetic linkage analysis of epidermolysis bullosa simplex, Kobner type. *Am J Med Gene.* 1984;19:573–577.

71. McKenna KE, Hughes AE, McLean WHI, Nevin NC. Linkage analysis of Weber-Cockayne epidermolysis bullosa simplex. *Br J Dermatol.* 1991;125(suppl 38):88.

72. Ryynanen M, Knowlton RG, Sawamura D. Li K-h, Giudice G, Diaz L, Uitto J. Molecular genetics of human bullous pemphigoid antigens: polymorphic genes for 230-kd and 180-kd proteins are excluded as the candidate genes in a large kindred with dominant simplex epidermolysis bullosa. *J Invest Dermatol.* 1991;96:535.

73. Bonifas JM, Rothman AL, Epstein Jr E. Linkage of epidermolysis bullosa simplex to probes in the region of keratin gene clusters on chromosomes 12q and 17q. *J Invest Dermatol.* 1991;96:550.

74. Ito M, Okuda C, Shimizu N, Tazawa T, Sato Y. Epidermolysis bullosa simplex (Koebner) is a keratin disorder: ultrastructural and immunohistochemical study. *Arch Dermatol.* 1991;127:367–372.

75. Jenkinson HA, Baere JM, Burrows D, Nevin N. Increased incidence of spontaneous abortions in two families with epidermolysis bullosa—is there an associated chromosomal abnormality? *Br J Dermatol.* 1984;111(suppl 26):33–34.

76. Sutherland GR, Hinton J. Heritable fragile sites on human chromosomes. VI. Characterization of the fragile site at 12q13. *Hum Genet.* 1981;57:217–219.

77. Savolainen ER, Kero M, Pihlajaniemi T, Kivirikko KL. Deficiency of galactosyl-hydroxylysyl glucosyltransferase, an enzyme of collagen synthesis, in a family with dominant epidermolysis bullosa simplex. *N Engl J Med.* 1981;304:197–204.

78. Sanchez G, Seltzer JL, Eisen AZ, Stapler P, Bauer EA. Generalized dominant epidermolysis bullosa simplex: decreased activity of a gelatinolytic protease in cultured fibroblasts as a phenotypic marker. *J Invest Dermatol.* 1983;81:576–579.

79. Winberg J-O, Gedde-Dahl Jr T. Gelatinase expression in generalized epidermolysis bullosa simplex fibroblasts. *J Invest Dermatol.* 1986;87:326–329.

80. Nazzaro V, Berti E, Cavalli R, Brusasco A, Caputo R. Very late antigen (VLA) expression in various forms of epidermolysis bullosa simplex. *Arch Dermatol Res.* 1991;283:1–4.

81. Dowling GB, Meara RH. Epidermolysis bullosa resembling juvenile dermatitis herpetiformis. *Br J Dermatol.* 1954;66:139–143.

82. McGrath JA, Ishida-Yamamoto A, Schofield OMV, Tidman MJ, Leigh IM,

Eady RAJ. A clinico-pathological review of 14 cases or the Dowling-Meara variant of epidermolysis bullosa simplex. *Br J Dermatol.* 1991;125(suppl 38):14.

83. Hacham-Zadeh S, Rappersberger K, Livshin R, Konrad K. Epidermolysis bullosa herpetiformis Dowling-Meara in a large family. *J Am Acad Dermatol.* 1988;18:702–706.

84. Coburn PR, Tidman MJ, Eady RAJ, Scott OLS. Epidermolysis bullosa herpetiformis (Dowling-Meara). *Br J Dematol.* 1983;109(suppl 24):58.

85. Caldwell I. Epidermolysis bullosa simplex with tylosis plantaris. *Br J Dermatol.* 1955;67:315.

86. Medenica-Mojsilovic L, Fenske NA, Espinoza CG. Epidermolysis bullosa herpetiformis with mottled pigmentation and an unusual punctate keratoderma. *Arch Dermatol.* 1986;122:900–908.

87. Tidman MJ, Wells RS, MacDonald DM. Epidermolysis bullosa simplex (Dowling-Meara). In: Wilkinson DS, Mascaro JM, Orfanos CE, Albers J, eds. *Clinical Dermatology, The CMD Case Collection, World Congress of Dermatology.* Stuttgart: Schattauer; 1987: 16–17.

88. Archer CB, Holden CA, Wells RS. Epidermolysis bullosa (Dowling-Meara). *Br J Dermatol.* 1983;109(suppl 24):58.

89. Bonnetblanc JM, Bouquier JJ. Response to pipamperone in case of epidermolysis bullosa herpetiformis. *Lancet.* 1986;1:1327–1328.

90. Gedde-Dahl Jr T, Anton-Lamprecht I. Epidermolysis bullosa. In: Emery AEH, Rimion DL, eds. *Principles and Practice of Medical Genetics.* Edinburgh: Churchill-Livingstone; 1983: 672–687.

91. Anton-Lamprecht I, Gedde-Dahl Jr T, Schnyder UW. Ultrastructural characterization of a new dominant epidermolysis genotype. *J Invest Dermatol.* 1979;72:280.

92. Anton-Lamprecht I, Schnyder UW. Epidermolysis bullosa herpetiformis Dowling-Meara: report of a case and pathomorphogenesis. *Dermatologica.* 1982;164:221–235.

93. Ishida-Yamamoto A, McGrath JA, Chapman SJ, Leigh IM, Eady RAJ. Distribution and significance of tonofilament clumping in the Dowling-Meara form of epidermolysis bullosa simplex (DM-EBS). *Br J Dermatol.* 1990;123:834.

94. Schofield OMV, McGrath J, Ishida-Yamamoto A, Barker J, Macdonald DM, Eady RAJ. Dowling-Meara epidermolysis bullosa simplex. *Br J Dermatol.* 1991;125(suppl 38):44–45.

94a. Ishida-Yamamoto A, McGrath JA, Chapman SJ, Leigh IM, Lane EB, Eady RAJ. Epidermolysis bullosa simplex (Dowling-Meara type) is a genetic disease characterized by an abnormal keratin-filament network involving keratins K5 and K14. *J Invest Dermatol.* 1991;97:959–968.

95. Wojnarowska F, Tidman MJ, Eady RAJ. Epidermolysis bullosa herpetiformis (Dowling-Meara). *Br J Dermatol.* 1983;109(suppl 24):56.

96. Niemi K-M, Kanerva L, Kero M, Dammert K. Signs of erythrodermia ichthyosiforme congenita and epidermolysis bullosa simplex in the same patient, twenty years follow-up. *J Cutan Pathol.* 1983;10:414.

97. Tidman M.J, Allen MH, Leigh IM, Eady RAJ, McDonald DM. Epidermolysis bullosa simplex (Dowling-Meara): an immunohistochemical study of keratin expression. *J Invest Dermatol.* 1986;87:171.

98. Tidman MJ, Eady RAJ, Leigh IM, McDonald DM. Keratin expression in epidermolysis bullosa simplex (Dowling-Meara). *Acta Derm Venereol (Stockh)*. 1988;68:15–20.

99. Coulombe PA, Hutton ME, Letai A, Herbert A, Paller AS, Fuchs E. Point mutations in human keratin 14 genes of epidermolysis bullosa simplex patients: genetic and functional analyses. *Cell*. 1991;66:1301–1311.

100. Fischer T, Gedde-Dahl Jr T. Epidermolysis bullosa simplex and mottled pigmentation: a new dominant syndrome. I. Clinical and histological features. *Clin Genet*. 1979;15:228–238.

101. Gedde-Dahl Jr T, Anton-Lamprecht T. Ultrastructural studies of a new syndrome: epidermolysis bullosa simplex and mottled pigmentation. *J Cutan Pathol*. 1981;8:161.

102. Bruckner-Tuderman L, Vogel A, Ruegger S, Odermatt B, Tonz O, Schnyder UW. Epidermolysis bullosa simplex with mottled pigmentation. *J Am Acad Dermatol*. 1989;21:425–432.

103. Boss JM, Matthews CNA, Peachey RDG, Summerly R. Speckled hyperpigmentation, palmo-plantar punctate keratoses and childhood blistering: a clinical triad, with variable associations, a report of two families. *Br J Dermatol*. 1981;105:579–585.

104. Matthews CNA, Peachey RDG. Epidermolysis bullosa with pigmentation and palmar and plantar keratoses. *Br J Dermatol*. 1977;97(suppl 15):44–46.

105. Bart BJ, Gorlin RJ, Anderson VE, Lynch FW. Congenital localized absence of skin and associated abnormalities resembling epidermolysis bullosa. *Arch Dermatol*. 1966;93:296–304.

106. Bart BJ. Congenital localized absence of skin, blistering and nail abnormalities, a new syndrome. *Birth Defects: Original Article Series*. 1971;VII:118–120.

107. Pearson RW. Clinicopathologic types of epidermolysis bullosa and their non-dermatological complications. *Arch Dermatol*. 1988;124:718–725.

108. Joensen HD. Epidermolysis bullosa dystrophica dominans in two families in the Faroe Islands: a clinico-genetic study of 56 living individuals. *Acta Derm Venereol (Stockh)*. 1973;53:53–60.

109. Wojnarowska FT, Eady RAJ, Wells RS. Dystrophic epidermolysis bullosa presenting with congenital localized absence of skin: report of four cases. *Br J Dermatol*. 1983;108:477–483.

110. Haber RA, Hana W, Ramsay CA, Boxall LBH. Hereditary epidermolysis bullosa. *J Am Acad Dermatol*. 1985;13:252–278.

111. Smith SZ, Cram DL. A mechanobullous disease of the newborn, Bart's syndrome. *Arch Dermatol*. 1978;114:81–84.

112. Briggaman RA. Hereditary epidermolysis bullosa with special emphasis on newly recognized syndromes and complications. *Dermatol Clin*. 1983;1:263–280.

113. Sybert VP. Aplasia cutis congenita: report of 12 new families and review of the literature. *Pediatr Dermatol*. 1985;3:1–14.

114. Butler DF, Berger TG, James WD, Smith TL, Stanley JR, Rodman OG. Bart's syndrome: microscopic, ultrastructural, and immunofluorscent mapping features. *Pediatr Dermatol*. 1986;3:113–118.

115. Butler DF. Bart's syndrome [letter]. J Am Acad Dermatol. 1986;15:130–131.

116. Bavinck JNB, van Haeringen A, Ruitter D, van der Schroeff JG. Autosomal dominant epidermolysis bullosa dystrophica: are the Cockayne-Touraine, the

Pasini and the Bart-types different expressions of the same mutant gene? *Clin Genet*. 1987;31:416–424.

117. Skoven I, Drzewiecki KT. Congenital localized skin defect and epidermolysis bullos hereditaria letalis. *Acta Derm Venereol (Stockh)*. 1979;59:533–537.

118. El Shafie M, Stidham GL, Klippel CH, Katzman GH, Weinfeld IJ. Pyloric atresia and epidermolysis bullosa letalis: a lethal combination in two premature newborn siblings. *J Pediatr Surg*. 1979;14:446–449.

119. Peltier FA, Tschen EH, Raimer SS, Kuo T-T. Epidermolysis bullosa letalis associated with congenital pyloric atresia. *Arch Dermatol*. 1981;117:728–731.

120. Cowton JAL, Beattie TJ, Gibson AAM, Mackie R, Skerrow CJ, Cockburn F. Epidermolysis bullosa in association with aplasia cutis congenita and pyloric atresia. *Acta Pediatr Scand*. 1982;71:155–160.

121. Gedde-Dahl Jr T. *Epidermolysis Bullosa: A Clinical, Genetic and Epidemiological Study*. Baltimore: The Johns Hopkins Press; 1971, 40–45.

122. Olaisen B, Gedde-Dahl Jr T. GPT-Epidermolysis bullosa simplex (EBS-Ogna) linkage in man. *Hum Hered*. 1973;23:189–196.

123. Olaisen B, Gedde-Dahl Jr T. Gpt-EBS1 linkage group, general linkage relations. *Hum Hered*. 1974;24:178–185.

124. Cavanaugh ML, Chan HS, Cohen IH, other members of the Howard Hughes Medical Institute Human Gene Mapping Library: New Haven Human Gene Mapping Library Chromosome Plots. Number 4, HGM9.5. Howard Hughes Medical Institute, 1988, p 18.

125. Salih MAM, Lake BD, El Hag MA, Atherton DJ. Lethal epidermolytic epidermolysis bullosa: a new autosomal recessive type of epidermolysis bullosa. *Br J Dermatol*. 1985;113:135–143.

126. Nielsen PG, Sjolund E. Epidermolysis bullosa simplex localisata associated with anodontia, hair loss and nail disorders: a new syndrome. *Acta Derm Venereol (Stockh)*. 1985;65:526–530.

127. Woerdeman MJ. Dystrophia bullosa hereditaria. Typus maculatus. Proceedings of the Second International Congress of Dermatology. *Acta Derm Venereol (Stockh)*. 1957;678:111–116.

128. Geerts ML, Overbeke J, Kint A, Cormane RH. Comparative electron microscopic study between Mendes da Costa's disease and recessive epidermolysis bullosa dystrophica. *Br J Dermatol*. 1978;98:529–536.

129. Pegum JS, Ramsay CA. X-linked epidermolysis bullosa (Mendes de Costa), poikiloderma, retarded growth. *Proc R Soc Med*. 1973;66:234–236.

130. Niemi K-M, Kero M, Kanerva L, Mattila R. Epidermolysis bullosa simplex: a new histologic subgroup. 1983;119:138–141.

131. Eisenberg M, Shorey CD, De Chair-Baker W. Epidermolysis bullosa—a new subgroup. *Austr J Dermatol*. 1986;27:15–18.

132. Taieb A, Surleve-Bazeille J-E, Sarlangue J, Maleville J. Epidermolysis bullosa with congenital fusion of the toes and eyelids. In: Wilkinson DS, Mascaro JM, Orfanos CE, eds. *Clinical Dermatology, the CMD Case Collection*. Stuttgart: Schattauer 1987: 128–130.

133. Taieb A, Legrain V, Surleve-Bazeille JE, Sarlangue J, Maleville J. Generalized epidermolysis bullosa with congenital synechiae, assorted malformations and unusual ultrastructure: a new entity? *Dermatologica*. 1988;176:76–82.

8
Junctional Epidermolysis Bullosa: A Clinical Overview

ANDREW N. LIN and D. MARTIN CARTER

Junctional epidermolysis bullosa is an autosomal recessive disorder characterized by the formation of blisters at the lamina lucida, an electron-lucent zone located between the basal cell plasma membrane and the lamina densa (Fig. 8.1). Like other forms of epidermolysis bullosa (EB), several subtypes are recognized (Table 8.1). These are differentiated mainly on the basis of clinical manifestations, and it is unclear if they represent varying expressivity of a single defective gene, or diseases caused by abnormalities at different genetic loci. Staining with monoclonal antibodies directed at various basement membrane zone antigens is useful in characterizing certain forms of junctional EB,[1] and this is topic is discussed in detail in Chapter 3. Abnormalities of hemidesmosomes have been observed in skin biopsy specimens from patients with junctional EB, especially those with the "letalis" form.[2] Reduced numbers of morphologically ill-defined "hemidesmosomelike structures" have been observed in cultured keratinocytes obtained from junctional EB patients.[3] In another study, cultured keratinocytes obtained from three patients with a nonletalis type of junctional EB showed altered structural, adhesive, and functional abnormalities.[4] Compared with normal keratinocytes, junctional EB cells showed elongated refractile appearance, diminished cell–stratum adhesion, and were slow growing.[4] A condition similar to junctional EB has been described in the toy poodle.[5]

Generalized Junctional EB, Gravis Variant
(EB letalis of Herlitz-Pearson)

The gravis variant of generalized junctional EB is characterized by widespread cutaneous blistering that often presents at birth or shortly thereafter. Death during infancy is common, but some patients may live to adulthood. Oral blistering is usually present.

In 1935, Herlitz[6] defined a syndrome based on a review of 16 cases previously reported and eight new cases of his own. He named the syndrome "EB letalis" because it was characterized by death in infancy usually before the

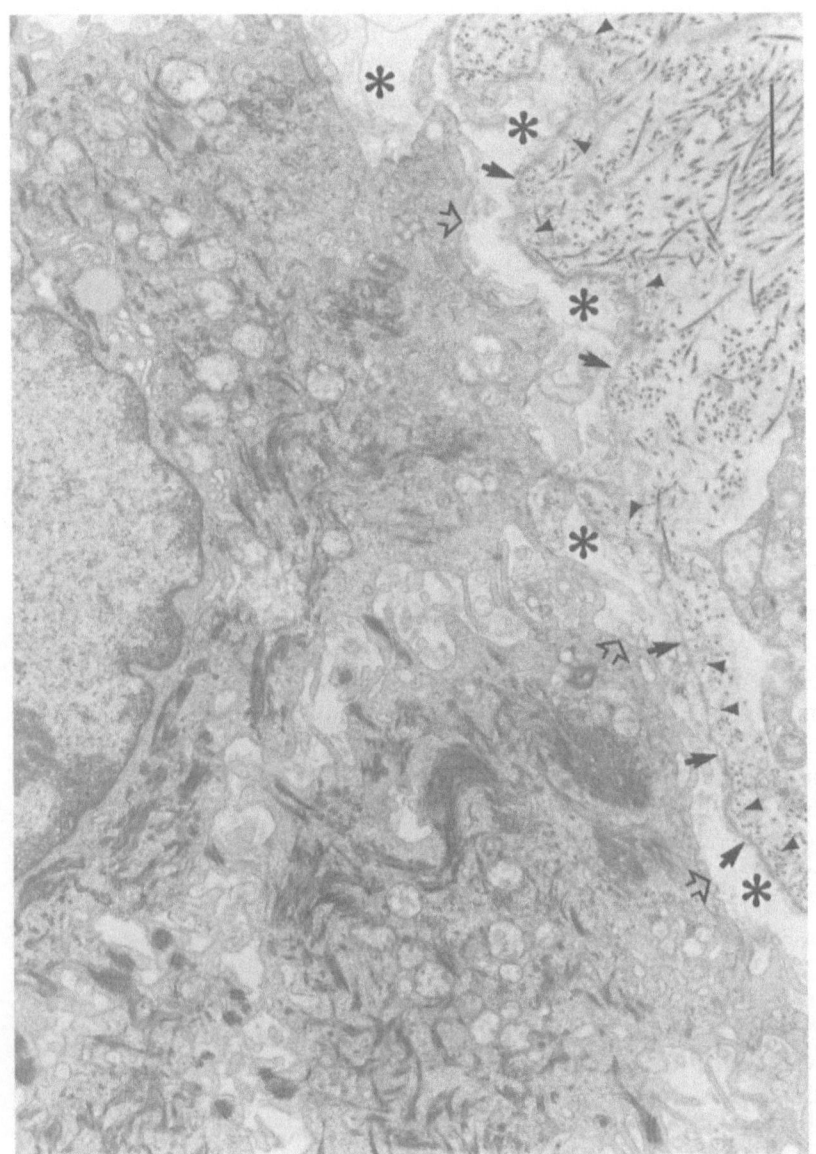

FIGURE 8.1. Electron micrograph of junctional EB. Separation (*) has occurred between the basal cell plasma membrane (*open arrows*) and the lamina densa (*black arrows*) of the dermal–epidermal junction. Hemidesmosomes are not apparent, but anchoring fibrils (*arrowheads*) extend from the lamina densa in the uppermost compartment of the papillary dermis. (Bar = 1 µm; 11,560X.) (Electron micrograph courtesy of Lynne T. Smith, Seattle, WA.)

TABLE 8.1. Clinical types of junctional EB.

Type	Characteristics
Generalized junctional EB, gravis variant	Severe widespread blistering
	Exuberant granulation tissue, especially on face, around mouth
	Severe extracutaneous involvement
	May be fatal in neonatal period
Generalized atrophic benign EB	Atrophy at sites of blistering
	Alopecia of scalp, pubic, and axillary areas
	May improve with age
Localized junctional EB	Predilection for pretibial areas
EB progressiva	Progressive nail and skin involvement
	Hearing loss in some cases
Inverse junctional EB	Predilection for inverse sites, such as groin and axilla
	"Albostriate" lesions in some cases
Cicatricial junctional EB	Flexion deformities of fingers
	Blisters heal with scarring

age of 3 months. Other features were appearance of blisters on skin and mucosa at or soon after birth, presence of hemorrhagic blisters, nail dystrophy, and absence of scarring. These features, especially early death, were felt to be sufficiently distinctive from EB simplex and dystrophic EB that the syndrome was recognized as a "third form" of EB.[7] Based on these criteria, many similar cases have since been described under various names, including "lethal EB," "EB letalis of Herlitz-Pearson," and "Herlitz disease." A review of the world literature in 1968 yielded 106 cases.[8] Some cases, however, were diagnosed solely on clinical grounds without benefit of histologic examination,[9-13] whereas others were studied only with light microscopy. Among the latter, many cases showed separation between the epidermis and dermis,[7,8,14-19] whereas others showed vacuolization of basal cells,[8,20,21] intraepidermal blistering,[22] or nonspecific features that were not helpful diagnostically.[23,24] Considerable controversy thus existed about whether Herlitz disease was a distinctive entity, and it was suggested that some cases of "lethal EB" were actually a severe variant of dystrophic EB,[25-27] especially the recessive type.[28,29] Clarification came when electron microscopy was used to study biopsy specimens. Early ultrastructural studies localized the site of blister formation in Herlitz disease to the "intermembrane space," located at the "junction" between the basal cell plasma membrane and the basement membrane.[30] This criterion has since been one of several standards by which Herlitz disease is defined.[31-34] Herlitz disease thus became known as "junctional EB," and the two terms have often been used interchangeably. This is misleading, for careful clinical observations have shown the existence of other types of EB in which separation occurs at the same ultrastructural level but whose clinical features are different. As a result, different clinical subtypes of junctional EB were recognized, and Herlitz disease came to be considered as one of several types of junctional EB.

Judging from the number of reported cases, Herlitz disease is by far the most common type of junctional EB. However, many early cases of "lethal Herlitz disease" did not include electron microscopic examination, and it is impossible to tell if they all represented junctional EB as we define it today. Furthermore, some cases of "lethal EB" survived as long as 35 years,[35] violating the cardinal criterion of death in infancy, as implied in the designation "letalis." For these reasons, it is best to consider cases of "Herlitz disease" as those having junctional EB with widespread involvement and high infant mortality, but that in some cases can survive to adulthood. Fine et al. proposed renaming the syndrome as "gravis variant of generalized junctional EB" to reflect better the prognosis and histology and to separate it from other forms of junctional EB.[1] Nevertheless, the name "lethal Herlitz disease" (and its variants) is so entrenched in the EB literature that it is useful to review these cases as a group, bearing in mind that some cases may not actually fulfill the electron microscopic criteria of junctional separation.

In 1968, Cross et al. reviewed the pattern of inheritance in 79 cases of "EB letalis," and concluded that increased parental consanguinity and results of segregation analysis were consistent with autosomal recessive pattern of transmission.[36]

Death in infancy has long been considered a hallmark of Herlitz disease, but the cause of death is not always apparent.[35] Most patients presumably die of overwhelming sepsis caused by extensive cutaneous blistering, but extracutaneous involvement could well have contributed to early demise. Autopsy reports have documented the presence of clinically inapparent involvement of extracutaneous organs. For example, gross examination at autopsy in one patient showed erosions in the esophagus and stomach, while microscopic blisters were seen in the jejunum, ileum, colon, rectum, gall bladder, vagina, urinary bladder, and trachea.[37] Similar autopsy findings in another patient were documented by Pearson et al.; this patient had esophageal erosion, epithelial–subepithelial separation in the jejunum and gall bladder, friable mucosa in the mouth, pharynx, and anus, and the surface of the teeth was noted to be pitted.[35] In other patients, vesicles have been found in the bronchioles,[38] bile ducts,[39] and pancreatic ducts.[39] Various ocular abnormalities including complete retinal detachment was seen at autopsy in one patient.[40] In some cases, however, necropsy failed to show any specific changes that could be directly attributed to EB.[16,41]

Among those who survive beyond infancy, various forms of systemic involvement have been reported. The most common site is the gastrointestinal tract, and most patients have oral blisters[13,42,43] at least some of the time. The presence of granulation tissue or crusting in perioral erosions is said to be a distinctive feature of Herlitz disease[31,36,44,45] (Fig. 8.2). One patient with junctional EB had erosions around the mouth and nose that led to scarring of the perinasal skin, causing obstructive sleep apnea.[46]

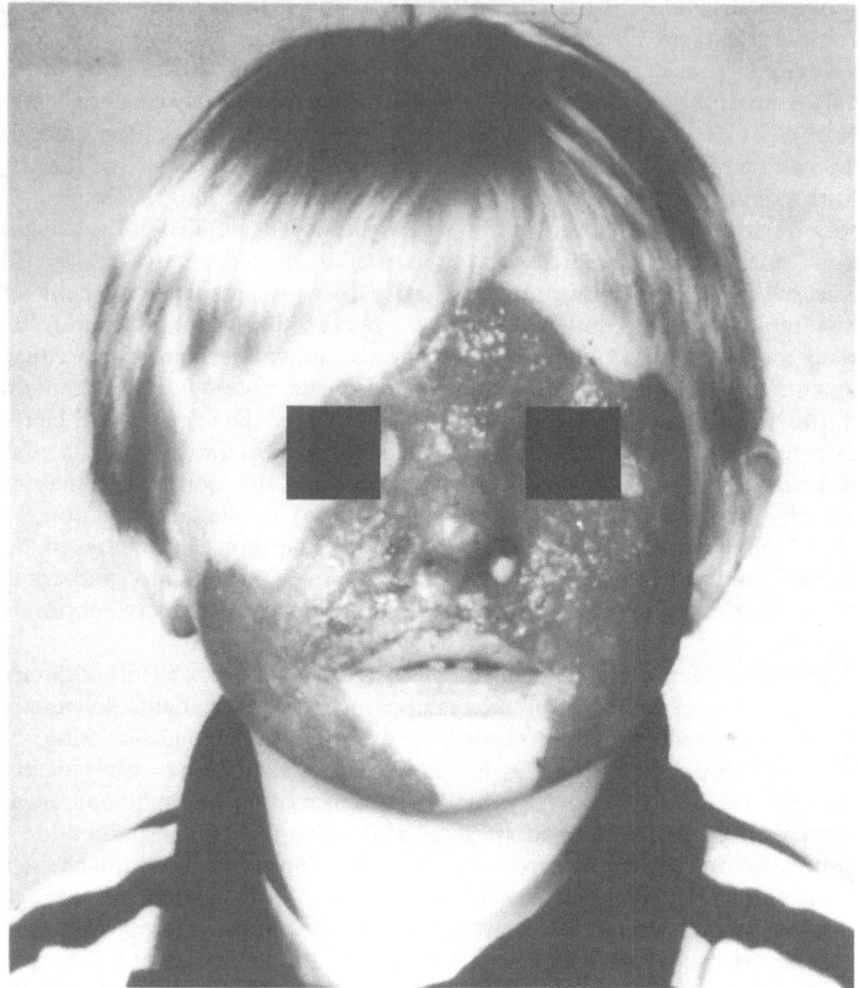

FIGURE 8.2. Gravis variant of junctional EB of Herlitz-Pearson: erosion and granulation tissue around the mouth is considered a pathognomonic feature.

A rare but serious condition that can be seen with Herlitz disease is pyloric atresia.[47-50] The mothers of affected infants almost always have polyhydramnios during pregnancy, and the infant often has widespread blistering at birth. Projectile vomiting develops soon after birth, and radiologic investigation shows the "single-bubble sign"[51] indicative of gastric outlet obstruction. These patients are extremely ill from fluid and electrolyte imbalance due to vomiting and widespread erosions. Prompt surgical correction of the pyloric atresia is necessary for survival. One patient developed "acquired pyloric obstruction" at 1 month of age.[52] Pyloric atresia has also been reported in a patient who may have a "nonlethal" type of junctional EB,[53] and in patients with unspecified subtypes of junctional EB[54,55]. Because pyloric atresia and junctional EB are both rare conditions, such an association probably represents pleiotropic expression of a single defective gene.

A number of patients with junctional EB and pyloric atresia also have various urological abnormalities, such as hydronephrosis[56,57] and interstitial nephritis.[58] Hydronephrosis has also been noted in two patients with junctional EB and pyloric stenosis,[59] and one other with junctional EB and gastric antral atresia.[59] Pyloric atresia may not be unique to junctional EB, for it has also been reported in cases of presumed or probable recessive dystrophic EB,[51,60,61] and in one patient in whom junctional EB was diagnosed on light and electron microscopy but who showed "fusion" of the digits.[50]

Chronic anemia is common,[44] although it is usually not as severe as in recessive dystropohic EB. This is usually attributable to several factors, including iron deficiency from chronic blood loss from cutaneous wounds and poor intake, as well as anemia of chronic disease. Various teeth abnormalities, including enamel defects[62,63] and abnormal ameloblasts,[64] have been described. Laryngeal involvement is a rare but serious complication that can be life threatening,[65] and early tracheostomy has been advocated.[66] Other forms of systemic involvement include corneal erosions and cicatricial ectropion,[67] esophagitis,[68] and balanitis leading to stricture of the prepuce.[69] Fine observed "web formation" in the axilla in two patients with Herlitz disease, presumably caused by chronic presence of granulation tissue.[70] Faulk et al. reported a patient with unusual congenital findings that included webbing of the fingers and toes, abnormal facies, bilateral inguinal hernias, abnormal thymus, undeveloped peripheral lymphoid tissues, and immunohistologic abnormalities of cytotrophoblast and amniotic epithelium in the amniochorion.[71]

By obtaining fetal skin samples during fetoscopy and then studying them with electron microscopy and antibody probes, investigators have successfully ruled in[72,73] and ruled out[74,75] Herlitz disease in pregnancies at risk. Hausser et al. suggested sampling amniotic epithelia as an alternative to fetoscopy,[76] but others have expressed concern about the safety of this procedure[77] (see also Chapter 19).

Generalized Atrophic Benign EB

In 1982, Hintner and Wolff[78] described eight patients (ages 3 to 40 years) with junctional EB characterized by continuous blistering since birth, improvement with age, atrophy at sites of blistering (without milia, mutilation, or severe scarring), nail dystrophy, and atrophic alopecia involving the scalp, pubic, and axillary areas (Fig. 8.3). All patients had normal complete blood count. This condition differed from Herlitz disease because they all survived

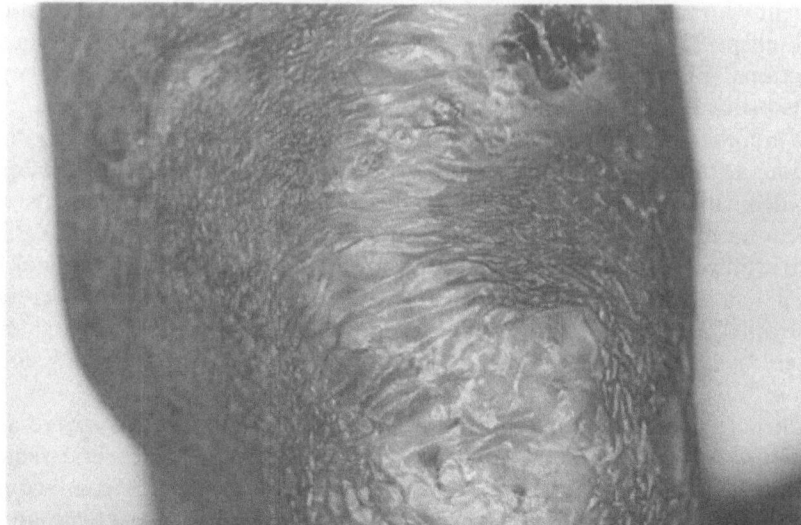

(A)

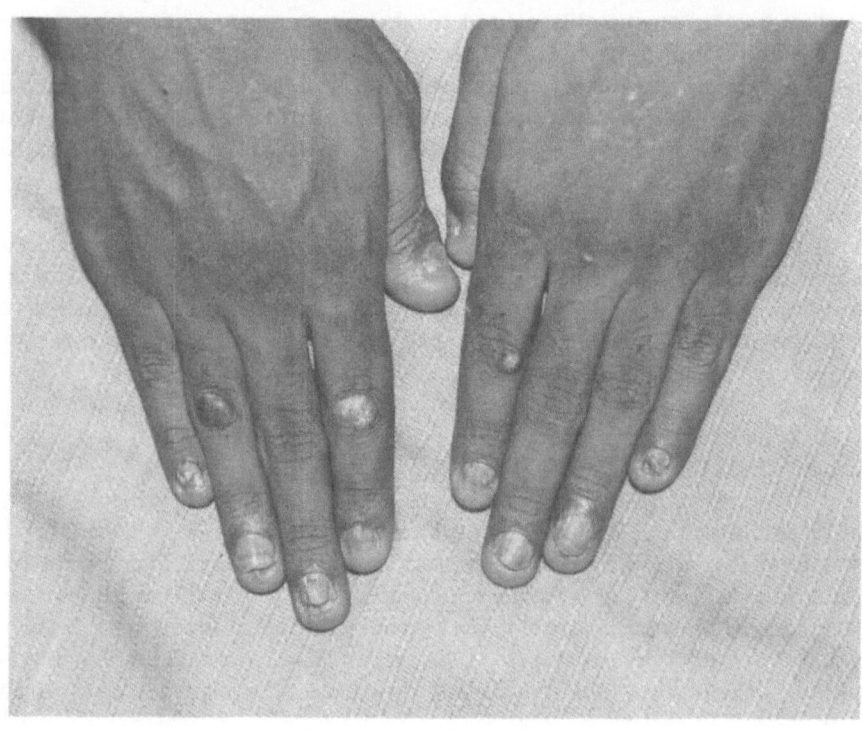

(B)

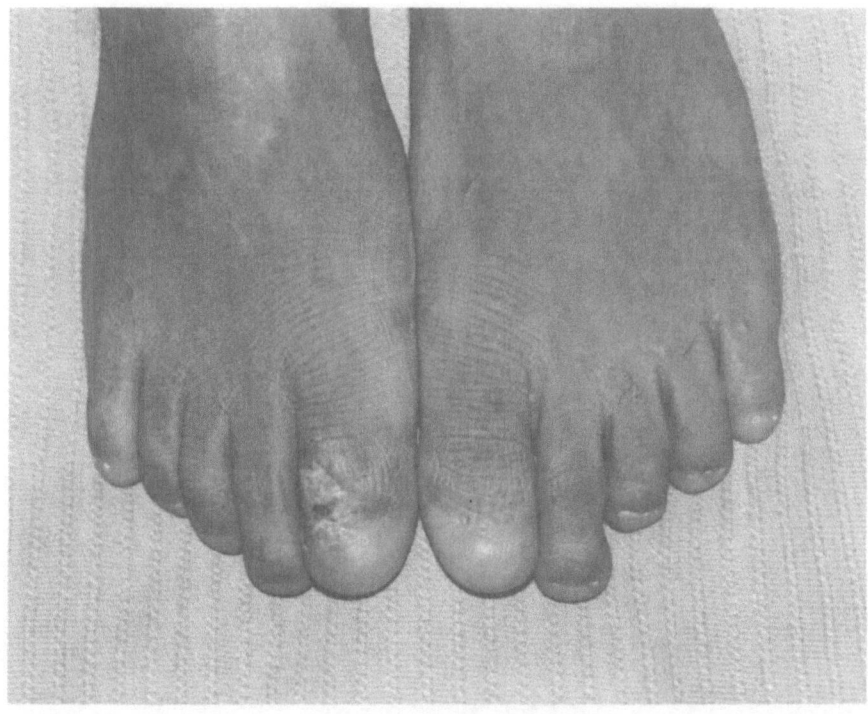

(C)

FIGURE 8.3. Generalized atrophic benign EB (GABEB): atrophic scarring on knee (A, facing page); dystrophy of finger nails (B, facing page) and toe nails (C); chronic erosion on leg (D, following page).

past infancy, extracutanoeus involvement was mild, and the prognosis appeared much better. They reviewed five other cases previously reported[79,80] whom they felt belonged to the same category, which they named generalized atrophic benign EB. One of these cases[79] has also been known as the "Disentis" type of EB[80a] (personal communication from I. Hashimoto, Hirosaki, Japan), named after the Swiss village where the patient lived. Since then, 16 additional cases have been reported,[81–87,87a,87b] bringing the total to 27, but this condition is probably more common than realized. Many patients have nevocytic nevi,[78,79,81,84] although the relation between the nevi and underlying EB remains unclear. Other associated features include esophageal stricture,[78] laryngeal involvement requiring tracheostomy,[81] oral erosions[78,81,86] corneal ulcers,[86] hypoacusis,[78,79] enamel defects,[78,86] keratoacanthoma,[85] urethral stricture,[87b] and cerebrotendinous xanthoma in unaffected siblings.[82] Intrafamilial variation in clinical severity was noted in two affected brothers.[87] Cases reported as "recessive-EB atrophicans mitis"[88–91] and "nonlethal junctional EB"[92] probably belong to this category. One $4\frac{1}{2}$-year-old boy was felt to have "features of benign junctional EB," but he also had serious systemic complications including pyloric atresia and bilateral hydronephrosis.[56]

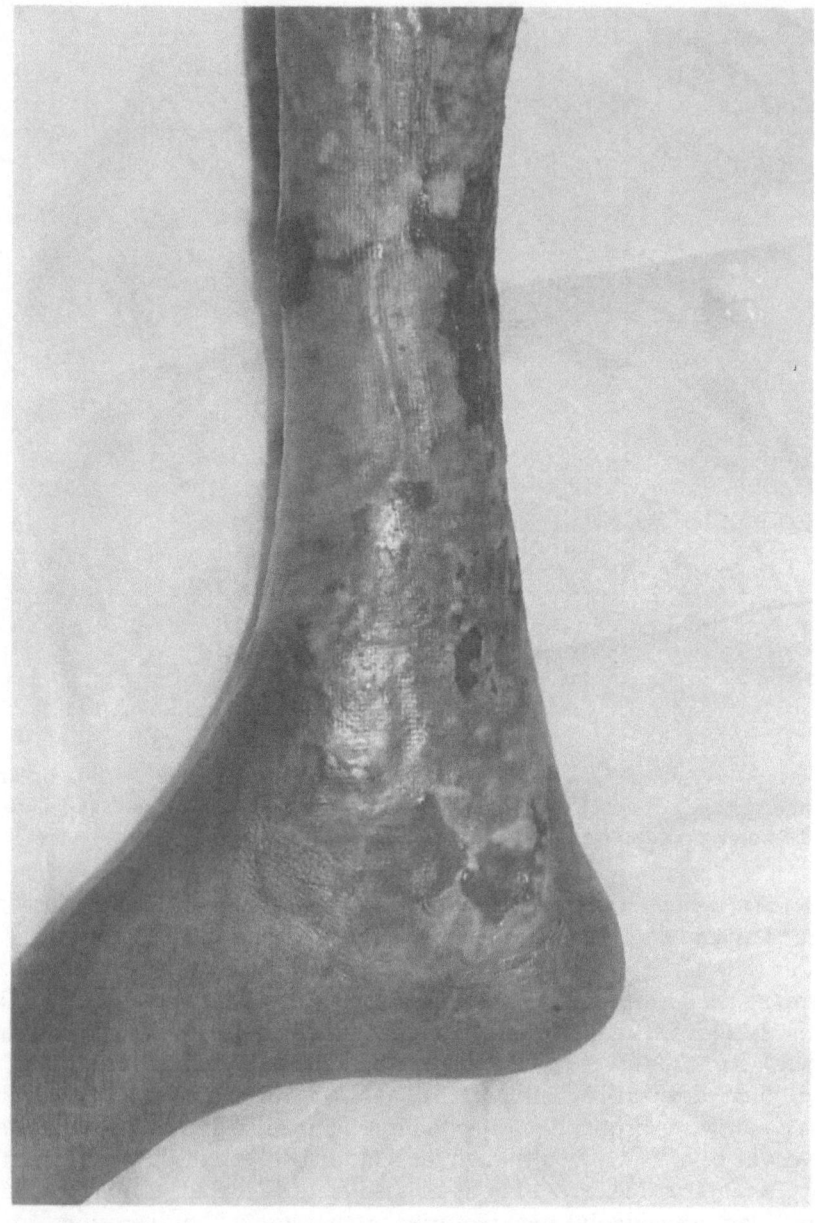

(D)

Localized Junctional EB

In some patients with junctional EB, blisters can appear anywhere on the skin but show predilection for the pretibial area. It is unclear if this represents a distinct disease or simply a continuum of generalized atrophic benign EB. This condition is infrequently reported, and the literature contains four such cases.

In 1983, Gedde-Dahl et al.[88] referred to a German paper[80] reporting a woman with junctional EB in whom blisters appeared only on the shins and soles. Her nails were involved and the teeth showed enamel hypoplasia. Others[93,94] reported two sisters (ages 20 and 21 years) with blistering mainly involving the legs. Teeth were not dysplastic, but nails and oral mucosa were involved, and tender hyperkeratotic lesions were present on the soles. Similarly, a 56-year-old man had blisters on the trunk and limbs but the pretibial area was particularly affected.[95,96] After a squamous cell carcinoma arising on normal skin on the hand was excised, he developed squamous cell carcinoma on a leg ulcer, which required amputation,[97,98] but transitional cell carcinoma of the bladder subsequently appeared.[96,98] These features are unusual because squamous cell carcinoma is known to occur in scars of dystrophic EB, but is very rare in junctional EB. The localized form of junctional EB should be distinguished from the "pretibial" form of dominant dystrophic EB.[99]

EB Progressiva

This uncommon condition is characterized by progressive appearance of nail and skin involvement starting in childhood. Nail dystrophy appears around age 5 to 8 years, followed by blisters, cutaneous atrophy, loss of finger ridge patterns, and mild finger contractures.[88] It was originally called "EB dystrophica neurotrophica" because some cases were associated with hearing loss.[100] However, it subsequently became clear that this is not a constant feature, occurring in only four of six Scandinavian kindreds.[101] Electron microscopy showed "widened lamina rara with deposits of amorphous material,"[88] and separation through the lamina lucida was documented in one case.[102]

Inverse Junctional EB

This is another uncommon type of EB that affects predominantly inverse sites such as the groin and axilla.[88,94] Perianal involvement can cause anal stenosis.[103] Oral mucosa, cornea, teeth, hair, and nails can also be involved).[88,94,103] Some patients develop "albostriate" lesions on the trunk and proximal extremities, showing small white atrophic spots or streaks that can be flat or elevated.[88] Separation through the lamina lucida has been confirmed by electron microscopy.[2] This form should be distinguished from inverse type of recessive dystrophic EB.[104]

Cicatricial Junctional EB

This condition was described in only three patients (two were siblings).[105] It is characterized by blisters that heal with scarring instead of atrophy. Flexion contractures and fusion of the digits resembling recessive dystrophic EB occurred in all patients, as did scarring of nasal mucosa with stenosis of the nares. Other features included oral blisters, dental caries, loss of nails, and laryngeal involvement. All cases were initially diagnosed on clinical grounds as dystrophic forms of EB, but electron microscopy showed separation through the lamina lucida. It has been suggested that this form may fit within the range of generalized atrophic benign EB.[106]

Others

Two siblings with junctional EB had mental retardation, enamel tooth defects, and dystrophic finger nails.[107] One of them also had subluxation of the lens. Mental retardation and subluxation of the lens are very uncommon in EB, and it is unclear if their occurrence in these patients represents coincidence or a distinctive syndrome.

Acknowledgments. Supported in part by a General Clinical Research Center grant (M01-RR00102) from the National Institutes of Health to The Rockefeller University Hospital; by a training grant (AR07525) from the National Institutes of Health to the Laboratory for Investigative Dermatology; by contracts AR62269 and AR62270 from the National Institutes of Health to the Laboratory for Investigative Dermatology; by a grant from the Dystrophic Epidermolysis Bullosa Research Association (D.E.B.R.A.) of America, Inc.; and with general support from the Pew Trusts.

References

1. Fine JD, Bauer EA, Briggaman RA, et al. Revised clinical and laboratory criteria for subtypes of inherited epidermolysis bullosa: a consensus report by the subcommittee on diagnosis and classification of the National Epidermolysis Bullosa Registry. *J Am Acad Dermatol.* 1991;24:119–135.
2. Tidman MJ, Eady RAJ. Hemidesmosome heterogeneity in junctional epidermolysis bullosa revealed by morphometric analysis. *J Invest Dermatol.* 1986;86: 51–56.
3. Chapman SJ, Leigh IM, Tidman MJ, Eady RAJ. Abnormal expression of

hemidesmosome-like structures by junctional epidermolysis bullosa keratino-cytes in vitro. *Br J Dermatol.* 1990;123:137–144.

4. Krueger JG, Lin AN, Leong I, Carter DM. Junctional epidermolysis bullosa keratinocytes in culture display adhesive, structural and functional abnormalities. *J Invest Dermatol.* 1991;97:849–861.

5. Dunstan RW, Sills RC, Wilkinson JE, Paller AS, Hashimoto KH. A disease resembling junctional epidermolysis bullosa in a toy poodle. *Am J Dermatopathol.* 1988;10:442–447.

6. Herlitz H. Kongenitaler nicht syphilitischer pemphigus. Eine ubersicht nebst beschreibung einer neuen krankheitsform (Epidermolysis bullosa heredihria letalis). *Ach Paediat.* 1935;17:315–371.

7. Schaffer G. Two cases of epidermolysis bullosa hereditaira letalis. *Acta Derm Venereol (Stockh).* 1951;31:704–709.

8. Bergenholtz A, Olsson O. Epidermolysis bullosa hereditaria letalis: a survey of the literature and report of 11 cases. *Acta Derm Venereol (Stockh).* 1968;48:220–241.

9. Calnan CD. Epidermolysis bullosa letalis. *Great Ormond Street J.* 1954–55;8:113–117.

10. Silver HK. Epidermolysis bullosa hereditaria letalis: report of a case surviving for two and a half years. *Arch Dis Child.* 1957;32:216–219.

11. Waldrigues A, Pedro R de J, Gross C. Epidermolysis bullosa hereditaria letalis [letter]. *Lancet.* 1972;2:1372.

12. Hidano A. Epidermolysis bullosa hereditaria in two sisters: discussion of the Herlitz type. *Pediatr Dermatol Mod Probl Paediatr.* 1975;17:93–94.

13. Kahn S, Trieger N. Epidermolysis bullosa hereditaria letalis: a case report with special emphasis on oral manifestations. *J. Oral Med.* 1976;31:32–35.

14. Lenstrup J. Lethal herditary bullous epidermolysis: survey, and a typical case. *Acta Paediatr.* 1947;34:263–278.

15. Henderson AT. Epidermolysis bullosa hereditaria letalis: report of a case failing to respond to cortisone. *J Pediatr.* 1955;46:186–191.

16. Lewis IC, Steven EM, Farquhar JW. Epidermolysis bullosa in the newborn. *Arch Dis Child.* 1955;30:277–284.

17. Gilbert EF. Epidermolysis bullosa. *Clin Proc Children's Hosp. District Columbia.* 1956;12:115–119.

18. Rossett M. Epidermolysis bullosa of the newborn. *Can Med Assoc J.* 1956;75:507–509.

19. Fattah AA. Epidermolysis bullosa hereditaria letalis (Herlitz). *Dermatologica.* 1966;133:475–481.

20. Roberts MH, Howell DRS, Bramhall JL, Reubner B. Epidermolysis bullosa letalis: report of three cases with particular reference to the histopathology of the skin. *Pediatrics.* 1960;25:283–290.

21. Madhaven M, Aurora AL, Puri RD. Epidermolysis bullosa letalis: report of a case. *Indian J Pediatr.* 1977;44:192–194.

22. Davidson LT. Hereditary epidermolysis bullosa: report of a case with a resume of the literature. *Am J Dis Child.* 1940;59:371–378.

23. Black RA, Wilhelm E, Gilbert C, White CJ. Epidermolysis bullosa in the newborn. *J Am Med Assoc.* 1945;129:734–736.

24. Walther T. Epidermolysis bullosa hereditaria letalis: a review and report of two own cases. *Ann Ped Int Rev Pediatr.* 1953;180:382–392.

25. Frank DJ, Kern WH. Epidermolysis bullosa: a case report. *Ohio State Med J.* 1954;50:679–680.
26. Tamayo L, Ruiz-Maldonado R. Epidermolysis bullosa: clinical aspects. *Mod Probl Paediatr.* 1975;17:77–84.
27. Carnevale A, Ruiz-Maldonado R, Diez JF. Epidermolysis bullosa: a study of 22 Mexican cases. *Mod Probl Paediatr.* 1975;17:85–92.
28. Lowe Jr LB. Hereditary epidermolysis bullosa. *Arch. Dermatol.* 1967;95:587–595.
29. Sofatzis JA. Blistering and scaling dermatoses [letter]. *J. Pediatr.* 1971;79:341.
30. Pearson RW. Studies of the pathogenesis of epidermolysis bullosa. *J Invest Dermatol.* 1962;39:551–575.
31. Esterly NB, Hruby M. Epidermolysis bullosa letalis in two brothers. *Birth Defects: Original Article Series.* 1974;X:155–157.
32. Skoven I, Drzewiecki KT. Congenital localized skin defect and epidermolysis bullos hereditaria letalis. *Acta Derm Venereol (Stockh).* 1979;59:533–537.
33. Heijima M, Inoue S, Ogata K. A fatal case of junctional epidermolysis bullosa (Herlitz-Pearson). *J Dermatol.* 1981;8:483–486.
34. De Jong MCJM, Meijer P, Van Voorst Vader PC, Hollema H. Junctional epidermolysis bullosa letalis. *Br J Dermatol.* 1990;123:681–682.
35. Pearson RW, Potter B, Strauss F. Epidermolysis bullosa hereditaria letalis: clinical and histologic manifestations and course of the disease. *Arch Dermatol.* 1974;109:349–355.
36. Cross HE, Wells RS, Esterly JR. Inheritance in epidermolysis bullosa letalis. *J Med Genet.* 1968;5:189–196.
37. Schachner L, Lazarus GS, Dembitzer H. Epidermolysis bullosa hereditaria letalis: pathology, natural history and therapy. *Br J Dermatol.* 1977;96:51–58.
38. Maddison TG, Barter RA. Epidermolysis bullosa hereditaria letalis. *Arch Dis Child.* 1961;36:337–339.
39. Leland LS, Hirschl D. Epidermolysis bullosa hereditaria letalis in newborn twins: report of two case with failure to respond favourably to cortisone. *Am J Dis Child.* 1954;87:321–327.
40. Aurora AL, Madhavan M, Rao S. Ocular changes in epidermolysis bullosa letalis. *Am J Ophthalmol.* 1975;79:464–470.
41. Lamb JH, Halpert B. Epidermolysis bullosa of the newborn. *Arch Derm. Syphilol.* 1947;55:369–374.
42. Arwill T, Bergenholtz A, Olsson O. Epidermolysis bullosa hereditaria. IV: Histologic changes of the oral mucosa in the polydysplastic dystrophic and the letalis form. *Odontologisk Revy.* 1965;16:101–111.
43. Arwill T, Bergenholtz A, Thilander H. Epidermolysis bullosa hereditaria. V: The ultrastructure of oral mucsoa and skin in four cases of the letalis form. *Acta Pathol Microbiol Scand.* 1968;74:311–324.
44. Hruby MA, Esterly NB. Anemia in epidermolysis bullosa letalis. *Am J Dis Child.* 1973;125:696–699.
45. Hiejima M, Inoue S, Ogata K. A fatal case of junctional epidermolysis bullosa (Herlitz-Pearson). *J Dermatol.* 1981;8:483–486.
46. Oakley CA, Wilson N, Ross JA, Barneston R StC. Junctional epidermolysis bullosa in two siblings: clinical observations, collagen studies and electron microscopy. *Br J Dermatol.* 1984;111:533–543.
47. El Shafie M, Stidham GL, Klippel CH, Katzman GH, Weinfeld IJ. Pyloric

atresia and epidermolysis bullosa letalis: a lethal combination in two premature newborn siblings. *J Pediatr Surg.* 1979;14:446–449.

48. Adashi EY, Louis FJ, Vasquez M. An unusual case of epidermolysis bullosa hereditaria letalis with cutaneous scarring and pyloric atresia. *J Pediatr.* 1980; 96:443–446.

49. Peltier FA, Tschen EH, Raimer SS, Kuo T-T. Epidermolysis bullosa letalis associated with congenital pyloric atresia. *Arch Dermatol.* 1981;117:728–731.

50. Chang C-H, Perrin EV, Bove KE. Pyloric atresia associated with epidermolysis bullosa: special reference to pathogenesis. *Pediatr Pathol.* 1983;1:449–457.

51. de Groot WG, Postuma R, Hunter AGW. Familial pyloric atresia associated with epidermolysis bullosa. *J Pediatr.* 1978;92:429-430.

52. Honig P, Yoder M, Ziegler M. Acquired pyloric obstruction in a patient with epidermolysis bullosa letalis. *J Pediatr.* 1983;102:598–600.

53. Nazzaro V, Nicolini U, De Luca L, Berti E, Caputo R. Prenatal diagnosis of junctional epidermolysis bullosa associated with pyrloric atresia. *J Med Genet.* 1990;27:244–248.

54. Swinburne LM, Kohler HG. Familial pyloric atresia associated with epidermolysis bullosa. *J Pediatr.* 1979;44:162.

55. Cambazard F, Kanitakis J, Thivolet J. Junctional epidermolysis bullosa associated with congenital pyloric atresia. In: Wilkinson DS, Mascaro JM, Orfanos CE, eds. *Clinical Dermatology, The CMD Case Collection.* Stuttgart: Schattauer; 1987:18–19.

56. Berger TG, Detlefs RL, Donatucci CF. Junctional epidermolysis bullosa, pyloric atresia, and genitourinary disease. *Pediatr Dermatol.* 1986;3:130–134.

57. Bull MJ, Norins AL, Weaver DD, Weber T, Mitchell M. Epidermolysis bullosa —Pyloric atresia: an autosomal recessive syndrome. *Am J Dis Child.* 1983;137: 449–451.

58. Egan N, Ward R, Olmstead PM, Marks Jr JG. Junctional epidermolysis bullosa and pyloric atresia in two siblings. *Arch Dermatol.* 1985;121:1186–1188.

59. Reitelman C, Burbige KA, Mitchell M, Hensle TW. The urological manifestations of epidermolysis bullosa. *J Urol.* 1986;136:1320–1322.

60. Korber JS, Glasson MJ. Pyloric atresia associated with epidermolysis bullosa. *J Pediatr.* 1977;90:600–601.

61. Pedersen PV, Hertel J. Pyloric atresia in epidermolysis bullosa. *J Pediatr.* 1977; 91:852–853.

62. Arwill T, Bergenholtz A, Olsson O. Epidermolysis bullosa hereditaria. III. A histological study of changes in teeth in the polydysplastic dystrophic and lethal forms. *Oral Surg Oral Med Oral Pathol.* 1965;19:723–744.

63. Brain EB, Wigglesworth JS. Developing teeth in epidermolysis bullosa hereditaria letalis: a histological study. *Br Dent J.* 1968;124:255–260.

64. Gardner DG, Hudson CD. The disturbances in odontogenesis in epidermolysis bullosa hereditaria letalis. *Oral Surg.* 1975;40:483–493.

65. Glossop LP, Michaels L, Bailey CM. Epidermolysis bullosa letalis in the larynx causing acute respiratory failure: a case presentation and review of the literature. *Int J Pediatr Otorhinolaryngol.* 1984;7:281–288.

66. Gonzalez C, Roth R. Laryngotracheal involvement in epidermolysis bullosa. *Int J Pediatr Otorhinolaryngol.* 1989;17:305–311.

67. Gans LA. Eye lesions of epidermolysis bullosa: clinical features, management and prognosis. *Arch Dermatol.* 1988;124:762–764.

68. Hruby MA, Esterly NB. Epidermolysis bullosa hereditaria letalis [letter]. *Arch Dermatol.* 1975;111:527–528.
69. Turner TW. Two cases of junctional epidermolysis bullosa (Herlitz-Pearson). *Br J Dermatol.* 1980;102:97–107.
70. Fine J-D. Epidermolysis bullosa: clinical aspects, pathology, and recent advances in research. *Int J Dermatol.* 1986;25:143–157.
71. Faulk WP, Hsi B-L, Yeh C-JG, McIntyre JA, Stevens PJ. Epidermolysis bullosa letalis: an immunogenetic disease of extraembryonic ectoderm? *Am J Obstet Gynecol.* 1988;158:150–157.
72. Rodeck CH, Eady RAJ, Gosden CM. Prenatal diagnosis of epidermolysis bullosa letalis. *Lancet.* 1980;1:949–952.
73. Haegerty AHM, Eady RAJ, Kennedy AR, et al. Rapid prenatal diagnosis of epidermolysis bullosa letalis using GB3 monoclonal antibody. *Br J Dermatol.* 1987;117:271–275.
74. Loftberg L, Anton-Lamprecht I, Michaelsson G, Gustavii B. Prenatal exclusion of Herlitz syndrome by electron microscopy of fetal skin biopsies obtained at fetoscopy. *Acta Derm. Venereol (Stockh).* 1983;63:185–189.
75. Haegerty AHM, Kennedy AR, Gunner DB, Eady RAJ. Rapid prenatal diagnosis and exclusion of epidermolysis bullosa using novel antibody probes. *J Invest Dermatol.* 1986;86:603–605.
76. Hausser I, Anton-Lamprecht I, Gustavii B. Prenatal diagnosis of junctional epidermolysis bullosa Herlitz type [letter]. *Lancet.* 1989;2:1035–1036.
77. Eady RAJ, Schofield OMV, Nicolaides KH, Rodeck CH. Prenatal diagnosis of junctional epidermolysis bullosa [letter]. *Lancet.* 1989;2:1453.
78. Hintner H, Wolff K. Generalized atrophic benign epidermolysis bullosa. *Arch Dermatol.* 1982;118:375–384.
79. Hashimoto I, Schnyder UW, Anton-Lamprecht I. Epidermolysis bullosa hereditaria with junctional blistering in an adult. *Dermatologica.* 1976;152:72–86.
80. Schnyder UW, Anton-Lamprecht I. Zur Klinik der epidermolysen mit junktionaler Blasenbildung (English abstract). *Dermatologica.* 1979;159:402–406.
80a. Braun-Falco O, Plewig G, Wolff HH, Winkelman RK. Vesicular and Bullous Diseases. In: Dermatology. Springer-Verlag, Berlin. 1991, p 473.
81. Paller AS, Fine J-D, Kaplan S, Pearson RW. The generalized atrophic benign form of junctional epidermolysis bullosa: experience with four patients in the United States. *Arch Dermatol.* 1986;122:704–710.
82. Hacham-Zadeh S. Benign junctional epidermolysis bullosa in three related Moroccan families [letter]. *J Am Acad Dermatol.* 1986;14:508–509.
83. Foldes C, Wallach D, Aubiniere E, Vignon-Pannamen M-D, Cottenot F. Generalized atrophic benign form of junctional epidermolysls bullosa. *Dermatologica.* 1988;176:83–90.
84. Grubauer G, Hintner H, Klein G, Fritsch P. Erworbene, flachige Riesen-Navuszellnavi bei generalisierter, atrophisierender, benigner Epidermolysis bullosa [English abstract]. *Hautarzt.* 1989;40:523–526.
85. Pellicano R, Fabrizi G, Cerimele D. Multiple keratoacanthomas and junctional epidermolysis bullosa. *Arch Dermatol.* 1990;126:305–306.
86. Schofield OMV, Eady RAJ. Generalized atrophic benign epidermolysis bullosa. In: Priestley GC, Tidman MJ, Weiss JB, Eady RAJ, eds. *Epidermolysis Bullosa: A Comprehensive Review of Classification, Management and Laboratory Studies.*

Crowthorne, England: Dystrophic Epidermolysis Bullosa Research Association; 1990:97–102.

87. Judge M, Phillips R, Blake B, Harper JI. Junctional epidermolysis bullosa in two brothers: survival and intrafamilial variation. *Br J Dermatol.* 1991;125 (suppl 38):43–44.

87a. Yamada Y, Dekio S, Jidoi J, Ishimoto T, Yoshioka T. Epidermolysis bullosa atrophicans generalisata mitis: report of a case with renal dysfunction. *J. Dermatol.* 1990;17:690–695.

87b. Mikio I, Mamoru K, Hiroshi H, Yoichiro S. Junctional epidermolysis bullosa with urethral stricture. *Dermatologica.* 1987;175;244–248.

88. Gedde-Dahl Jr T, Anton-Lamprecht I. Epidermolysis bullosa. In: Emery AEH, Rimion DL, eds. *Principles and Practice of Medical Genetics.* Edinburgh: Churchill-Livingstone; 1983:672–687.

89. Kero M. Epidermolysis bullosa in Finland: clinical features, morphology and relation to collagen metabolism. *Acta Derm. Venereol (Stockh).* 1984; suppl 110:1–51.

90. Kero M, Palotie A, Peltonen L. Collagen metabolism in two rare forms of epidermolysis bullosa. *Br J Dermatol.* 1984;110:177–184.

91. Kero M. Occurence of epidermolysis bullosa in Finland. *Acta Derm Venereol (Stockh).* 1984;64:57–62.

92. Tidman MJ, Eady RAJ, Marsden RA. Non-lethal junctional epidermolysis bullosa. *Br J Dermatol.* 1985;113(suppl 29):83.

93. Haegerty AHM, Tidman MJ, Bor S, Eady EAJ. Non-lethal junctional epidermolysis bullosa in two adult sisters. *J R Soc Med.* 1985;78(suppl. 11):32–33.

94. Eady RAJ, Tidman MJ. Junctional epidermolysis bullosa. In: Wojnarowski F, Briggaman RA, eds. *Management of Blistering Diseases.* New York: Raven Press; 1990:213-223.

95. Goodwin P, Eady RAJ. A case of ?epidermolysis bullosa. *Clin Exp Dermatol.* 1977;2:409–412.

96. Parker SC, Schofield OMV, Black MM, Eady RAJ. Non-lethal junctional epidermolysis bullosa complicated by squamous cell carcinoma. In: Priestley GC, Tidman MJ, Weiss JB, Eady RAJ, eds. *Epidermolysis Bullosa: A Comprehensive Review of Classification, Management and Laboratory Studies.* Crowthorne, England: Dystrophic Epidermolysis Bullosa Research Association; 1990: 103–106.

97. Monk BE, Pembrook AC. Epidermolysis bullosa with squamous cell carcinoma. *Clin Exp Dermatol.* 1987;12:373–374.

98. Parker SC, Eady RAJ, Black MM. Junctional epidermolysis bullosa and squamous cell carcinoma. *Br J Dermatol.* 1988;119(suppl 33):107–108.

99. Lichtenwald DJ, Hann W, Sauder DN, Jakubovic HR, Rosenthal D. Pretibial epidermolysis bullosa: report of a case. *J Am Acad Dermatol.* 1990;22:346–350.

100. Gedde-Dahl Jr T. *Epidermolysis Bullosa: A Clinical, Genetic and Epidemiological Study.* Baltimore: The Johns Hopkins Press; 1971, 119.

101. Gedde-Dahl Jr T. The epidermolysis bullosa progressiva-hypoacusis (EBR3-HOAC) linkage. *Cytogenet Cell Genet.* 1984;37:474.

102. Haber RM, Hanna W. Epidermolysis bullosa progressiva. *J Am Acad Dermatol.* 1987;16:195–200.

103. Ridley CM. Epidermolysis bullosa with unusual features: inverse type. *Proc R Soc Med.* 1977;70:576–577.

104. Pearson RW, Paller AS. Dermolytic (dystrophic) epidermolysis bullosa inversa. *Arch. Dermatol.* 1988;124:544–547.
105. Haber RM, Hanna W, Ramsay CA, Boxall L. Cicatricial junctional epidermolysis bullosa. *J Am Acad Dermatol.* 1985;12:836–844.
106. Tabas M, Gibbons S, Bauer EA. The mechanobullous Diseases. *Dermatol Clin.* 1987;5:123–136.
107. Nakar S, Ingber A, Kremer I, Hodak E, Garty B-Z, Ben-David E, David M, Shohat M. Late onset localized junctional epidermolysis bullosa and mental retardation: a distinct autosomal recessive syndrome. *Am J Med Genet.* (in press).

9
Recessive Dystrophic Epidermolysis Bullosa: A Clinical Overview

ROBERT A. BRIGGAMAN

Recessive dystrophic epidermolysis bullosa (EB) is defined as a mechanobullous disease with dermolytic separation (i.e., separation at the basement membrane zone deep to the lamina densa) and recessive inheritance. Ultimately, the diagnosis depends on confirmation of the level of separation by ultrastructural examination (Fig. 9.1), antigen mapping, or preferably both.[1-6] This disorder has also been called dermolytic EB to emphasize the importance of the level of separation on the dermal side of the lamina densa.[3] Dystrophic scarring is a distinctive feature in these patients and serves as a useful clinical marker. It must be remembered, however, that dystrophic scarring may be seen in some of the other types of EB, particularly in junctional EB in areas of healed granulation tissue and in some special subvariants of that disease.[7] All forms of dystrophic EB follow simple mendelian inheritance patterns being either autosomal dominant or autosomal recessive. It is traditional to classify dystrophic EB into recessive and dominant types. A clear-cut inheritance pattern can be recognized in many families by the presence of multiple affected siblings in a family with normal parents. History of consanguinity further supports recessive inheritance. However, sporadic cases are common, in which case it is often difficult to distinguish between recessive inheritance and spontaneous mutation in a dominantly inherited disease. For example, distinguishing between dominant epidermolysis bullosa dystrophica (EBD) and localized recessive EBD may be particularly difficult.

Among the patients that we designate recessive dystrophic EB based on the features noted above, considerable variability of the clinical phenotype has been noted, particularly regarding severity, extent, and distribution of the disease.[8-15] This has led to a trend to subclassify further recessive dystrophic EB into subtypes as indicated in Table 9.1. It is well to remember that these subtypes represent more quantitative than qualitative alterations and their definition is somewhat arbitrary. Even so, specific subtypes of recessive dystrophic EB tend to breed true. Cases conforming to localized, severe generalized, or the inversa subtypes rarely occur in the same kindred. Based on

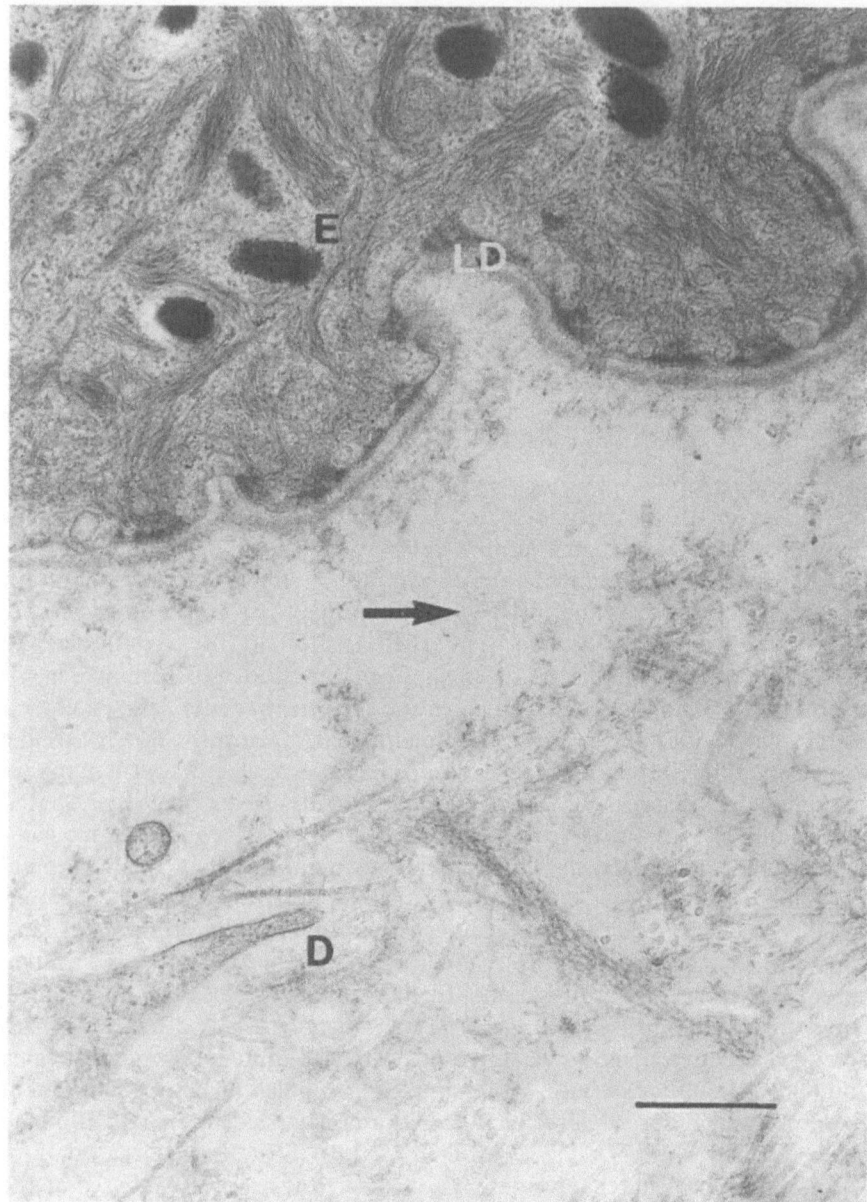

FIGURE 9.1. Recessive dystrophic EB (generalized gravis). Electron micrograph of skin showing separation (*arrow*) between the epidermis (*E*) and dermis (*D*) beneath the lamina densa (*LD*). This level of separation is characteristic of dermolytic EB. (Bar = 0.5 μm.)

TABLE 9.1. Classification of recessive dystrophic EB.

Scarring EB with dermolytic separation and recessive inheritance
(EBD—recessive group)
   EBD recessive (Hallopeau-Siemens).
      Generalized gravis (sublethal, mutilans)
      Generalized mitis type
      Localized type
   EBD inversa

---

clinical and inheritance data, Gedde-Dahl has suggested that these diseases result from mutations at two different gene loci, EBD-HS and EBD-I, corresponding to the generalized and inversa subtypes.[8] Gedde-Dahl has further proposed that localized and generalized recessive dystrophic EB are caused by different mutations at the same gene locus.[9] It is well to point out that uncertainty still exists regarding the relationship of these diseases and that this uncertainty will be settled only by characterization and cloning of the involved genes.

Clinical Features

Skin fragility is a feature in all patients with recessive dystrophic EB and leads to the formation of blisters after even minimal mechanical trauma. The blisters may be either clear fluid–filled or hemorrhagic. Blisters commonly extend laterally with pressure and may become huge. Eventually, the blisters rupture and form superficial ulcerations that are slow to heal (Fig. 9.2). In some skin areas that are subjected to repeated trauma, ulcerations can persist for months and even years. Healing always results in some degree of scarring. Initially, the scars may be relatively superficial, giving the involved skin an atrophic, wrinkled appearance (Fig. 9.3). Repeated cycles of blisters, ulcers, and healing result in the characteristic dystrophic scarring of this disease. The most characteristic dystrophic scarring is usually found at sites of repeated trauma such as on the elbows, knees, hands, and feet (Fig. 9.4). Milia are usually present and may be seen in great numbers in some healed lesions.

Some patients with dystrophic EB have distinctive ulcerations present at birth. This has been termed "congenital localized absence of skin" and may be seen in other forms of EB as well.[12] In recessive dystrophic EB, the skin defect is usually limited in severity and extent and most commonly found on the lower leg and foot, where it may be either unilateral or bilateral (Fig. 9.5).

We will continue our discussion of the clinical features by focusing on the special features of each of the subtypes of dystrophic recessive EB.

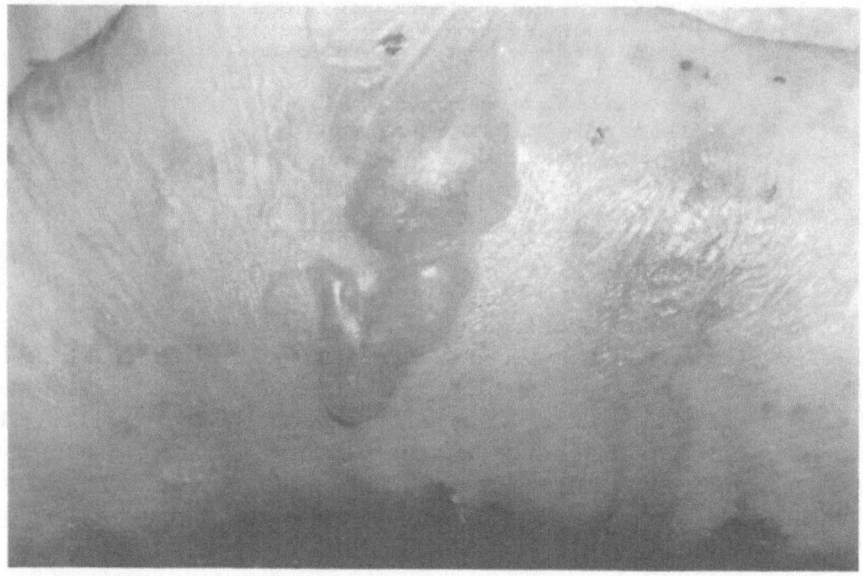

FIGURE 9.2. Recessive dystrophic EB (generalized gravis). Superficial ulcerations are seen in an area of chronically traumatized, scarred skin.

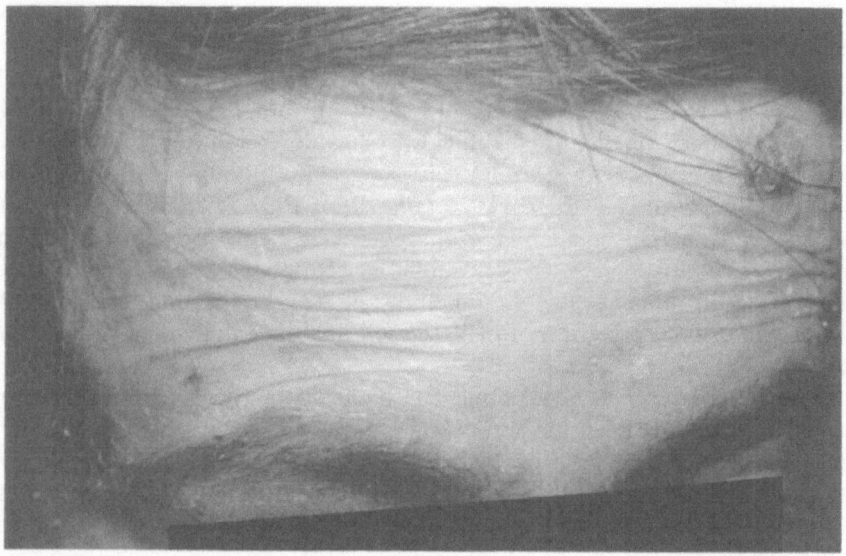

FIGURE 9.3. Recessive dystrophic EB (generalized gravis). Superficial scarring is evident as atrophic wrinkled appearance of the skin in an occasionally involved area on the forehead.

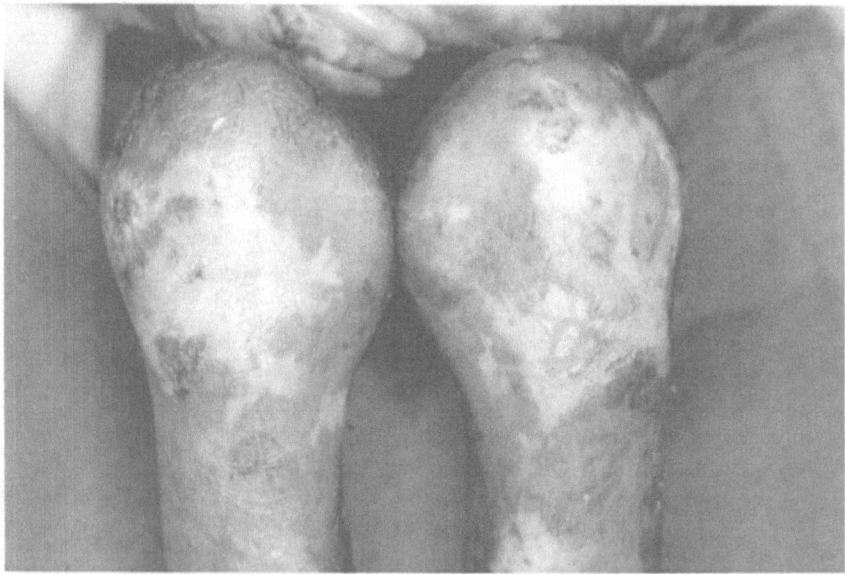

FIGURE 9.4. Recessive dystrophic EB (generalized gravis). Dystrophic scarring is seen at the site of repeated trauma on the patient's knees.

Dystrophic Recessive EB of the Generalized Gravis Subtype

This disorder represents the most severe subtype of dystrophic recessive EB (Hallopeau-Siemens) and has also been designated sublethal or mutilans. Marked skin fragility characterizes this disease, which also involves other stratified squamous epithelia including the oral, esophageal, ocular, and anal mucous membranes. Onset is always in the neonatal period with blisters and ulcerations commonly present at birth. Sites of predilection vary with the age of the patient but correspond to areas of most significant mechanical trauma. In infancy, the medial surface of the legs and the medial surface of the arms, the lateral sides of the abdomen and chest, as well as the knees, elbows, buttocks, and occiput are involved. These sites doubtless represent the sites of friction and rubbing in the day-to-day life of these infants. In early childhood and thereafter, involvement shifts to the knees (Fig. 9.4), elbows, hands, and feet. Other areas may also be the sites of significant involvement, including nape of the neck (Fig. 9.6), shoulder, buttocks, and back, particularly over the spine. Pruritus is a variable feature in this disease and may be a significant problem in some patients leading to worsening of the clinical features because of excessive scratching. The scalp is commonly involved; scarring and eventual cicatricial alopecia may result (Fig. 9.7). The toe nails and finger nails are usually lost early and are replaced by scarred nail beds.

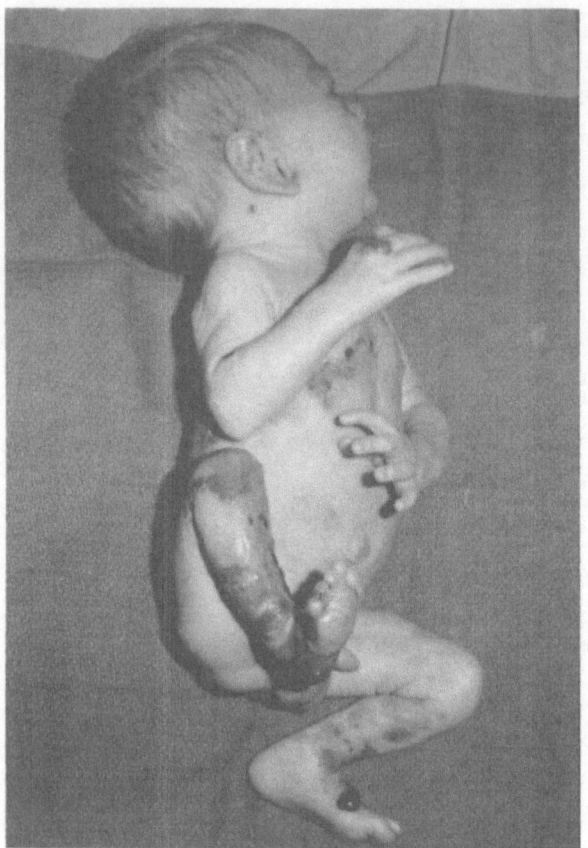

FIGURE 9.5. Recessive dystrophic EB (generalized gravis). This infant exhibits an area of congenital skin defect on the lower leg, ankle, and foot. In addition, blisters and superficial erosions are seen on the medial chest wall and on the medial aspects of the legs and foot, common sites of involvement during infancy.

Over a period of time, continued dystrophic scarring of the hands and feet leads to deformity and functional impairment. Progressive hand involvement is shown in the same patient over a period of years in Fig. 9.8. Syndactyly occurs between adjacent fingers, followed by encasement of the fingers and thumb in a mittenlike enclosure that is a distinctive feature in many patients with this disease. With time, advanced hand deformities result and cause major functional hand impairment. Similar changes may be seen on the feet.

Mucosal involvement is a constant feature in these patients. Oral blisters and erosions are present from the onset of the disease and may be severe. With time and continued involvement, scarring results. Loss of papillae on the tongue and ankyloglossia are commonly seen. Microstomia is also a

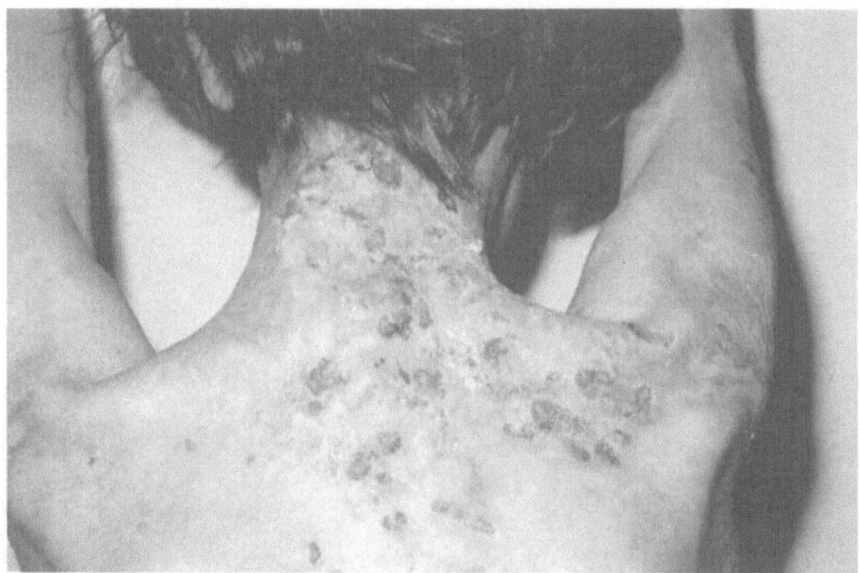

FIGURE 9.6. Recessive dystrophic EB (generalized gravis). Extensive blisters and superficial erosions are present over the neck, upper back, and shoulders.

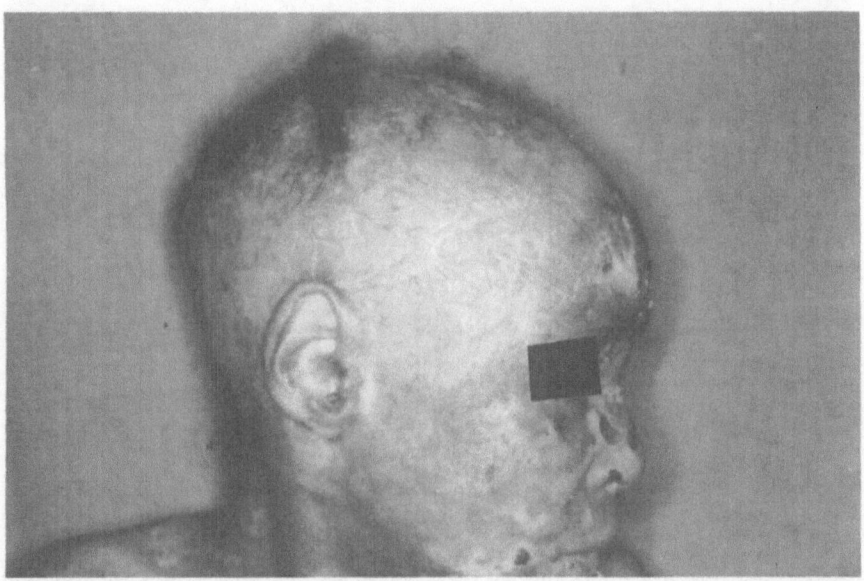

FIGURE 9.7. Recessive dystrophic EB (generalized gravis). Cicatricial alopecia is present in this patient as a result of repeated blistering and superficial ulceration. This patient experienced severe pruritus of her skin, particularly over the scalp and face, which significantly accentuated involvement in these area.

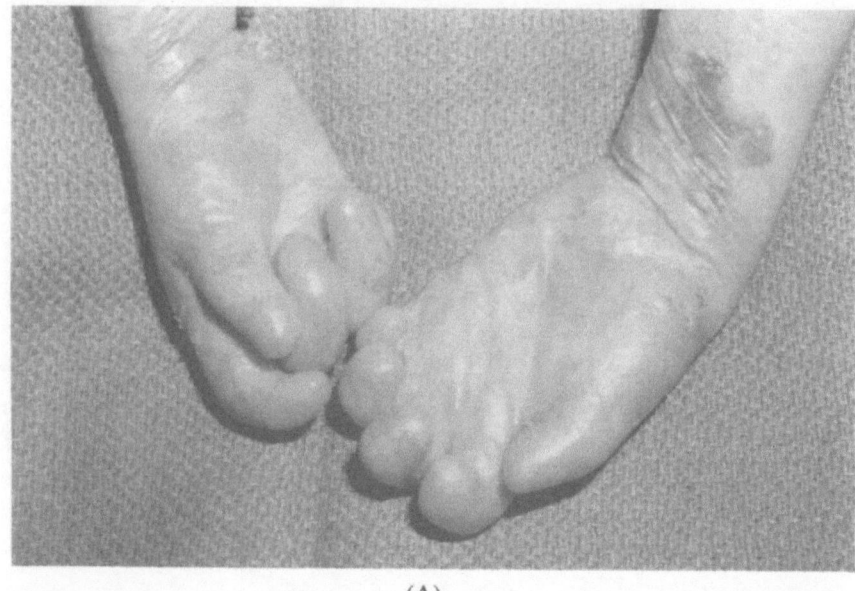

(A)

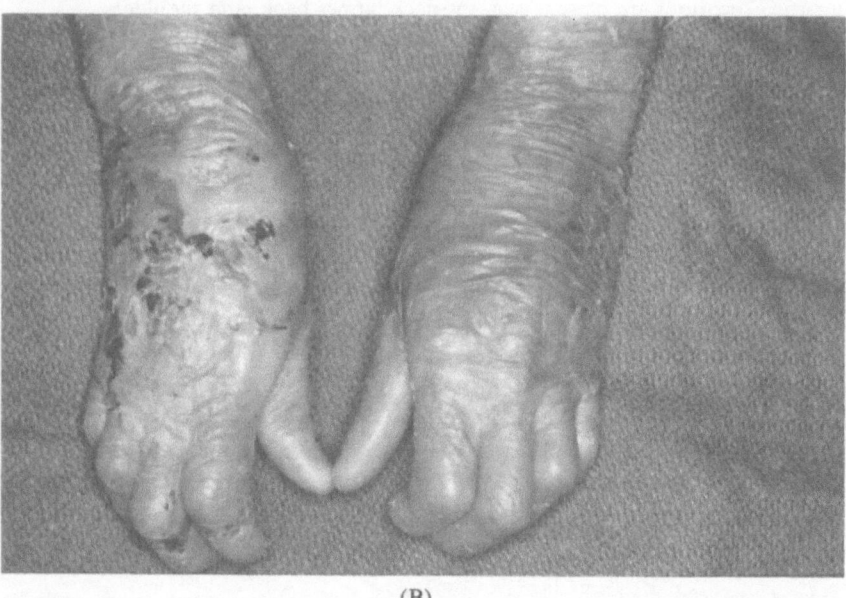

(B)

FIGURE 9.8. Recessive dystrophic EB (generalized gravis). This series of photographs taken over a period of time in the same patient demonstrates the progressive development of severe incapacitating hand defects. **A:** At 4 years old, early scarring of the fingers and palms with nail loss is present. **B:** Progressive changes with increased scarring and early syndactyly at age 16. **C:** At age 21 years, significant syndactyly and mittenlike encasement of the hand enclosing the thumb and fingers in a mittenlike epithelial enclosure is evident.

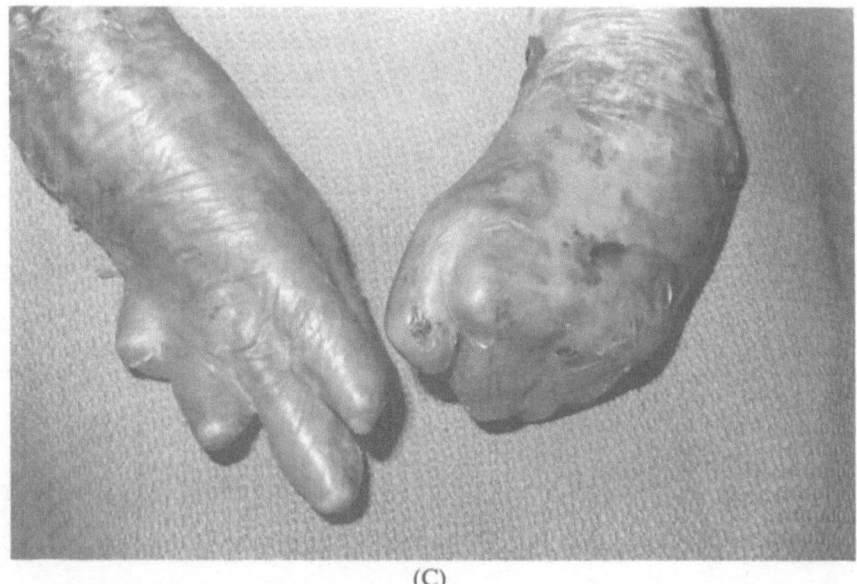

(C)

feature. The gums are fragile and erosions are common, giving a picture of marginal gingivitis. The tooth surface may appear normal initially and lacks the distinctive cobblestone or pitted appearance of the enamel defect in junctional EB.[16-18] However, cavities appear, particularly at the marginal areas where the dentine is exposed, and may result in extensive caries and ultimately tooth destruction (Fig. 9.9).

Ocular involvement is relatively common, predominantly involving the lids and conjunctivae. Blisters and erosions of the lids may lead to scarring and, if severe, to ectropion.[19] Sometimes tear ducts may be occluded by the scarring process and result in excessive tearing. The lashes may also be lost. Corneal erosions and scarring are uncommon but occasionally produce decreased visual acuity.

Gastrointestinal mucous membranes are frequently the site of impairment. Esophageal involvement is a constant feature in this severe generalized type and is a major source of disability.[20-26] Onset may occur early within the first year or so, although symptomatic involvement usually occurs later. The entire esophagus may be involved, although the upper third is the most commonly affected. Initially epithelial separation produces ulceration and later scarring. Occasionally pieces of epithelium may be regurgitated and rarely an entire cast of the esophageal mucous membrane may be produced. Subsequent scarring results in esophageal stenosis, which commonly worsens with time and may progress to complete esophageal obstruction. Usually, the course is punctuated by episodes of partial obstruction that resolve after a week or so, probably associated with acute separation of an area of esopha-

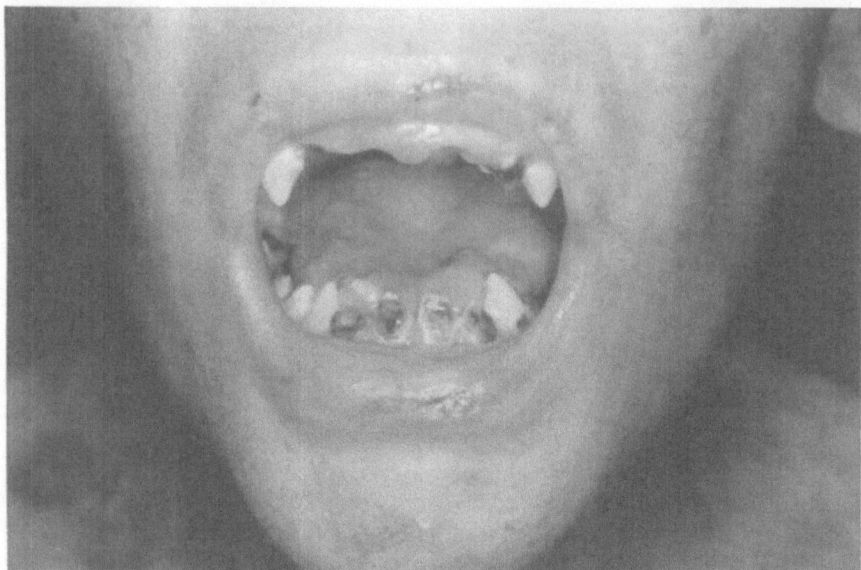

FIGURE 9.9. Recessive dystrophic EB (generalized gravis). The teeth show extensive caries and tooth destruction. Loss of papillae is evident on the tongue.

geal mucosa, followed by healing. Esophageal webs[25,26] and acquired double-barrel esophageal defects[24] have been reported in these patients.

Growth retardation is seen in nearly all of the patients with the severe generalized subtype. These patients are nearly always of small stature and below normal in weight. Anemia is a common systemic complication and probably multifactorial in origin. Hypoalbuminemia is also seen. Nephrotic syndrome caused by secondary amyloidosis and post-infectious glomerulonephritis presumably secondary to chronic skin infection caused by nephritogenic strains of Streptococcus pyogenes have been reported.[26a]

Squamous cell carcinomas may develop in any of the dystrophic forms of EB.[27-33] The tumors are most frequent in the more severe recessive forms where the more severely scarred areas of skin are the predominant sites of involvement (Fig. 9.10). Squamous cell carcinomas have also been reported in mucosal sites including the mouth and esophagus. Several features of these tumors are particularly noteworthy. They occur at an earlier age than most squamous cell carcinomas. The frequency is greatest in the third to fifth decades of life. This is similar to the duration from injury to carcinoma development seen in other scar carcinomas such as thermal burns. Another feature of these tumors is the high frequency of multiple primary tumors being in the order of 75%.[32] Another particularly ominous feature of these tumors is their aggressive biologic behavior. They tend to recur frequently and to metastasize. Death has resulted in a high proportion of these cases

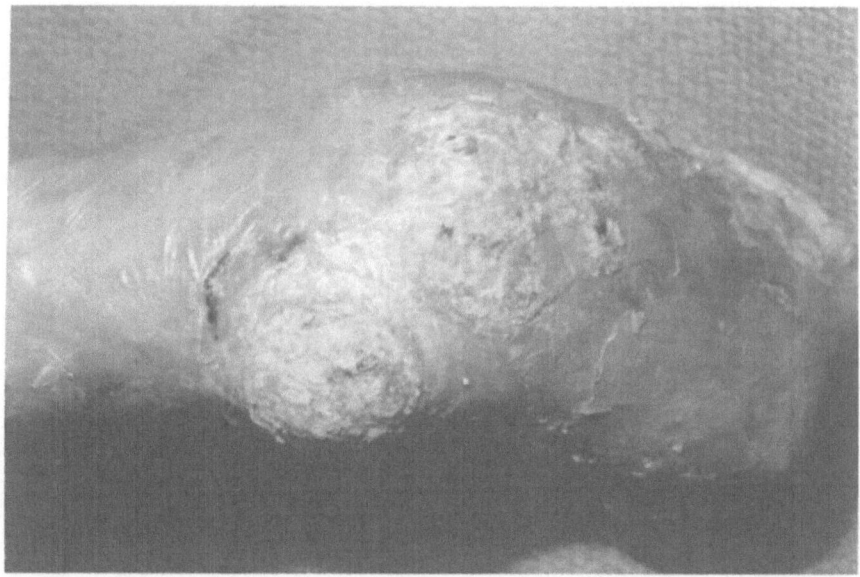

FIGURE 9.10. Recessive dystrophic EB (generalized gravis). This squamous cell carcinoma present on the wrist in an area of chronic scarring later metastasized to the regional lymph nodes in the axilla, spread locally to the lateral chest wall and ultimately metastasized to the lung. Two other primary squamous cell carcinomas had previously been present on the other hand and elbow.

from widespread metastasis of the tumor. We have seen several recent cases, both with aggressive and debilitating regional metastasis as well as distant metastasis to the lung and other organs. This aggressive biologic behavior occurs without regard for the histopathologic type of the tumor, which varies from well differentiated in most of the cases to poorly differentiated or spindle-cell types. Our own recent experience suggests that squamous cell carcinoma is a major cause of death in patients with more severe forms of recessive dystrophic EB.

Recessive Dystrophic EB of the Generalized Mitis Subtype

This disorder represents a continuum with the previously discussed gravis subtype. The distinction between the two is somewhat arbitrary. Nevertheless, it is useful to distinguish a group of recessive dystrophic EB patients with more mild involvement.[34-36] Skin fragility is present in these patients but is more difficult to demonstrate objectively by experimentally inducing skin separation. The overall pattern of lesions and scarring is similar to that seen

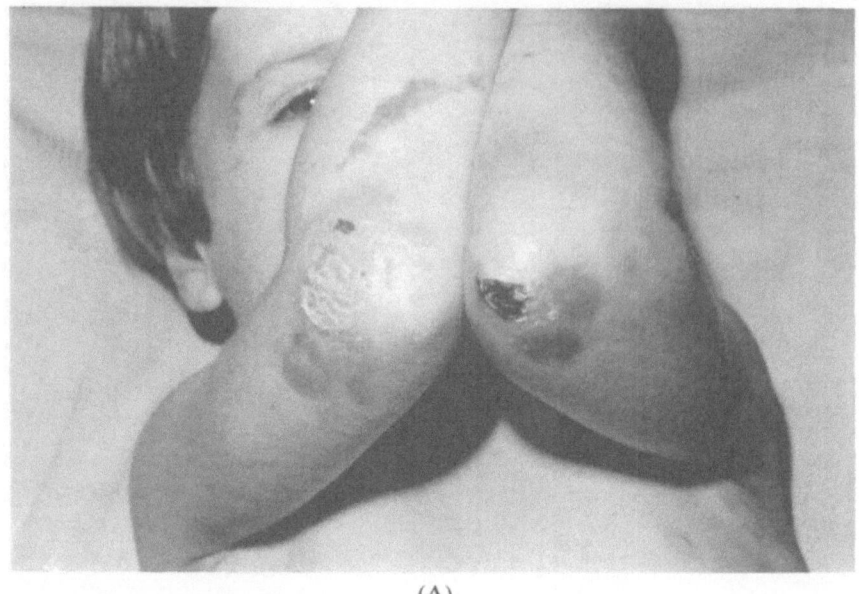

(A)

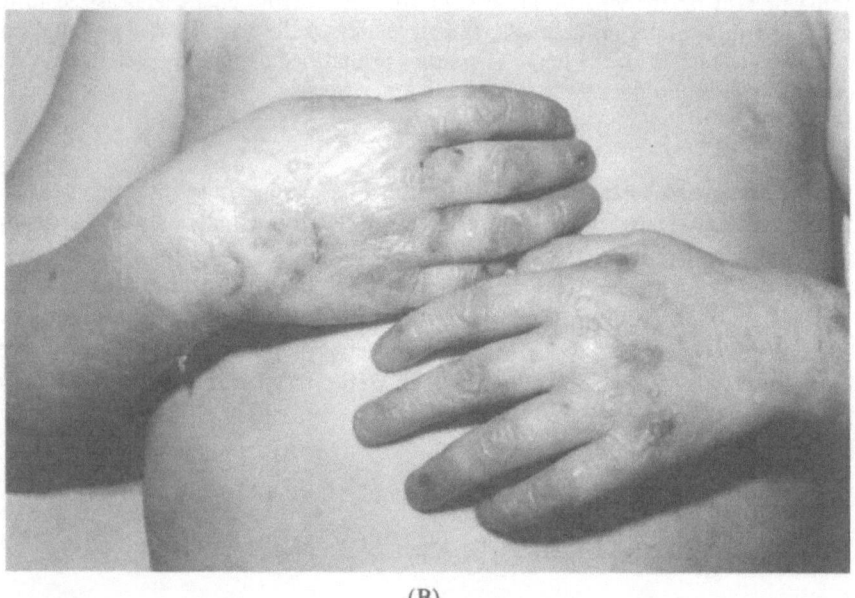

(B)

FIGURE 9.11. Recessive dystrophic EB (generalized mitis). This series of pictures demonstrates cutaneous abnormalities seen in a patient with this disease. Dystrophic scarring is present about the elbows (**A**, top), hands (**B**), knees (**C**, top, facing page), and feet (**D**). The nails are absent. In addition, the patient had mild oral blistering and ulceration.

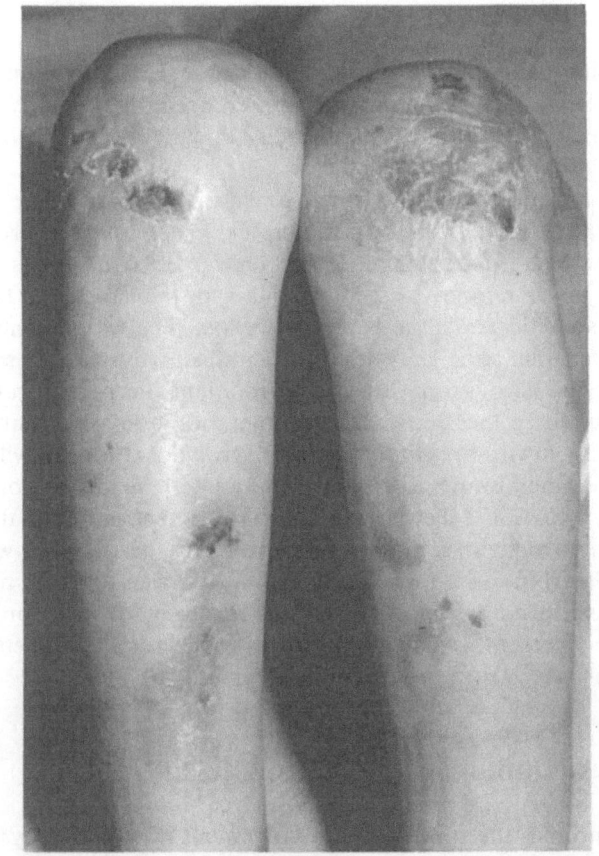

(C)

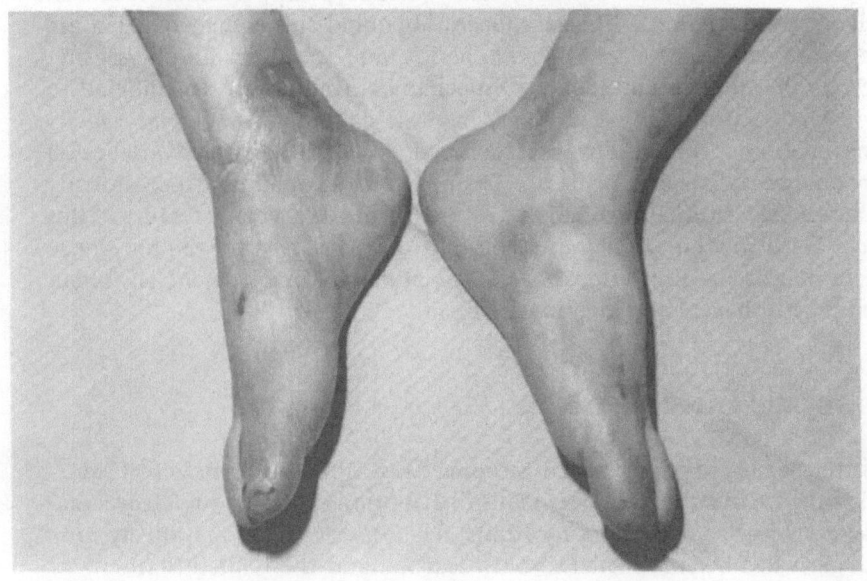

(D)

in other dystrophic EB subtypes. The entire skin surface may be involved. Phenotypically, these patients resemble the generalized dominant dystrophic EB. Features of a patient with the generalized mitis subtype are shown in Fig. 9.11.

The disease is usually present at birth or soon thereafter. The sites of predilection are the knees, elbows, hands, and feet. These patients are spared the mutilating hand and foot deformities that characterize the gravis variant. Some degree of syndactyly may be seen. The nails of the hands and feet may be dystrophic or sometimes nails are completely lost. The scalp is usually not involved. Repeated blistering may lead to significant dystrophic scarring, particularly over the elbows and knees and indolent ulcers may take long periods to heal in these locations. Mucous membrane involvement is also much less than is seen with the gravis variants. Oral ulcerations may be seen. Scarring of mucous membranes is usually minimal with an absence of microstomia and ankyloglossia. Likewise, dental involvement is minimal. Other extracutaneous involvement is also significantly less than is seen with the gravis variety. Gastrointestinal involvement may be seen in some patients; however, the severe esophageal stenosis and resultant obstruction of the esophagus is rarely present. In addition, growth retardation and anemia that characterize the gravis variety are usually absent.

Recessive Dystrophic EB of the Localized Subtype

This disorder continues the spectrum of involvement in recessive dystrophic EB. These patients can be included with the mitis subtype described above or distinguished as a separate category. They phenotypically resemble localized dominant dystrophic EB. Blisters, ulcerations, and subsequent scarring are largely confined to the elbows, knees, hands, and feet. Skin fragility is suggested by the localization at sites of mechanical trauma yet it is difficult to demonstrate skin fragility objectively in these patients. The disease usually begins in infancy but is always much milder than the other varieties of dystrophic recessive EB. Nails are frequently dystrophic and occasionally lost completely. Mutilating hand and foot deformities are not a feature of this disease. Occasional oral mucous membrane erosions may be seen but severe scarring is absent. Likewise, other extracutaneous involvement is absent, including esophageal and anal involvement.

Dystrophic EB–Inversa

The inversa subtype of recessive dystrophic EB was first recognized by Gedde-Dahl[8] because of its unique cutaneous distribution centering on flexural and trunk areas rather than acral locations. This disease is comparatively rare, although it has been reported in both Europe and the United States.[37-41]

Onset is in infancy with generalized skin involvement similar to other types of recessive dystrophic EB. Blisters, ulcers, and, subsequently, superficial scarring are noted in these patients during the first years of life. Later the generalized involvement considerably lessens but severe involvement persists and actually progresses in flexural and truncal locations. This disease concentrates on the inguinal folds, perineum, axillae, inframammary area, and a beltlike area involving the lower abdomen and buttocks as well as the upper thighs. These patients are spared severe acral scarring and deformity. The nails are affected but less than in the Hallopeau-Seimans type. Initially, milia were said to be absent in this disease, but have been present in several recently reported cases.[40,41]

Severe oral and esophageal involvement has been a constant feature of this disease. Ankyloglossia and microstomia are usually present, however, the teeth are usually spared the severe dental abnormality seen in the generalized gravis Hallopeau-Siemans subtype. Esophageal stenosis is often severe and may be a major source of disability. Frequent traumatic corneal erosions were reported in the initial cases but appear to be a variable expression of this disease, present in some patients and absent in others. Patients with the inversa subtype usually are of normal stature and usually lack hematologic abnormalities.

References

1. Pearson RW. Studies on the pathogenesis of epidermolysis bullosa. *J Invest Dermatol.* 1962;39:551–575.
2. Eady RA, Tidman MJ. Diagnosing epidermolysis bullosa. *Br J Dermatol.* 1983;108:621–626.
3. Pearson RW. The mechanobullous diseases (epidermolysis bullosa). In: Fitzpatrick TB, Arndt KA, Clark W, eds. *Dermatology in General Medicine.* New York: McGraw-Hill; 1971:621–643.
4. Fine JD, Hintner H, Katz SI. Immunofluorescence studies in epidermolysis bullosa utilizing polyclonal and monoclonal antibodies. In: Beutner EH, Chorzelski TP, Kumar V, eds. *Immunopathology of the Skin.* New York: John Wiley & Sons; 1987:399–405.
5. Hintner H, Stingl G, Schuler G, et al. Immunofluorescence mapping of antigenic determinants within the dermal-epidermal junction in mechanobullous diseases. *J Invest Dermatol.* 1981;76:113–118.
6. Kero M, Peltonen L, Foidart JM, et al. Immunohistological localization of three basement membrane components in various forms of epidermolysis bullosa. *J Cutan Pathol.* 1982;9:316–328.
7. Haber RM, Hanna W, Ramsay CA, et al. Cicatricial junctional epidermolysis bullosa. *J AM Acad Dermatol.* 1985;12:836–844.
8. Gedde-Dahl T Jr. *Epidermolysis Bullosa: A Clinical, Genetic and Epidemiological Study.* Baltimore: The Johns Hopkins University Press, 1971.
9. Gedde-Dahl T, Anton-Lamprecht I. Epidermolysis bullosa. In: Emery AEH, Rimoin DL, eds. *Principles and Practice of Medical Genetics.* Edinburgh, London, Melbourne, New York: Churchill Livingstone, 1983:672–687.

10. Gedde-Dahl T. Sixteen types of epidermolysis bullosa: on their clinical discrimination, therapy and prenatal diagnosis. *Acta Dermatovenereol (Stockh).* 1981; (suppl) 95:74–87.

11. Cooper TW, Bauer EA, Briggaman RA. The mechanobullous diseases (epidermolysis bullosa). In: Fitzpatrick TB, Eisen AZ, Wolf KW, et al., eds. *Dermatology in General Medicine.* New York: McGraw-Hill, 1987:610–626.

12. Briggaman RA. Hereditary epidermolysis bullosa with special emphasis on newly recognized syndromes and complications. *Dermatol Clin.* 1983;1:263–280.

13. Fine JD. Epidermolysis bullosa: clinical aspects, pathology, and recent advances in research. *Int J Dermatol.* 1986;25:143–157.

14. Tabas M, Gibbons S, Bauer EA. The mechanobullous diseases. *Dermatol Clin.* 1987;5:123–136.

15. Gedde-Dahl T Jr. Classification of epidermolysis bullosa. In: Herzbert JJ, ed. *Padiatrische Dermatologie.* Stuttgart: FK Shattauer-Verlag; 1978:65–91.

16. Crawford EG Jr, Burkes J, Briggaman R. Hereditary epidermolysis bullosa: oral manifestations and dental therapy. *Oral Surg.* 1976;42:490–500.

17. Gorlin RJ. Epidermolysis bullosa. *Oral Surg.* 1971;32:760–766.

18. Hitchin AD. The defects in cementum in epidermolysis bullosa dystrophica. *Br Dent J.* 1973;135:437–442.

19. Hill JC, Rodrique D. Cicatricial ectropion in epidermolysis bullosa and in congenital ichthyosis: its plastic repair. *Can J Ophthalmol.* 1971;6:89–97.

20. Nix TE Jr, Christianson HB. Epidermolysis bullosa of the esophagus; report of two cases and review of literature. *South Med J.* 1965;58:612–620.

21. Bergenholtz A, Olsson 0, Arwill T. Epidermolysis bullosa hereditaria: II. Esophageal changes in epidermolysis bullosa hereditaria dystrophica. *Pract Otorhinolaryngol.* 1965;27:219–224.

22. Berkmen Y. Esophageal involvement in epidermolysis bullosa. *Am J Gastroenterol.* 1974;62:145–147.

23. Orlando RC, Bozymski EM, Briggaman RA, et al. Epidermolysis bullosa: gastrointestinal manifestations. *Ann Intern Med.* 1974;81:203–206.

24. Warren RB, Warner TF, Gilbert EF, et al. Acquired double-barrel oesophagus in epidermolysis bullosa dystrophica. *Thorax.* 1980;35:472–476.

25. Hillemeir C, Touloukian R, McCallum R, et al. Esophageal web: a previously unrecognized complication of epidermolysis bullosa. *Pediatrics.* 1981;67:678–682.

26. Marsden R, Sambrook Gowar F, MacDonald A, et al. Epidermolysis bullosa of the esophagus with esophageal web formation. *Thorax* 1974;29:287–295.

26a. Mann JFE, Zeier M, Zilow E, et al. The spectrum of renal involvement in epidermolysis bullosa dystrophica hereditaria: report of two cases. *Am J Kidney Disease.* 1988;11:437–441.

27. Reed WB, College J, Francis MJO, et al. Epidermolysis bullosa dystrophica with epidermal neoplasms. *Arch Dermatol.* 1974;110:894–902.

28. Reed W, Roenigk H, Dorner W, et al. Epidermal neoplasms with epidermolysis bullosa dystrophica with the first report of carcinoma with the acquired type. *Arch Dermatol Res.* 1975;253:1–14.

29. Didolkar M, Gerner R, Moore G. Epidermolysis bullosa dystrophica and epithelioma of the skin. *Cancer.* 1974;33:198–202.

30. Wetteland P, Houding G. Squamous cell carcinoma in epidermolysis bullosa. *Acta Dermatovenereol (Stockh).* 1956;36:27–36.

31. Edland RW. Dystrophic epidermolysis bullosa. Tolerance of the bed and response of multifocal squamous cell carcinomas to ionizing radiation: report of a case. *Am J Roentgenol.* 1969;105:644–647.

32. Goldberg GI, Eisen AZ, Bauer EA Tissue stress and tumor promotion. *Arch Dermatol.* 1988;124:737–741.

33. Smoller BA, McNutt S, Carter DM, et al. Recessive dystrophic epidermolysis bullosa skin displays a chronic growth-activated immunophenotype. *Arch Dermatol.* 1990;126:78–83.

34. Tidman MJ, Eady RAJ. Evaluation of anchoring fibrils and other components of the dermal-epidermal junction in dystrophic epidermolysis bullosa by a quantitative ultrastructural technique. *J Invest Dermatol.* 1985;84:374–377.

35. Ramelet AA, Boillat C. Autosomal recessive albopapuloid dystrophic epidermolysis bullosa. *Dermatologica.* 1986;171:397–406.

36. Smith EB, Michener WM. Vitamin E in the treatment of dermolytic bullous dermatosis: a controlled study. *Arch Dermatol.* 1973;108:254–256.

37. Hashimoto I, Anton-Lamprecht I, Hofbauer M. Epidermolysis bullosa dystrophica inversa: report on two sisters. *Hautarzt.* 1976;27:532–537.

38. Hashimoto I, Schnyder UW, Anton-Lamprecht I, et al. Ultrastructural studies in epidermolysis bullosa hereditaria III. Recessive dystrophic types with dermolytic blistering (Hallopeau-Siemens types and inverse type). *Arch Dermatol Res.* 1976;256:137–150.

39. Stevanovic D, Lalevic B, Jovovic D, et al. The inverse type of polydysplastic epidermolysis bullosa (Gedde-Dahl). *Ann Dermatol Venereol.* 1979;106:65–67.

40. Pearson R, Paller A. Dermolytic (dystrophic) epidermolysis bullosa inversa. *Arch Dermatol.* 1988;124:544–547.

41. Bruckner-Tuderman L, Niem K-M, Kero M, et al. Type VII collagen is expressed but anchoring fibrils are defective in dystrophic epidermolysis bullosa inversa. *Br J Dermatol.* 1990;122:383–390.

10
Dominant Dystrophic Epidermolysis Bullosa: A Clinical Overview

ANDREW N. LIN and D. MARTIN CARTER

Dominant dystrophic epidermolysis bullosa (DDEB) is characterized by formation of blisters below the lamina densa and by autosomal dominant inheritance. Patients often present with trauma-induced blisters at birth or shortly thereafter. In contrast to epidermolysis bullosa simplex (EBS), blisters heal with scarring (Fig. 10.1), but the severe mittenlike scars of the hands and feet so characteristic of recessive dystrophic EB do not occur in DDEB. Nails are often dystrophic (Fig. 10.2). Extracutaneous involvement is usually mild and is often limited to the mouth.

Electron microscopic examination of a blister will show that separation occurs below the lamina densa (Fig. 10.3). Using a quantitative ultrastructural technique, investigators showed that structurally normal anchoring fibrils were significantly reduced in number in DDEB and localized recessive dystrophic EB, when compared with site-matched samples from healthy adults.[1] In contrast, anchoring fibrils were not detected at all in samples from patients with severe generalized recessive dystrophic EB.[1] In DDEB, structural abnormalities of anchoring fibrils have also been noted.[2,3]

Based primarily on clinical features, four types of DDEB are recognized (Table 10.1). The literature contains many cases reported as DDEB with no particular subtype specified.[4-14] Among these, four patients had squamous cell carcinoma,[8,10,12] highlighting the observation that DDEB is similar to recessive dystrophic EB in predisposing patients to squamous cell carcinoma at sites of blisters and scarring. Another patient presented with the unusual finding of an esophageal web.[13,14] Esophageal strictures were described in two siblings whose clinical presentation "fits with the dystrophic form of epidermolysis bullosa, transmitted by an autosomal dominant gene"[15]; however, it is unclear on what basis the condition was believed to be transmitted as an autosomal trait in that kindred, and how the possibility of autosomal recessive transmission was ruled out. One report described the occurrence of two different types of DDEB (Pasini and Cockayne-Touraine types) in the same kindred,[16] highlighting the difficulty in precise classification, and calling into question the validity of differentiating these subtypes. Congenital localized absence of the skin resembling Bart's syndrome was observed in one

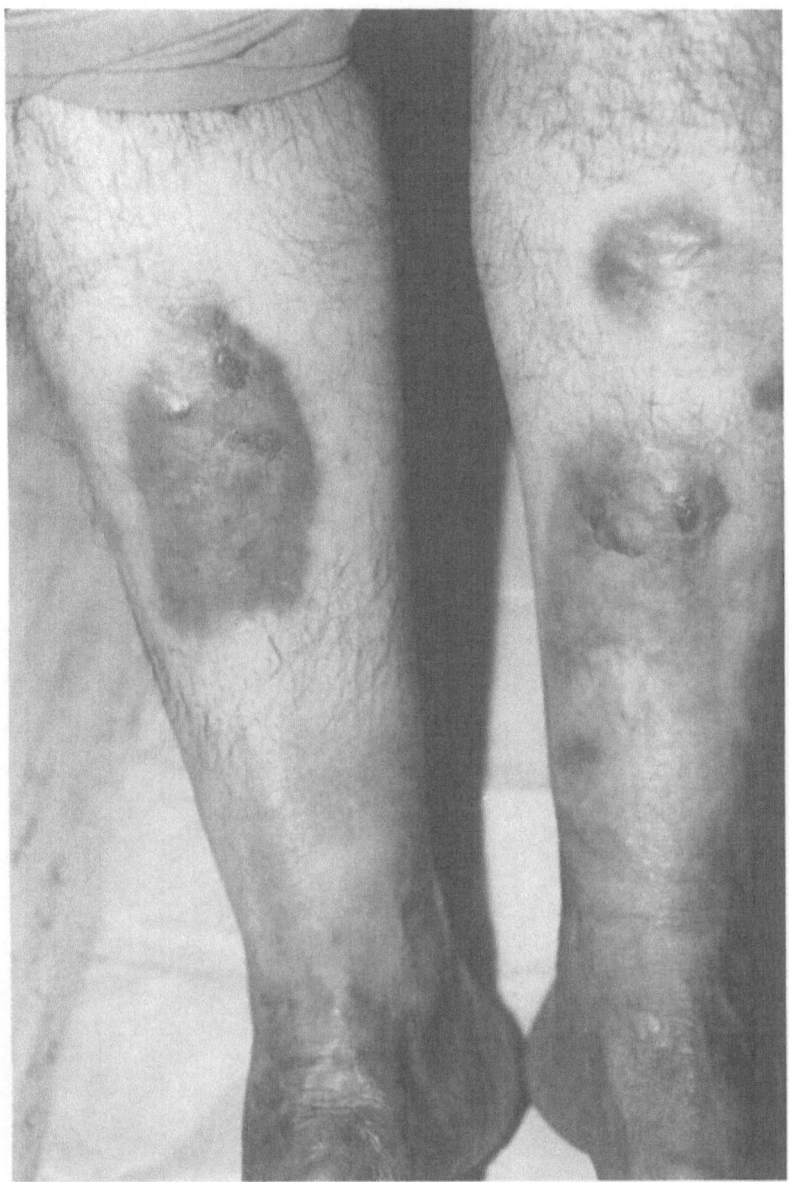

FIGURE 10.1. Lesions in dominant dystrophic EB heal with scarring.

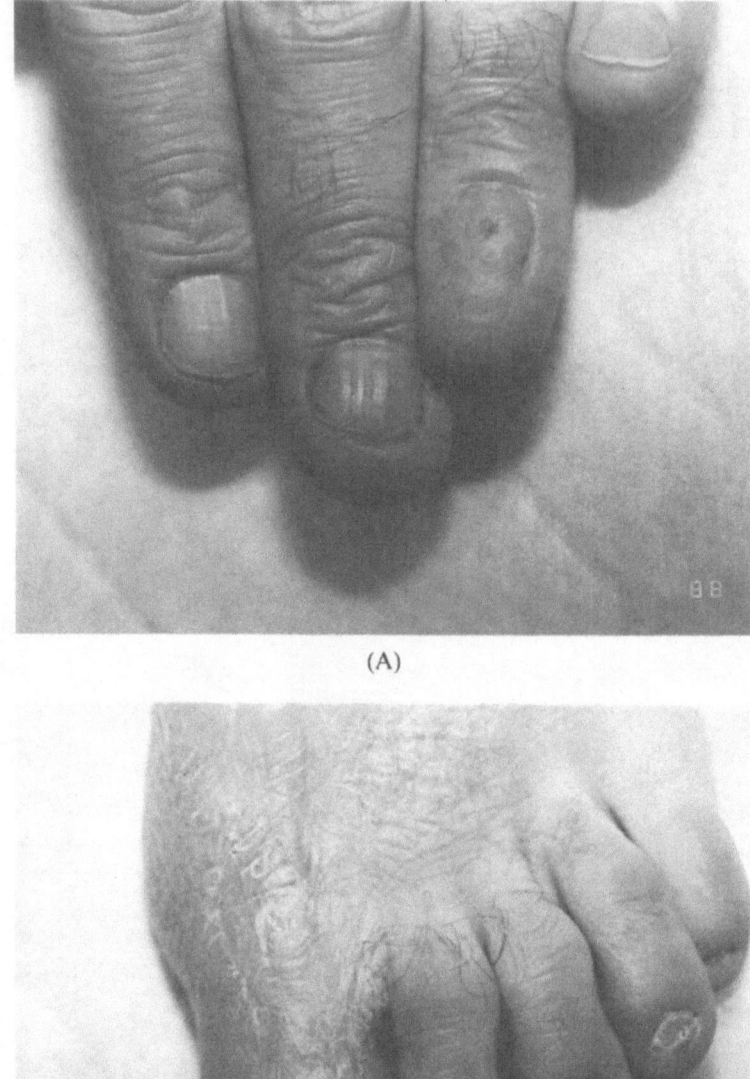

(A)

(B)

FIGURE 10.2. Dominant dystrophic EB: dystrophy of the finger nails (**A**) and toe nails (**B**).

family with DDEB.[17] In one kindred with dominant dystrophic EB of unspecified subtype, there was strong evidence for genetic linkage of the EB phenotype to a collagenous gene locus that was tentatively identifed as type VII collagen gene.[18]

Albopapuloid Dominant Dystrophic EB of Pasini

In 1928 Pasini described two patients with a blistering disorder characterized by numerous white papules that he called "albo-papuloid" lesions.[19] Since then albopapuloid lesions have been considered the hallmark of the "Pasini" type of dominant dystrophic EB. However, despite the importance of albopapuloid lesions as a diagnostic marker, the exact histologic and clinical nature of these lesions has yet to be fully clarified.

Albopapuloid lesions can best be defined as ivory-white papules that characterize at least a subset of patients with dominant dystrophic EB (Fig. 10.4). They most commonly occur on the trunk,[20-23] especially the lumbosacral area,[24,25] but have also be seen on the upper limbs,[20,22] fingers,[25] toes,[25] and neck.[25] They are usually small and multiple, but sometimes coalesce to form plaques up to 3 cm in size.[23,25] Some patients cannot remember how long they have had these lesions,[20] but onset during chlldhood[22] and even infancy[25] has been documented. They have been noted to occur spontaneously without relation to previous blistering,[20,22] but similarity to scars has been noted.[21] Occurrence in a linear arrangement as in Köbnerization has also been seen.[26] Histologic examination of albopapuloid lesions has yielded various findings,[20-22,24-26] including flattening of the epidermis, changes in dermal collagen and elastin, and presence of milia (Table 10.2). Although albopapuloid lesions are cited as a useful diagnostic marker of the Pasini type of DDEB, it is unclear how specific they are. Such lesions have been described in three patients (from two different kindreds) with recessive dystrophic EB[27,28] and in patients with the pretibial form of DDEB.[29,30] Lesions clinically indistinguishable from albopapuloid lesions have also been reported in one patient with the generalized Köbner form of EB simplex.[31] One patient with "slightly elevated, pale-white elements with a pronounced follicular pattern" was reported as "recessive EB et albopapuloidea without nail dystrophy and scarring."[32] In this patient, however, blistering occurred "between the plasma membrane of the basal cells and the basement membrane,"[32] features that together with the presumed recessive inheritance are more consistent with junctional rather than dominant dystrophic EB.

Patients with albopapuloid type of DDEB often have dystrophic nails and oral blisters, but teeth are usually normal.[33] In one series of 10 patients with Pasini DDEB, only one had corneal erosions.[34] Cutaneous blisters often heal with atrophic scars,[35] and areas of scarring are at risk for development of squamous cell carcinoma.[23] Electron microscopic studies have shown that a structural defect of anchoring fibrils is present in involved as well as intact

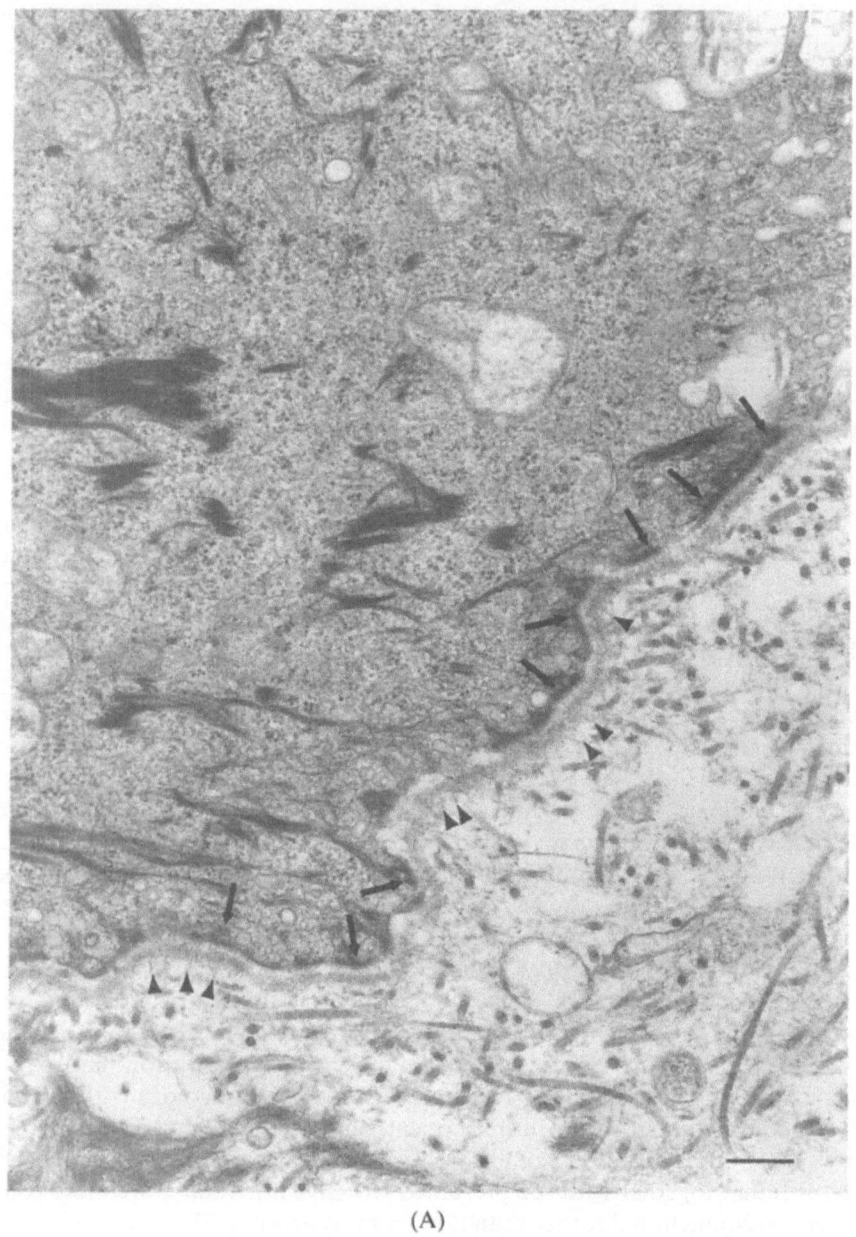

(A)

skin.[2] Increased amounts of degraded chrondroitin sulfates in the skin has been described.[22] The major urinary glycosaminoglycan in one patient was shown to be partially degraded chondroitin sulfate B, and the amounts of partially degraded chrondroitin sulfates C and/or A were decreased.[36] Fibro-blast cultures from affected individuals also showed increased amounts of

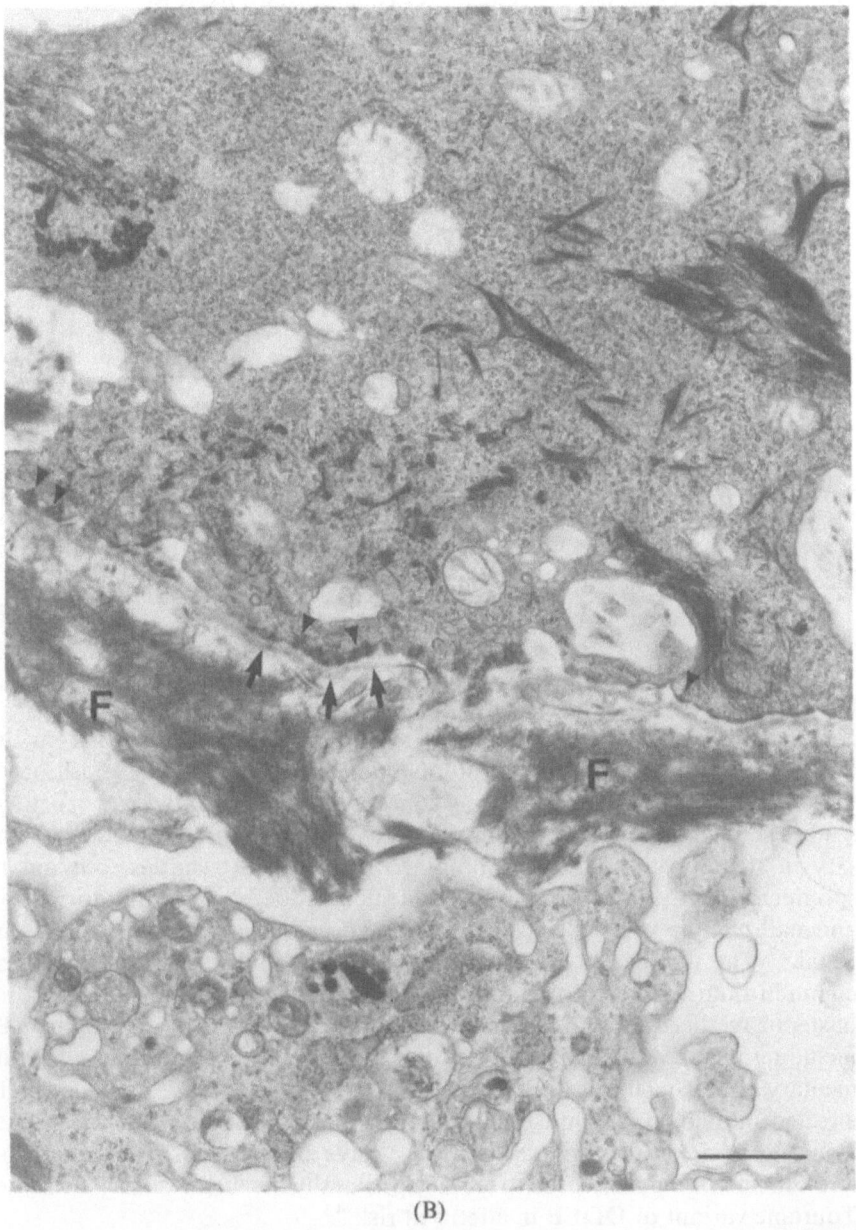

(B)

FIGURE 10.3. Electron micrographs of dominant dystrophic EB. **A**, facing page: Hemidesmosomes are normal in structure and numbers (*arrows*), but anchoring fibrils are sparse and hypoplastic (*arrowheads*). (Bar = 0.5 μm; 17,100 ×.) **B**: Where a blister cavity has formed, fibrin (*F*) is present below the lamina densa (*arrows*) of the dermal–epidermal junction. Hemidesmosomes are indicated by arrowheads. (Bar = 0.5 μm; 28,080 ×.) (Electron micrographs courtesy of Lynne T. Smith, Seattle, WA.)

TABLE 10.1. Clinical types of dominant Dystrophic EB (DDEB).

Type	Clinical Characteristics
Albopapuloid DDEB of Pasini	Generalized blistering Albopapuloid lesions Defective anchoring fibrils in blistered and intact skin
DDEB of Cockayne-Touraine	Blistering may be generalized, with predilection for extremities Anchoring fibril defects may be confined to sites of predilection for blistering Absence of albopapuloid lesions
Pretibial DDEB	Predilection for pretibial area
Transient bullous dermolysis of the newborn	Blistering stops after 1 year of age

sulfated glycosaminoglycans.[37] In one study, however, glycosaminoglycan production by cultured fibroblasts from patients with Pasini dominant dystrophic EB did not show "exceptional features" when compared with fibroblasts from patients with Cockayne-Touraine dominant dystrophic EB.[38]

Dominant Dystrophic EB of Cockayne-Touraine

Dominant dystrophic EB of Cockayne-Touraine is distinguished from the Pasini variant by the absence of albopapuloid lesions and predisposition of the extremities to blistering.[33] This concept is supported by ultrastructural studies showing that anchoring fibrils were reduced in number and rudimentary in structure in specimens obtained from the extremities, but not in specimens from sites of nonpredilection such as the back.[3] Milia formation and nail changes have been noted,[26] but oral blisters are said to be unusual.[33] The number of reported cases is small, and it appears to be less common than the Pasini variant. Teeth are generally not affected, but oral blisters have been noted.[39] Distinction from other forms of dystrophic EB, including recessive dystrophic EB, can be difficult.[40] In one kindred, rudimentary anchoring fibrils were seen in the normal-appearing skin of one mildly affected individual,[41] while ultrastructural similarities between Cockayne-Touraine and Pasini variants of DDEB have been noted.[42] Transmission electron microscopy was used to exclude prenatally the diagnosis of Cockayne-Touraine variant of DDEB in a fetus at risk.[43]

Genetic linkage analysis has been done in several kindreds with DDEB of Cockayne-Touraine. In one study, examination of 91 individuals from one single kindred failed to demonstrate linkage to any of 27 markers studied.[44]

FIGURE 10.4. **A, B:** Albopapuloid lesions in dominant dystrophic EB of Pasini.   ▷

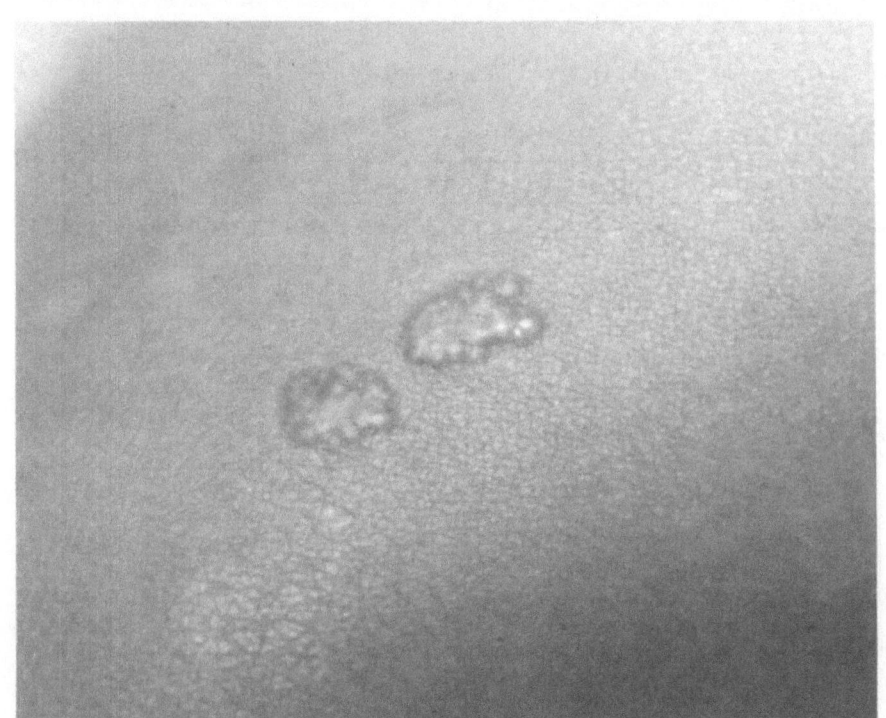

(A)

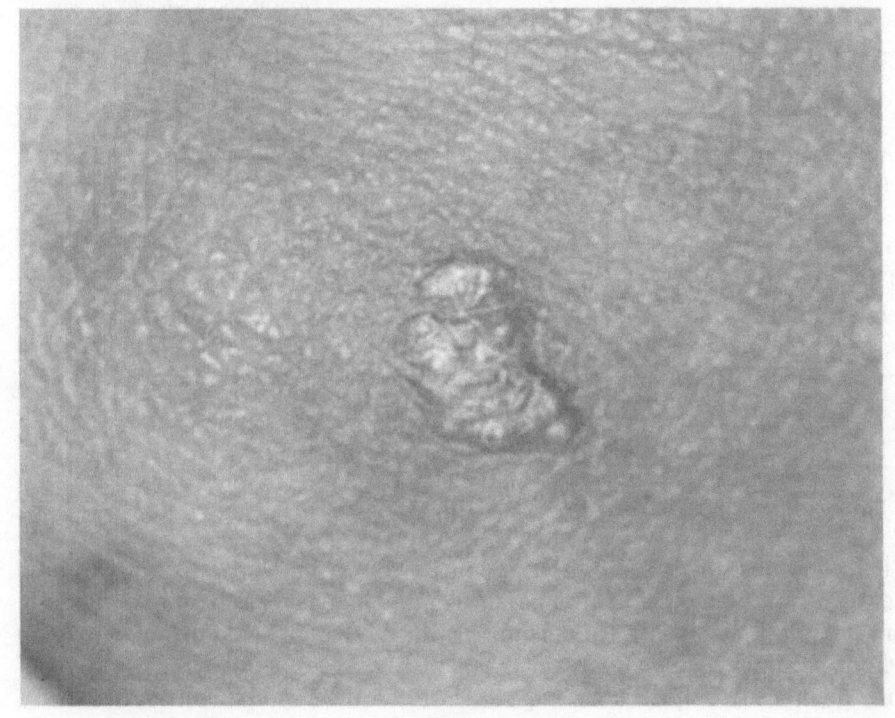

(B)

TABLE 10.2. Histology of albopapuloid lesions.

Author	Epidermal changes	Dermal changes
Ilic and Stevanovic[21]	Invaginated Enlarged follicular orifices Pronounced keratinous layer Granular layer "hardly noticeable"	Sweat gland hypertrophy
Rehtijarvi et al.[26]	Weak hyperkeratosis	Hyalinized, broadened fibrotic papillae Milia seen in some sections
Menter and Patz[20]	Mildly atrophic	Extremely fine collagen Attenulated fibrocytes Flat rete ridges Upper dermal edema Increased capillaries Mild lymphocytic infiltrate
Kumar and Kumar[25]	Thinned	Hyperplasia and homogenization of collagen
Sasai et al.[22]	Slight hyperkeratosis Focal follicular plugging Slightly thinned epidermis	Slightly homogenous Decreased elastic and oxytalen fibers that were fine and parallel to skin surface
The and Murk[24]		Papillary layer rich in collagen Nonspecific lymphohistiocytic infiltrate

Similarly, another study did not yield significant evidence to support linkage with any of 19 loci examined.[45]

In a study of human leukocyte antigens (HLA) involving one kindred with 11 affected individuals, five of seven affected individuals who were tested for HLA antigens had the same haplotype (Aw24 and B5), but two healthy relatives did not have it.[46] A previous study, however, reported that "close genetic linkage, and therefore, true association to HLA" was excluded for five dominant (including both Cockayne-Touraine and Pasini types) and three recessive types of EB.[47]

Pretibial Dominant Dystrophic EB

This refers to a subset of DDEB patients in whom blistering affects predominantly the pretibial area. Only a handful of patients have been reported under this designation.[29,30,48–51] One family with DDEB included one member in whom pretibial involvement was a salient feature, but other members had only toe nail dystrophy.[9] One report described the simultaneous occurrence of pretibial EB, hereditary nephritis, and beta-thalassemia minor in each of two siblings[52]; this syndrome was felt to be transmitted as an autosomal recessive trait, and it is unlikely to be related to dominant dystrophic EB. Since albopapuloid lesions have been observed in members of kindreds diagnosed as pretibial DDEB,[29,30] this condition may represent a localized form of the Pasini variant of DDEB. Others, however, believe that families with predominantly pretibial involvement cannot be clearly separated from the Cockayne-Touraine type of DDEB.[33] In one study of three affected families, investigators noted that cases with onset before 1 year of age showed pretibial blistering during childhood, whereas cases in which onset occurred after 10 years of age showed nail dystrophy with pruritic papulonodular lesions at pretibial sites.[30]

Transient Bullous Dermolysis of the Newborn

This is an uncommon entity that is tentatively classified as a subtype of DDEB.[53] It is characterized by the cessation of blisters beyond 1 year of age, and cleavage below the basal lamina.

In 1985, Hashimoto et al.[54] described a black male newborn with friction-induced blisters that healed rapidly with hypopigmentation, but without scarring or milia. Electron microscopy showed separation below the basal lamina. Blistering stopped after 4 months of age, and reexamination at the time of reporting when the patient was 1 year old showed only residual hypopigmentation. Several similar cases have since been reported. One neonate had friction-induced blisters with cleavage below the basal lamina that quickly healed with milia and fine reticulated scars.[55] Trauma-induced skin blisters stopped after age 4 months, but tongue lesions and nail dystrophy was noted when he was examined at age 5 years at the time of reporting. He was treated with oral phenytoin until the age of 2 years, but the dose (up to 15 mg daily) was felt to be subtherapeutic and likely unrelated to his clinical improvement. Hashimoto et al.[56] then reported two additional patients. One patient had blisters that healed without scars, and was almost free of new lesions by 4 months of age. The other patient had oral erosions, and blisters healed with milia and depigmentation, but new blistering stopped after $1\frac{1}{2}$ months of age. The first of these two patients was subsequently studied by Fine et al. in a report that included three additional cases.[57] In all four cases, blistering ceased within the first year of life. In two patients, family history established a dominant mode of inheritance while the possibility of recessive inheritance in the other two sporadic cases could not be ruled out. In all four patients, indirect immunofluorescence staining with LH 7:2 monoclonal antibody (directed against type VII collagen) showed granular basilar keratinocyte intracytoplasmic deposits, and indirect immunoelectron microscopy showed these deposits were primarily perinuclear. These findings were interpreted to indicate a defect in the intracytoplasmic packaging or transport of type VII collagen withing basilar keratinocytes.[57] In a separate report of three additional cases, indirect immunofluorescence and immunoelectron microscopy in one patient demonstrated the presence of type VII collagen in vacuoles within basal keratinocytes, suggesting a secretion abnormality.[58]

Acknowledgments. Supported in part by a General Clinical Research Center grant (M01-RR00102) from the National Institutes of Health to The Rockefeller University Hospital; by a training grant (AR07525) from the National Institutes of Health to the Laboratory for Investigative Dermatology; by contracts AR62269 and AR62270 from the National Institutes of Health to the Laboratory for Investigative Dermatology; by a grant from the Dystrophic Epidermolysis Bullosa Research Association (D.E.B.R.A.) of America, Inc.; and with general support from the Pew Trusts.

References

1. Tidman MJ, Eady RAJ. Evaluation of anchoring fibrils and other components of the dermal-epidermal junction in dystrophic epidermolysis bullosa by a quantitative ultrastructural technique. *J Invest Dermatol.* 1985;84:374–377.
2. Anton-Lamprecht I, Hashimoto I. Epidermolysis bullosa dystrophica dominans (Pasini)—A primary structural defect of the anchoring fibrils. *Hum Genet.* 1976;32:69–76.
3. Hashimoto I, Gedde-Dahl Jr T, Schnyder UW, Anton-Lamprecht I. Ultrastructural studies in epidermolysis bullosa hereditaria. II. Dominant dystrophic type of Cockayne and Touraine. *Arch Dermatol Res.* 1976;255:285–295.
4. Lewis IC, Steven EM, Farquhar JW. Epidermolysis bullosa in the newborn. *Arch Dis Child.* 1955;30:277–284.
5. Ibezi GC, Antia AU, Allenby CF. Epidermolysis bullosa dystrophica: a report of 3 cases in Nigerian children. *West African Med J.* 1967;16:114–117.
6. Moore JR. Epidermolysis bullosa. *Proc R Soc Med.* 1971;64:26–27.
7. Kennedy C. Epidermolysis bsullosa dystrophica (Dermolytic bullous dermatoses). *Proc R Soc Med.* 1974;67:1240–1241.
8. Reed WB, Roenigk Jr H, Dorner Jr W, Welsh O, Martin FJO. Epidermal neoplasms with epidermolysis bullosa dystrophica with the first report of carcinoma with the acquired type. *Arch Dermatol Res.* 1975;253:1–14.
9. Jones RR. Epidermolysis bullosa: report of a family and discussion of the dominant dystrophic types. *Clin Exp Dermatol.* 1979;4:303–308.
10. Schwartz RA, Birnkrant AP, Rubenstein DJ, et al. Squamous cell carcinoma in dominant type epidermolysis bullosa dystrophica. *Cancer.* 1981;47:615–620.
11. Chalmers RJG, Shuster S. Dominant dystrophic epidermolysis bullosa (letter). *Arch Dermatol.* 1984;120:707–708.
12. Song IC, Dicksheet S. Management of squamous cell carcinoma in a patient with dominant-type epidermolysis bullosa dystrophica: a surgical challenge. *Plast Reconstr Surg.* 1985;75:732–736.
13. Tidman MJ, Marsden RA. Severe dominant dystrophic epidermolysis bullosa. *Br J Dermatol.* 1985;113(Suppl 29):80–81.
14. Tidman MJ, Martin IR, Wells RS, Marsden RA, Eady RAJ. Oesophageal web

formation in dystrophic epidermolysis bullosa. *Clin Exp Dermatol.* 1988;13:279–281.

15. Gnanapragasam A. Oesophageal involvement in epidermolysis bullosa. *J Laryngol Otol.* 1977;41:271–274.

16. Kero M. Epidermolysis bullosa in Finland: clinical features, morphology and relation to collagen metabolism. *Acta Dermatol Venereol (Stockh).* 1984;Suppl. 110:1–51.

17. Bavinck JNB, van Haeringen A, Ruitter D, van der Schroeff JG. Autosomal dominant epidermolysis bullosa dystrophica: are the Cockayne-Touraine, the Pasini and the Bart-types different expressions of the same mutant gene? *Clin Genet.* 1987;31:416–424.

18. Uitto J, Ryynanen M, Parente G, Chung L, Chu M-l, Knowlton R. Epidermolysis bullosa: evidence for genetic linkage to a collagenous (tentative type VII collagen) gene in a family with dominant dystrophic subtype. *J Invest Dermatol.* 1991;96:539.

19. Pasini A. Dystrophie cutanee bulleuse atrophiante et albo-papuloide: essai clinique. *Ann Dermatol.* 1928;VI Serie. T. IX. No. 12:1044–1066.

20. Menter MA, Patz IM. The pattern of epidermolysis bullosa in the Bantu. *Br J Dermatol.* 1971;85(Suppl 7):32–36.

21. Ilic S, Stevanovic D. Atrophic and albo-papuloid dystrophy of Pasini: a variant of epidermolysis bullosa. *Acta Genet Stat Med.* 1960;10:27–33.

22. Sasai Y, Saito N, Seiji M. Epidermolysis bullosa dystrophica et albo-papuloidea. *Arch Dermatol.* 1973;108:554–557.

23. Reed WB, Torres-Rodriguez V, Francis MJO, Ryan T, Torres C. Dystrophic epidermolysis bullosa with epidermal neoplasm with emphasis on a dermal collagen defect. *Birth Defects: Original Article Series.* 1975;XI:153–166.

24. The L, Murk HFM. Dystrophic and albopapuloid epidermolysis bullosa. *Br J Dermatol.* 1979;101:219.

25. Kumar K, Kumar R. Epidermolysis bullosa dystrophica et albo-papuloidea Pasini in an Indian: a case report. *Dermatologica.* 1973;147:137–143.

26. Rehtijarvi K, Dammert K, Niemi K-M, Kuokkanen K. Dermatological meetings 1966: reports of cases of particular interest, University of Oulu. *Acta Derm Venereol (Stockh).* 1968;48.370–376.

27. Ramelet AA, Boillat C. Epidermolyse bulleuse dystrophique albopapuloid autosomique recessive (English abstract). *Dermatologica.* 1985;171:397–406.

28. Prigent F. Autosomal recessive epidermolysis bullosa of the albopapuloid type. *Dermatologica.* 1986;173:16.

29. Garcia-Perez A, Crapeto FJ .Pretibial epidermolysis bullosa: report of two families and review of the literature. *Dermatologica.* 1975;150:122–128.

30. Burrows NP, Jones RR. Pretibial epidermolysis bullosa: a report of three families. *Br J Dermatol.* 1990;123(Suppl 37):53–67.

31. Fine J-D. Changing clinical and laboratory concepts in inherited epidermolysis bullosa (editorial). *Arch Dermatol.* 1988;124:523–526.

32. Neering H, Wasseldijk W. Recessive epidermolysis bullosa et albopapuloidea without nail dystrophy and scarring. *Dermatologica.* 1974;149:180–184.

33. Gedde-Dahl Jr T, Anton-Lamprecht I. Epidermolysis bullosa. In: Emery AEH, Rimion DL, eds. *Principles and Practice of Medical Genetics.* Edinburgh: Churchill-Livingstone; 1983: 672–687

34. Gans LA. Eye lesions of epidermolysis bullosa: clinical features, management and prognosis. *Arch Dermatol.* 1988; 124: 762–764.
35. Whittle CH, Lyell A. Epidermolysis bullosa dystrophica (with Albo-papuloid dystrophy of Pasini). *Br J Dermatol.* 1948; 61: 175–176.
36. Endo M, Yamamoto R, Yosizawa Z, Sasai Y, Saito N. Urinary chondroitin of epidermolysis bullosa dystrophica et albo-papuloidea (Pasini). *Clin Chim Acta.* 1974; 57: 249–253.
37. Bauer EA, Fiehler WK, Esterly NB. Increased glycosaminoglycan accumulation as a genetic characteristic in cell cultures of one variety of dominant dystrophic epidermolysis bullosa. *J Clin Invest.* 1979; 64: 32–39.
38. Priestley GC. Glycosaminoglycans production by cultured skin fibroblasts from the Pasini and Cockayne-Touraine forms of dominant dystrophic epidermolysis bullosa. *J Invest Dermatol.* 1991; 96: 168–171.
39. Gorlin RJ, Pindborg JJ, Cohen MM. *Syndromes of the Head and Neck.* 2nd. ed. New Yrok: McGraw-Hill; 1976, 281–288.
40. Burkhart CG, Ruppert ES. Dystrophic epidermolysis bullosa. *Clin Pediatr.* 1981; 20: 493–496.
41. De Raevd L, De Dabbeleer G, Song M, Achten G. Dominant dystrophic epidermolysis bullosa of Cockayne-Touraine in father and son: clinical and ultrastructural similarities. *Dermatologica.* 1988; 176: 91–94.
42. Oakley CA, Gawkrodger DJ, Ross JA, Hunter JAA. The Cockayne-Touraine type of dominant dystrophic epidermolysis bullosa—ultrastructural similarities to the Pasini variant. *Acta Derm Venereol (Stockh).* 1984; 64: 253–256.
43. Fine J-D, Eady RAJ, Levy ML, et al. Prenatal diagnosis of dominant and recessive dystrophic epidermolysis bullosa: application and limitations in the use of KF-1 and LH 7:2 monoclonal antibodies and immunofluorescence mapping technique. *J Invest Dermatol.* 1988; 91: 465–471.
44. Mulley JC, Turner T, Nicholls C, Propert D, Sutherland GR. Genetic linkage analysis of epidermolysis bullosa dystrophica, Cockayne-Touraine type. *Clin Genet.* 1985; 28: 31–35.
45. Joensen HD, Hansen HE, Kenningsen K, Svejgaard A, Andersen I. A study of the linkage relations of epidermolysis bullosa dystrophica. *Hum Hered.* 1979; 29: 221–225.
46. Ozawa A, Matsuo I, Niizuma K, Ohkido M, Nose Y, Tsuji K. HLA antigens and dominant dystrophic epidermolysis bullosa in a famlly study. *Tissue Antigens.* 1978; 12: 233–235.
47. Gedde-Dahl Jr T, Thorsby E. HLA and epidermolysis bullosa. *Arch Dermatol.* 1977; 113: 1722–1723.
48. Harper JI, Copeman PWM. Pretibial epidermolysis bullosa: the use of homograft skin dressings. *Br J Dermatol.* 1983; 109(Suppl 24): 60–62.
49. Furue M, Ando I, Inoue Y, Tamaki K, Oohara K, Kukita A. Pretibial epidermolysis bullosa: successful therapy with a skin graft. *Arch Dermatol.* 1986; 122: 310–313.
50. Lichtwenwald DJ, Hanna W, Sauder DN, Jakubovic HR, Rosenthal D. Pretibial epidermolysis bullosa: report of a case. *J Am Acad Dermatol.* 1990; 22: 346–350.
51. Gassia V, Bazex J, Ortonne J-P. Pretibial epidermolysis bullosa (letter). *J Am Acad Dermatol.* 1991; 24: 663–664.
52. Kagan A, Feld S, Chemke J, Bar-Khayim Y. Occurrence of hereditary nephritis,

pretibial epidermolysis bullosa and beta-thalassemia minor in two siblings with end-stage renal disease (letter). *Nephron.* 1988;49:331–332.

53. Fine J-D, Bauer EA, Briggaman RA, et al. Revised clinical and laboratory criteria for subtypes of inherited epidermolysis bullosa: a consensus report by the sub-committee on diagnosis and classification of the National Epidermolysis Bullosa Registry. *J Am Acad Dermatol.* 1991;24:119–135.

54. Hashimoto K, Matsumoto M, Iacobelli D. Transient bullous dermolysis of the newbom. *Arch Dermatol.* 1985;121:1429–1438.

55. Fisher GB, Greer KE, Cooper PH. Congenital self-healing (transient) mechano-bullous dermatosis. *Arch Dermatol.* 1988;124:240–243.

56. Hashimoto K, Burk JD, Bale GF, et al. Transient bullous dermolysis of the newborn: two additional cases. *J Am Acad Dermatol.* 1989;21:708–713.

57. Fine J-D, Horiguchi Y, Stein DH, Esterly NB, Leigh IM. Intraepidermal type VII collagen: evidence for abnormal intracytoplasmic processing of a major basement membrane protein in rare patients with dominant and possibly localized recessive forms of dystrophic epidermolysis bullosa. *J Am Acad Dermatol.* 1990;22:188–195.

58. Schofield OMV, Yamamoto A, McGrath J, Bowers W, Dahl M, Eady RAJ. Transient bullous dermolysis of the newborn: a disorder of type VII collagen secretion? *Br J Dermatol.* 1991; 125(Suppl 38):89.

IV
Extracutaneous Manifestations and Their Management

11
Gastrointestinal Aspects of Epidermolysis Bullosa

GULCHIN ERGUN and ROBERT A. SCHAEFER

The gastrointestinal complications of epidermolysis bullosa (EB) are a major cause of symptoms and morbidity and contribute substantially to the nutritional problems and growth retardation of these patients. The most severe problems are related to involvement of the proximal gut, oropharynx, and esophagus. However, anal lesions and altered colonic function lead to frequent difficulties with bowel function. In one study of 101 EB patients representing simplex, junctional and dystrophic forms of EB,[1] a wide variety of upper gastrointestinal symptoms were seen in 68 patients. These consisted of oral blisters, odynophagia, dysphagia, dental anomalies, microstomia and pyrosis. Forty six patients had lower gastrointestinal manifestations, consisting of hematochezia, anal pain, constipation, perianal blisters and tenesmus. Management of these gastrointestinal complications is difficult and must be approached cautiously because of the danger of further injury to the squamous mucosa.

Oropharyngeal Lesions

The oral manifestations of EB are expressed differently according to the type of disorder. In some cases, the oral findings are minimal or absent, whereas in others, the oral manifestations are severe enough to become major management problems.

The oral cavity epithelia as well as the teeth are involved in all types of EB. There are no epidemiologic studies describing the incidence and frequency of lesions appearing in the oral cavity; however, the lesions are most common and most extensive in patients with recessive-dystrophic EB and junctional EB.[1a] The lips, tongue, lingual frenulum, palate, pharynx, and uvula are often involved and the epithelia can develop bullae that rupture, become eroded, and heal with resultant scarring.[1a] The buccal mucosa, tongue, and lips are the most frequent sites of bullae formation in the mouth, with the gingiva and hard palate less frequently involved.[2,3]

Mucosal involvement in afflicted patients appears to increase with time.

Initial examination of the oropharynx of infants with severe dystrophic EB may reveal normal mucosa with uninhibited tongue movement and normal oral opening. As the child grows, nonnutritive sucking and oral action predominate. The diet is changed to include coarser foods, and the employment of eating utensils is begun. These factors are all implicated in an increase in bullae formation.[3] This may lead to tissue contraction and microstomia with lingual frenulum shortening, tongue immobility, and tongue surface and papillae atrophy. Fusion of the alveolar ridge to the buccal mucosa and obliteration of the vestibular sulci and the pillars of the tonsillar fauces by scarring and adhesion of tissues may also result. With the repeated cycles of blistering and healing, there is reduction in mandibular mobility and the oral functions of mastication, swallowing, and even speaking are reduced.[3]

Oral hygiene is further jeopardized because of the difficulty of toothbrush manipulation and fear of blister formation. With the coincident problem of poor dentition, optimal nutritional intake and the preservation of intact oral mucosa is compromised.

Esophageal Lesions

Extracutaneous involvement in patients with EB simplex (EBS) is not common. Bullae can occur, however, on any mucosal surface in patients with junctional and dystrophic EB. The most common extracutaneous site is the gastrointestinal tract.[4]

In the gastrointestinal tract, the esophagus is particularly vulnerable to damage because it is lined by stratified squamous epithelium like the skin. It can therefore be the site of bullae formation, erosion, and scarring. When comparing the various types of EB, esophageal involvement is most common in patients with recessive dystrophic EB.[4,5]

Esophageal disease becomes symptomatic at any age and patients may develop symptoms well under the age of 2 years. In a review of 24 patients with recessive dystrophic EB, Nix and Christianson noted that dysphagia began early in life in most cases and nearly all patients were symptomatic by the third decade of life.[6] Although dysphagia usually starts insidiously in the first decade of life, delay until the fifth decade of life has been reported.[7]

Odynophagia (painful swallowing) and dysphagia (difficulty in swallowing) are the major symptoms of esophageal involvement in EB. The extent and nature of the esophageal involvement vary but the spectrum encompasses formation of bullae, erosions or ulcerations, webs, and strictures. True odynophagia usually signifies active mucosal lesions such as bullae or erosions, although this may be difficult to distinguish from the pain of esophageal spasm, which may accompany any of these lesions. The occurrence of mucosal bullae often coincides with the presence of active skin lesions but can arise independently. The bullae can be precipitated by the ingestion of coarse or very hot food. Dysphagia, on the other hand, generally implies more

TABLE 11.1. Esophageal radiologic findings.

Bullae
Ulcers/erosions
Webs
Strictures
Pseudo-diverticula
Stenosis

chronic disease due to scarring such as web or stricture formation. Despite histologically proven EB, however, the complaint of dysphagia does not necessarily indicate stricture formation. Dysphagia may result from bullae and accompanying reversible inflammatory reactions.

Roentgenographic or fluoroscopic examination of the esophagus is a useful means of demonstrating esophageal lesions (Table 11.1). Nonspecific inflammatory changes may be seen early in the course of the disease and may be manifested as mucosal edema and areas of inconstant spasm.[7] Bullae may be demonstrated as small, constant, nodular, filling defects if barium studies are done early in the course of the disease or during a recurrent bullous episode. Occasionally, superficial erosions or ulcerations secondary to rupture of bullae may be seen. Radiographically, these ulcers heal slowly with extensive surrounding scar tissue. In patients examined during quiescent stages of the disease, mucosal irregularities due to scarring are commonly seen. Pseudo-diverticula and esophageal intramural diverticulosis have been reported.[8]

In 1974, Marsden et al.[9] reported the presence of fine, weblike projections in the postcricoid area of four patients with recessive dystrophic EB and in 1977, Hillemeier et al.[10] recognized esophageal webs as a complication of EB in three patients. In two patients, weblike constrictions in the upper esophagus or cricopharyngeal regions were associated with the gradual development of severe dysphagia. In both patients the dysphagia resolved when they noted a "pop" in the neck after ingestion of food. In the third patient the web was mechanically ruptured during surgery for a colonic interposition.

Seaman reviewed a series of 53 patients with esophageal webs of all causes and found most lesions in the cervical esophagus near the cricopharyngeal region and only four lesions in the hypopharynx.[11] A web was found in only one patient with recessive dystrophic EB but subsequent case reports have described esophageal webs complicating EB.[7] The more assiduous the search for esphageal webs, the more commonly they are found; therefore, they may indeed be more common in EB than the existing case reports would indicate (Figs. 11.1, 11.2).

The advent of cineradiography has markedly increased reporting of hypopharyngeal and cervical webs.[12] Since barium passes through the upper esophagus rapidly, the cine-esophagram may demonstrate lesions missed by conventional barium studies. If a proximal lesion is suspected, it is preferable

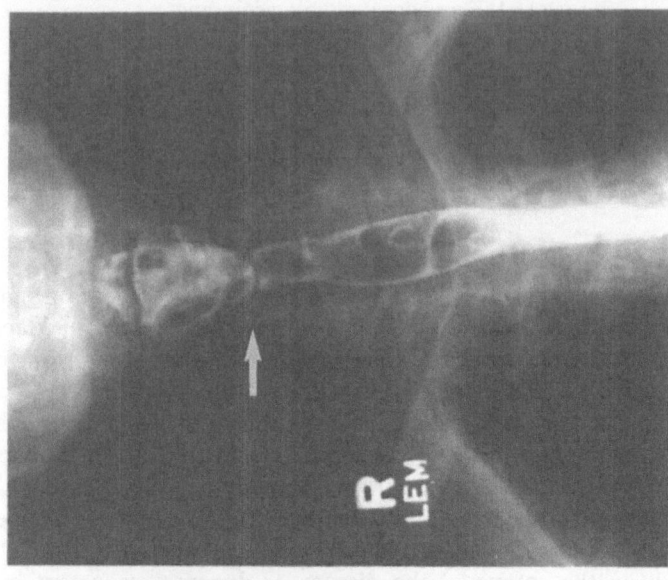

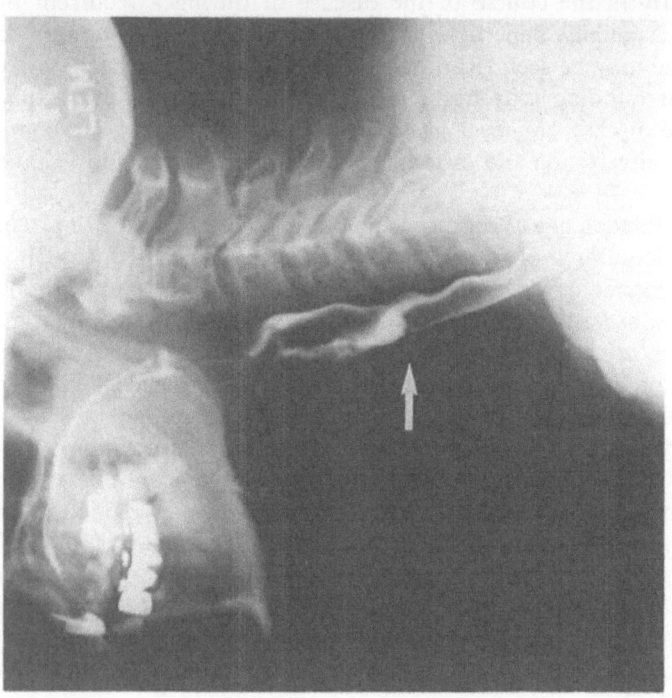

FIGURE 11.1. Cervical web. This radiograph was taken from a 60-year-old woman with a clinical diagnosis of recessive-dystrophic EB and 20 years of intermittent meat and pill impactions. The web was demonstrated on video-esophagram.

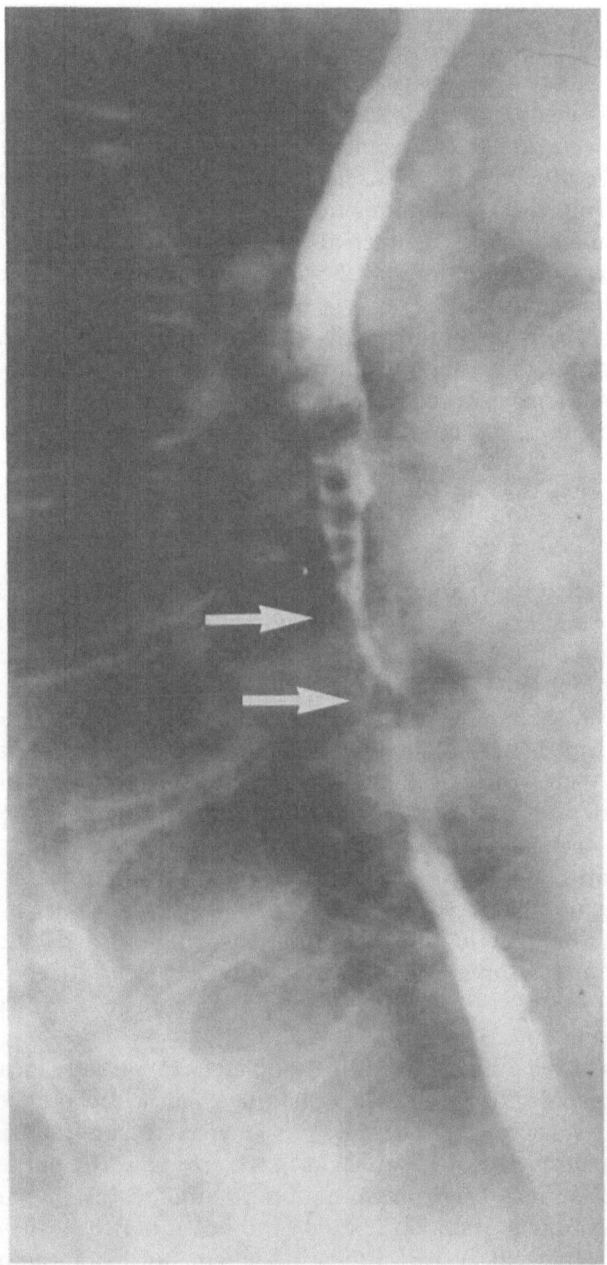

FIGURE 11.2. Multiple cervical webs. This radiograph was taken from a 66-year-old woman with a clinical diagnosis of recessive-dystrophic EB and many years of intermittent solid food dysphagia. A cervical web was first demonstrated at age 25 years and dilated using Eder-Puestow dilators. Since then she has had multiple cervical webs demonstrated and at least nine dilations in her lifetime. She was most recently dilated 1 month before this examination. This barium esophagram demonstrates two partially disrupted cervical webs.

to study the patient with a video-esophagram first and complement the study with a barium swallow if necessary.

The Plummer-Vinson (Paterson-Kelly) eponym refers to the association of webs occurring in the upper 2 to 4 cm of the esophagus and dysphagia.[13] In many patients described, an iron-deficiency anemia was demonstrated, and symptoms were improved by administration of iron and esophageal dilatation. Since common features between the Plummer-Vinson syndrome and selected EB patients are often found, the question of a relationship between the two is sometimes raised.

Unlike EB, however, the pathogenesis of the Plummer-Vinson syndrome is not clear. Since the Plummer-Vinson syndrome and EB are likely distinct in etiology and pathogenesis, the likelihood of resolution of an EB web with just iron supplementation is improbable and not recommended.

Strictures

The irritation of the pharynx and esophagus by the passage of food causes separation of the epithelial layer from the lamina propria with formation of vesicles that rupture, leaving ulcers that heal with scarring and eventual stricture formation (Fig. 11.3). Strictures occur throughout the entire esophagus at any time in the course of the disease, and occur twice as frequently in males as in females, although this may reflect the nature of sampling performed.[14] In their review of 26 patients, Nix et al. have shown that 50% of cases have strictures in the upper one third of the esophagus, 25% in the lower one third, and the remaining 25% involve multiple sites.[6] The average length of strictures was 2 to 6 cm, although longer strictures as well as complete narrowing of the esophagus was described. Mauro et al. in 1987 reported the radiographic features of 16 patients with EB and described a similar distribution of esophageal strictures, with eight (50%) of the esophageal strictures in this series occurring in the proximal third, and five (31%) multiple in location.[15]

The strictures of the upper third of the esophagus are usually localized to the level of the cricoid cartilage and cricopharyngeal muscle where the caliber of the esophagus is narrowest. These lesions may result from the trauma of ingested food as it traverses the esophagus in the area of aortic pulsations. It is possible that food may exert pressure on the wall of the esophagus at the level of the arch of the aorta and the tracheal bifurcation where the esophagus is normally somewhat narrower than in the remainder of its course.[16]

Strictures in the distal third of the esophagus may reflect, in part, increased mucosal damage from gastric acid reflux. As cicatrization progresses, shortening of the esophagus leads to development of traction hiatal hernia and gastroesophageal reflux. Four patients with a predisposition to reflux were studied by Orlando et al.[5] using manometric and radiographic techniques. None of these patients, however, were found to have lower esophageal stric-

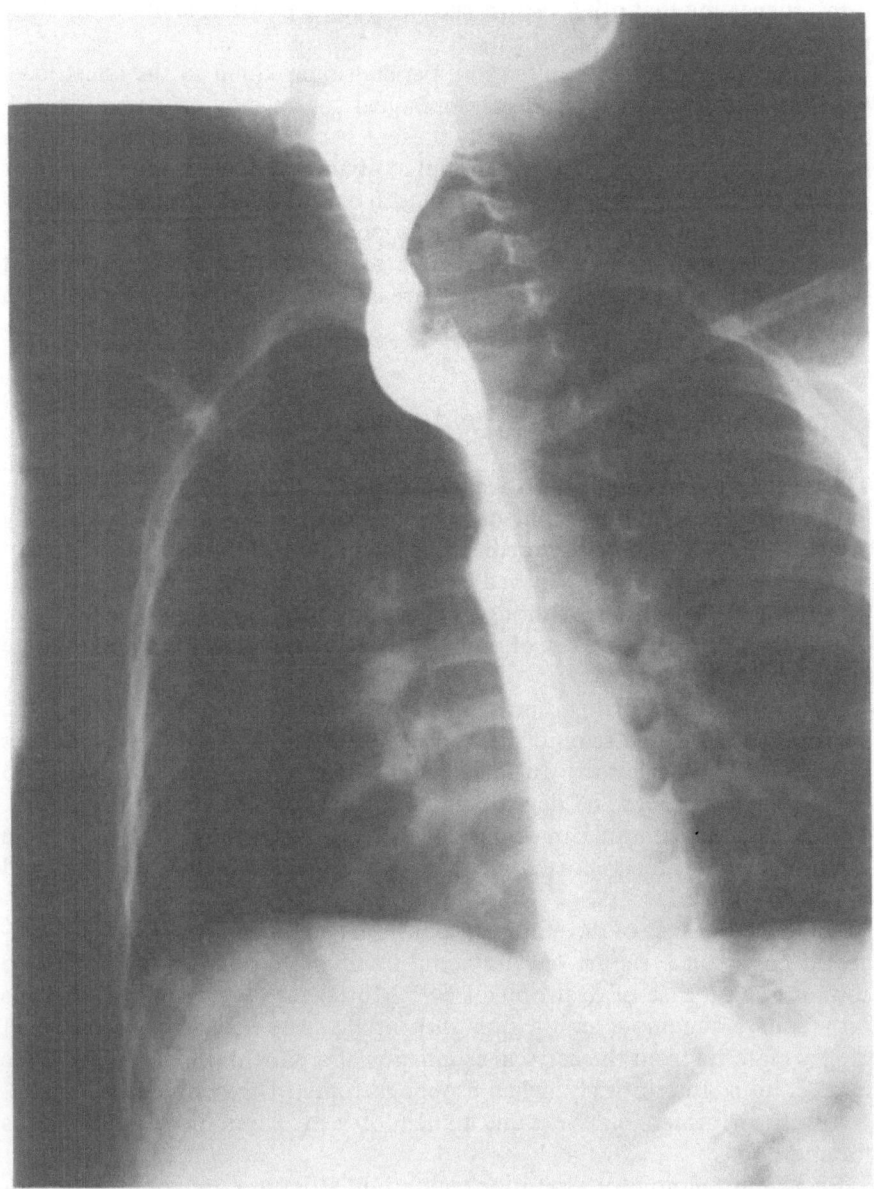

FIGURE 11.3. Barium swallow showing stricture in proximal third of esophagus in a 3-year-old boy with recessive dystrophic EB.

tures, suggesting that other factors such as trauma play a role in the development of strictures in these patients.[5]

During radiographic examination, peristalsis proximal to the constricted zone may be normal or signs of esophageal spasm may be demonstrated. Some prestenotic dilatation is usally present. At the proximal margin of the stricture, abrupt transition from normal to abnormal mucosa may be seen or gradual tapering in conjunction with smooth or scarred mucosa seen distally.

Stenosis or complete occlusion of the esophageal lumen may occur because of diffuse bullous and ulcerative lesions of the esophagus, or because of stricture. Obstruction due to multiple areas of stricture formation has also been described.[6]

Complications of Esophageal Lesions

The most common complication of epidermolysis bullosa of the esophagus is lodgement of food in the esophagus. If the bolus does not pass spontaneously or after a trial of antispastic medication such as nitrates or calcium channel blockers, it can usually be relieved by therapeutic endoscopy and removal of the impacting substance. Although fiberoptic endoscopy may be employed, a large bolus may require use of rigid endoscopy under anesthesia for its safe removal.

Similar to other skin disorders typified by recurrent injury and scarring, the cutaneous lesions and scars of EB are also susceptible to dysplastic changes that may be precancerous. In fact, patients with dystrophic EB appear to be especially prone to the development of cutaneous epidermal neoplasms. These cutaneous tumors can occur anywhere but extracutaneous sites where carcinoma have been reported include the tongue, stomach, bronchus, and pulmonary pleura.[4,17,18]

An increased risk of development of esophageal carcinoma has been suggested based on a report of carcinoma involving esophagus and stomach complicating a case of dystrophic EB.[19] Moreover, dysplasia, evidenced as proliferative squamous epithelium with atypia, has been demonstrated in biopsy material from the cervical esophagus of a patient undergoing colonic interposition. Interestingly, when esophagectomy of that bypassed esophagus was performed on the same patient 2 years later, no dysplasia was found.[20]

Recurrent pulmonary aspirations with tight strictures are common. Spontaneous perforation of the esophagus, a fatal complication, has been reported by Nix et al.[6] Esophageal hemorrhage has been reported but no fatalities described.[6]

The prognosis of EB of the esophagus is poor because of continued odynophagia and dysphagia with limited nutritional intake. Severe malnutrition, refractory anemia, and death from inanition or aspiration pneumonitis typify the disabling nature of these esophageal complications.

Treatment of Esophageal Lesions

Role of Endoscopy

Dysphagia in patients with EB most often has its onset in childhood. If it has not occurred by the middle of the third decade, it will rarely appear later in life without a specific traumatic incident.[14] The therapy of esophageal involvement in EB is often unsatisfactory, but begins with dietary and nutritional manipulation.

Treatment in the acute stage is symptomatic and aimed at decreasing the formation of bullae and preventing aspiration of food and secretions. Patients may be placed on a liquid or semiliquid diet for 10 to 14 days when suffering from odynophagia. Nutrition is a prime concern since most of these patients are frequently malnourished as well. They should be placed on enteral nutritional supplements during the acute episode and caloric needs should be estimated with the help of a clinical nutritionist.

There is no definitive medical management for the cutaneous manifestations of EB and similarly no definitive therapy exists for esophageal lesions. Prednisolone lozenges, oral corticosteroid elixirs, and large intravenous doses of corticosteroid have been advocated to reduce the edema and inflammation accompanying oral and esophageal bullae formation, but most experience has been anecdotal with no published randomized, controlled clinical trials.[21,22] Similarly, since phenytoin is known to inhibit collagenase activity, oral phenytoin has also been used to reduce epithelial detachment and blister formation. There has been some success with the skin lesions but only in open trials. No randomized double-blind studies have been performed demonstrating success with phenytoin in improving mucosal lesions. Only anecdotal improvement in esophageal lesions has been suggested.[23] In those patients with a significant component of esophageal spasm accompanying mucosal lesions, calcium channel blockers such as verapamil have been used to provide relief from chest discomfort.[24,25] Since any degree of gastric acid reflux may irritate existing esophageal lesions, antacids are often empirically used.

Treatment in the chronic stages is aimed at providing adequate nutritional support while reducing the risk of aspiration. Again, enlisting the aid of the dietician, the patient may be placed on a mechanical soft or pureed diet. Most patients tolerate soft diets remarkably well and can manage simple meals such as hamburgers adequately. Should patients require any medications, they should be given in liquid preparations.

Review of published reports shows most authors reluctant to recommend endoscopy as an investigative tool in the evaluation of dysphagia or odynophagia in these patients. Endoscopy may be difficult to perform because of microstomia caused by scarring of the oral cavity, and the trauma of even gentle passage of the endoscope may be hazardous in causing bullae, hemorrhage from ulcerations, or even esophageal perforation. On occasion, endoscopy becomes unavoidable and is reserved for patients with esophageal impaction failing conservative or medical management and those patients in whom the suspicion of esophageal neoplasm is high.

Until recently, the treatment of esophageal strictures has been largely conservative with dietary manipulation and occasionally gastrostomy placement for feedings. Invasive measures such as dilation were withheld as long as possible because even the most gentle dilation could result in formation of bullae or perforation or extension of stricture. Because tangential shearing forces, rather than vertical pressure, lead to detachment of skin and mucous membranes, any bougienage, for example with the Eder-Puestow or Malony dilators, has been discouraged by some authors. Instead, balloon dilation at different esophageal levels has been recommended.[23] To avoid greater injury to the esophagus, guide threads rather than wires have been used in the placement of the dilators. This remains a controversial area, however, since some centers recommend operative rigid esophagoscopy performed under general anesthesia because of the common occurrence of aspiration. A wide-bore esophagoscope is passed to the stricture, then flexible-tipped dilators are passed, stretching the esophagus until the rigid scope can be passed over the largest dilator. Routine bougie dilation is later performed to keep the stricture open.

Routine mercury bougie dilation has also been performed initially and it has been suggested that cervical strictures of EB are easily dilated with minimal morbidity or risk of perforation.[22] Diffuse esophageal involvement is more difficult to manage. In one study in which patients were studied 1 to 5 years after dilation, worsening of the strictures was reported.[26]

It is our opinion that balloon dilation at different esophageal levels should be attempted first, if possible, and followed by operative rigid esophagoscopy if balloon dilation cannot be performed. A barium esophagram is mandatory in the evaluation of dysphagia and before any attempt at therapeutic dilation.

Nutrition

The nutritional management, when dietary manipulation is inadequate, may necessitate other means of enteral supplementation such as feeding tube placement, percutaneous endoscopic gastrostomy placement when feasible, or even surgical gastrostomy.

Feurle et al. placed small nasogastric or nasoduodenal feeding tubes of increasing size introduced under general anesthesia in those patients they dilated using inflatable dilator balloons.[23] This method proved successful for months in some patients, facilitating a reduction of a tight stenosis so that the patient could swallow liquids alongside the tube.

Surgical gastrostomy provides a long-term method of nutritional support and is an effective way of maintaining nutrition in the young. It may decrease the risk of regurgitation or aspiration although prevention of these complications is, of course, never guaranteed.

Total parenteral nutrition and peripheral hyperalimentation are used only in acute or short-term settings such as severe malnutrition or in the perioperative period.

Colonic Interposition

Surgical treatment for esophageal stricture is indicated when the lesion is no longer responsive to dilation, if a complication of dilation such as perforation or further stricturing occurs, or if esophageal neoplasm is encountered.

Curative esophageal reconstruction using esophagocolonoplasty was first reported by Absolon et al. in 1969.[27] An isoperistaltic segment of right colon was interposed between the cervical esophagus and stomach with bypass or complete resection of the esophagus. Pyloroplasty and temporary feeding gastrostomy were usually performed. A 5-year follow-up of the procedure performed in two children demonstrated good results. Harmel in 1986 performed a reversed gastric tube for one of his two patients.[28] Kralik and Rapant have performed resection of a mucosal segment with reanastomosis through a longitudinal esophagomyotomy for a short annular stenosis just distal to the pharyngoesophageal junction.[29] Touloukian et al. favor an ileocolonic interposition since the lumina at the cervical anastomosis are nearly the same diameter.[20] They cite preservation of the ileocecal valve as an additional benefit since this prevents reflux of gastric contents into the mouth.

The two patients in their series had prolonged symptom-free periods. Early postoperative complications include cervical anastomotic leaks that occur spontaneously within several weeks, or the later complications of anastomotic stricture, which can be managed by dilation. Although esophageal reconstruction is an extensive and complicated surgical procedure, it has been done without mortality and relatively few complications.[30,31]

Since the entire esophagus is subject to repeated injury and subsequent scarring, colonic replacement appears to be the procedure most likely to provide permanent relief of esophageal obstruction (Fig. 11.4, Table 11.2).

Small Bowel Involvement

Pyloric atresia, or the complete luminal obstruction of the pyloric canal, is a rare congenital anomaly of the alimentary tract that represents about 1% of all intestinal atresias.[32] Prenatally, it is suspected with the detection of polyhydramnios, which occurs approximately 50% of the time, but vomiting within the first few days of life is usually the initial manifestation. Radiographically the stomach is seen to be distended with air but there is no gas beyond the pylorus. This is the so-called single-bubble sign. Pyloric atresia associated with EB was first described by Korber and Glasson in 1977.[33] Since then, at least 19 cases have been reported and support the association of junctional EB and pyloric atresia.[34-37]

The pathogenesis of the pyloric atresia is unclear but may occur as a

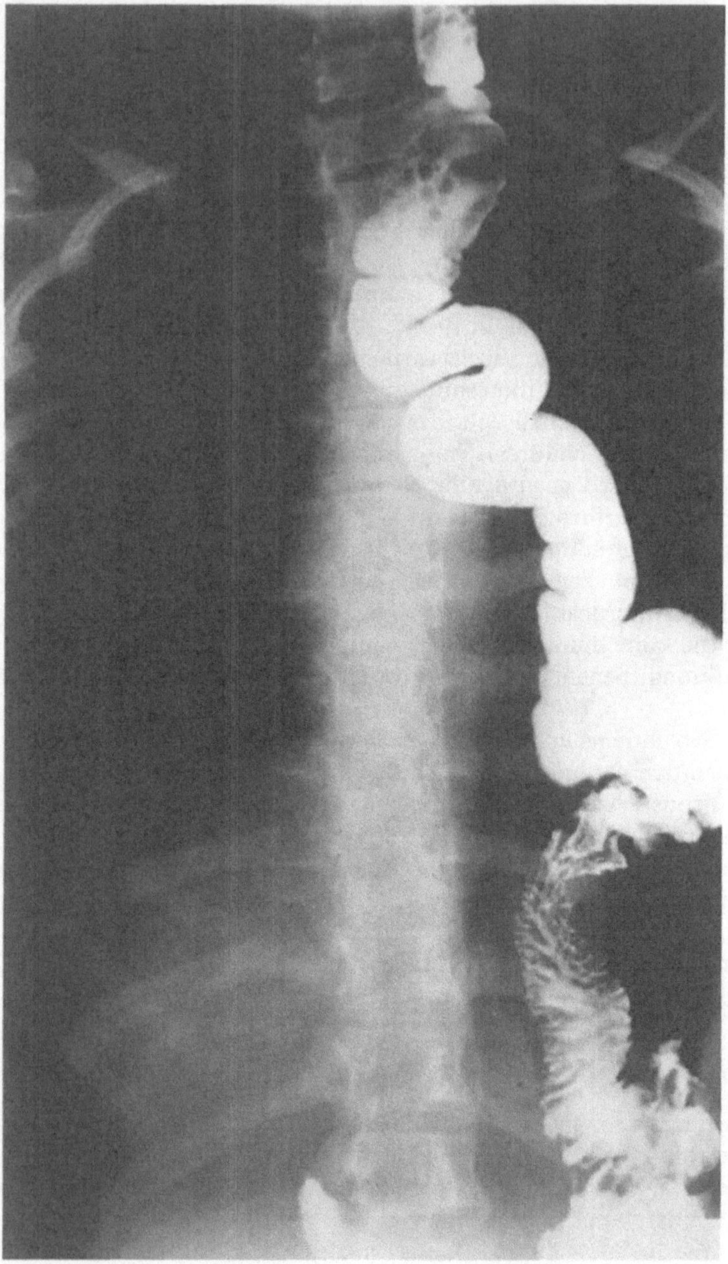

FIGURE 11.4. Colonic interposition. This barium swallow was performed on an 11-year-old patient with recessive dystrophic EB who underwent a colonic interposition at age 6 years. This barium swallow demonstrates the interposed colon. The bypassed esophagus is not visualized.

TABLE 11.2. Treatment of Odynophagia/Dysphagia.

Diet manipulation
Prednisolone lozenges or corticosteroid elixirs
Dilation
Feeding tube
Gastrostomy
Colonic interposition

consequence of excessive deposition of connective tissue, failure of the tube to canalize during development, or the formation of a diaphragmatic membrane across the lumen. It is thought that this complication results either from expression of a closely linked autosomal recessive gene or the pleiotropic effects of the same gene.

Malrotation of the intestine with a duodenal volvulus has been described in one patient with a "dominantly inherited, nonscarring form of EB" and the association of malrotation of the midgut with EB in this patient may suggest an association with various congenital gut abnormalities.[38] However, since the skin disease, as described, may not represent dystrophic, recessive EB, an association based on one case remains unproven.

Colonic Involvement

Colonic involvement in EB is rarely discussed and the frequency of colonic involvement is unknown. This may be directly related to infrequent investigation of possible colonic pathology coupled with probable infrequent involvement. The paucity of colonic disease reported in the literature may be explained by the difference in the tissue involved. Colon is typically columnar epithelium and would not be expected to be Involved in the bullous disease affecting squamous epithelium. It is common, however, to find an iron deficiency anemia in these patients, often with evidence of microscopic blood in the stool. This is most likely multifactorial and secondary to profound skin losses, decreased enteral intake, esophageal losses, and anal and perirectal disease. Although tissue examined postmortem in a child with EB and pyloric atresia has demonstrated denuded epithelium in the colon, case reports of patients undergoing colonic interposition have not described any colonic pathology.[39]

Anal Lesions

The occurrence of anal lesions in patients with EB is also infrequently discussed. Bullae, erosions, fissures, and scarring with stenosis can cause severe discomfort and may lead, especially in children, to withholding of stool, which may result in chronic constipation, encopresis, or even fecal impaction. These patients are at an increased risk of constipation with their limited oral

TABLE 11.3. Treatment of constipation.

Increase fluid intake
Increase fiber intake
Stool softener
Cathartics
Enemas

intake of fluid and fiber and the excessive fluid losses through their skin lesions.

Anal lesions may be treated locally using anesthetic creams, corticosteroid ointments, or suppositories. Effective treatment of constipation is necessary to prevent a vicious cycle of withholding, trauma from passing a bulky, hard stool, and further constipation. Commercial fiber preparations containing psyllium, stool softeners in large doses, and the mandatory increase in fluid intake to more than six to eight glasses of fluid daily should be encouraged. Routine use of orally administered mineral oil as a stool softener is to be avoided because of the increased risk of lipoid pneumonia from aspiration in patients with esophageal involvement. However, used with caution and supervision, large doses may be helpful in the management of severe obstipation. Other stimulant purgatives such as anthracine derivatives are not encouraged because of the risk of potential habituation and irritant effects on the colon, but their use may be unavoidable. If necessary, sodium docusate with senna in a pediatric liquid preparation, lactulose, glycerine suppositories, or mineral oil enemas can be used. The best therapy still remains preventative, with a regimen that avoids medications and supplies the diet with adequate fluid and fiber intake (Table 11.3).

References

1. Ergun GA, Lin AN, Dannenberg AJ, Carter DM. Gastrointestinal manifestations of epidermolysis bullosa: a study of 101 patients. Medicine, 1992 (in press).
1a. Holbrook KA. Extracutaneous epithelial involvement in inherited epidermolysis bullosa. *Arch Dermatol.* 1988;124:726–731.
2. Pratilas V, Biezvnski A. Epidermolysis bullosa manifested and treated during anesthesia. *Anesthesiology.* 1975;43:581–583.
3. Nowak AJ. Oropharyngeal lesions and their management in epidermolysis bullosa. *Arch Dermatol.* 1988;124:742–745.
4. Lin AN, Carter DM. Epidermolysis bullosa: when the skin falls apart. *J Pediatr.* 1989;112:349–355.
5. Orlando RC, Bozymski EM, Briggaman RA, et al. Epidermolysis bullosa: gastrointestinal manifestations. *Ann Intern Med.* 1974;81:203–206.
6. Nix TE, Christianson HB. Epidermolysis bullosa of the esophagus: report of two cases and review of the literature. *South Med J.* 1965;58:612–620.
7. Agha FP, Francis IR, Ellis CN. Esophageal involvement in epidermolysis bullosa

dystrophica: clinical and roentgenographic manifestations. *Gastrointest Radiol.* 1983;8:11–117.
8. Hahn AL. Esophageal epidermolysis bullosa dystrophica? *Ann Intern Med.* 1975; 82:427.
9. Marsden RA, Sambrook Gowar FJ, MacDonald AF. Epidermolysis bullosa of the esophagus with oesophageal web formation. *Thorax.* 1974;29:287–295.
10. Hillemeier C, Touloukian R, McCallum R, et al. Esophageal webs: a previously unrecognized complication of epidermolysis bullosa. *Pediatrics.* 1981;67:678–682.
11. Seaman WB. The significance of webs in the hypopharynx and upper esophagus. *Radiology.* 1967;89:32–38.
12. Nosher JL, Campbell WL, Seaman WB. The clinical significance of cervical esophageal and hypopharyngeal webs. *Radiology.* 1975;117:45–47.
13. Logan JS. The Plummer-Vinson stricture. *Ulster Med J.* 1978;47(Suppl 2):1.
14. Schuman BM, Areiniegas E. The management of esophageal complications of epidermolysis bullosa. *Digest Dis.* 1972;17:875–880.
15. Mauro MA, Parker CA, Hartley WS, Renner JB, et al. Epidermolysis bullosa: radiographic findings in 16 cases. *AJR.* 1987;149:925–927.
16. Bergenholtz A, Olsson O, Arwill T, et al. Oesophageal changes in epidermolysis bullosa hereditaria dystrophica. *Pract Oto-rhino-laryngol.* 1965;27:219–232.
17. Wetteland P, Hovding G. Squamous-cell carcinoma in dystrophic epidermolysis bullosa. *Acta Dermatoveneralcol.* 1956;36:27–36.
18. Wechsler HL, Krugh FJ, Domonkos AN, et al. Polydysplastic epidermolysis bullosa and development of epidermal neoplasms. *Arch Dermatol.* 1970;102:374–380.
19. Sonneck HJ, Hantzschel K. Uber einen fall von epidermolysis bullosa dystrophica mit oesophagusstenose, und kardiocarcinom. *Hautarzt.* 1961;12:124–125.
20. Touloukian RJ, Schonholz SM, Gryboski JD. Perioperative considerations in esophageal replacement for epidermolysis bullosa: report of two cases successfully treated by colon interposition. *Am J Gastroenterol.* 1988;83:857–861.
21. Katz J, Gryboski JD, Rosenbaum HM, et al. Dysphagia in children with epidermolysis bullosa. *Gastroenterology.* 1967;52:259–262.
22. Gryboski JD, Touloukian R, Campanella RA. Gastrointestinal manifestation of epidermolysis bullosa in children. *Arch Dermatol.* 1988;124:746–752.
23. Feurle GE, Weidauer H, Baldauf G, et al. Management of esophageal stenosis in recessive dystrophic epidermolysis bullosa. *Gastroenterology.* 1984;87:1376–1380.
24. Kern IB, Eisenberg M, Willis s. Management of oesophageal stenosis in epidermolysis dystrophica: *Arch Dis Child.* 1989;64:551–556.
25. Mitchell JD, Eisenberg M. Management of esophageal spasm in epidermolysis bullosa dystrophica using verapamil. *J Pediatr Gastroenterol Nutr.* 1989;8:133–134.
26. Manier JW, Kaplan AP. Polydysplastic epidermolysis bullosa with esophogeal stricture: report of a case. *Gastrointest Endosc.* 1972;19:19–20.
27. Absolon KB, Kinney LA, Waddill GM, et al. Esophageal reconstruction colon transplant in two brothers with epidermolysis bullosa. *Surgery.* 1969;65:832–836.
28. Harmel RP. Esophageal replacement in two siblings with epidermolysis bullosa. *J Pediatr Surg.* 1986;21:175–176.

184   Gulchin Ergun and Robert A. Schaefer

29. Kralik J, Rapant V. Radical surgical treatment of esophageal stenosis due to epidermolysis bullosa. *J Thorac Cardiovasc Surg.* 1975;69:790–792.
30. Sehhat S, Amirie A. Oesophageal reconstruction for complete stenosis due to dystrophic epidermolysis bullosa. *Thorax.* 1977;32:697–699.
31. Deleon R, Mispireta LA, Absolon KB. Five year follow up of colonic transplants in patients with epidermolysis bullosa producing esophageal obstruction. *Med Ann District of Columbia.* 1974;43:241–244.
32. Bronsther B, Nadeam MR, Abrams NW. Congenital pyloric atresia: a report of 3 cases and a review of the literature. *Surgery.* 1971;69:130–136.
33. Korber JS, Glasson MJ. Pyloric atresia associated with epidermolysis bullosa. *J Pediatr.* 1977;90:600–601.
34. Chang C, Perrin EV, Bore KE. Pyloric atresia associated with epidermolysis bullosa: special reference to pathogenesis. *Pediatr Pathol.* 1983;1:449–457.
35. Berger TG, Detlefs RL, Donatucci CF. Junctional epidermolysis bullosa, pyloric atresia, and genitourinary disease. *Pediatr Dermatol.* 1986;3:130–134.
36. Bull MJ, Norins AL, Weaver DD, et al. Epidermolysis bullosa-pyloric atresia. *Am J Dis Child.* 1983;137:449–451.
37. Egan N, Ward R, Olmstead M, et al. Junctional epidermolysis bullosa and pyloric atresia in two siblings. *Arch Dermatol.* 1985;121:1186–1188.
38. Rabinowitz BN, Coldwell JG, Jegatheson S. Epidermolysis bullosa and gastrointestinal anomalies. *J Pediatr.* 1979;94:488.
39. Adashi EY, Louis FJ, Vasquez M. An unusual case of epidermolysis hereditaria lethalis with cutaneous scarring and pyloric atresia. *J Pediatr.* 1980;96:443–446.

12
Ophthalmological Aspects of Epidermolysis Bullosa

Scott E. Brodie

Epidermolysis bullosa (EB) is known to affect virtually every epithelial structure in the body.[1] The epithelial surfaces of the eyelids, conjunctiva, and cornea are vulnerable to the disease process, producing a spectrum of ocular difficulties ranging from mild irritation and·corneal abrasion to severe scarring, which may cause permanent loss of vision.[2] This chapter reviews the epithelial structures of the eye, and describes the common patterns of ocular injury seen in the various major subtypes of EB. Surgical and nonsurgical therapies are also discussed.

The Ocular Surface

The skin of the eyelids is reportedly the thinnest in the body. Although the excellent vasculature of the lids permits facile free autografts of skin from elsewhere in the body, it is difficult to obtain a good cosmetic and functional match for lid skin, except by using skin from another eyelid. The inner surface of the eyelids is lined by the conjunctiva, a diaphanous membrane consisting of a nonkeratinizing squamous epithelium overlying a loose substantia propria. The normal conjunctiva is endowed with numerous mucous-secreting goblet cells, as well as accessory lacrimal glands that contribute to the aqueous layer of the tear film. The conjunctiva forms superior and inferior recesses known as fornices, and then is reflected onto the surface of the eyeball. The conjunctival epithelium merges with the epithelial surface of the cornea at the corneal limbus.

Maintenance of the clarity and smoothness of the ocular surface is dependent on normal functioning of the eyelids and normal dispersion of the tear film over the cornea. The tear film's stability on the eye is normally a result of its three-layered structure: adhesion to the eye is enhanced by a mucinous layer secreted by conjunctival goblet cells; the aqueous component, secreted by the lacrimal glands, adheres to hydrophilic moieties in the mucinous layer. Evaporation of the aqueous layer is inhibited by a superficial lipid layer, which is secreted by the meibomian glands at the lid margins and spread across the surface of the tear film with each blink. Disruption of any of these functions can compromise the ocular surface. Depending on the severity of the insult, the eyes may become merely irritated and injected, or may develop varying degrees of breakdown of the corneal epithelium. In severe cases, the unprotected ocular surface may undergo keratinization, precluding its effective function as an optical element of the eye.

EB in the Neonate

The eyes of infants born with EB are generally normal. [One report[3] of widespread focal necrosis throughout the eyes of an infant with junctional EB ("letalis") is difficult to interpret, as the child died at 13 days of age of overwhelming *Pseudomonas* septicemia.] The subsequent course depends strongly on the type of EB, with the most serious ocular sequelae generally occurring in individuals with the most severe cutaneous involvement.

EB Simplex

Patients with EB simplex seldom demonstrate serious ocular problems.[2] An occasional case of recurrent blepharitis has been reported. In one family,[4] a ringlike configuration of fine bullous lesions was seen in the midperiphery of the cornea, in the basal cell layer of the corneal epithelium (superficial to the basement membrane). In one patient, these occasionally broke through to the ocular surface. A mild inferior stromal infiltrate was present.

Junctional EB

Junctional EB typically causes more frequent corneal abrasions, and some stromal scarring is likely with advancing age.[2] A more difficult problem is cicatrization of the eyelids due to repeated blister formation within the lid skin. Small contractures have the effect of rotating the eyelid margin away from the globe (ectropion), preventing normal tear flow and interfering with ocular lubrication. If larger contractures develop, the lids fail to close during blinks, or even on deliberate forced lid closure (lagophthalmos). This can lead to more severe exposure problems, causing corneal surface breakdown. In the most severe cases, the skin over much of the face is replaced by hypertrophic granulation tissue.[5] The eyelids can be foreshortened to the point that they are virtually bound down to the orbital rims (Fig. 12.1). Forced attempts at lid closure merely cause the orbicularis muscles to evert the conjunctiva, causing further exposure of the mucosal surface, but scarcely protect the surface of the globe.

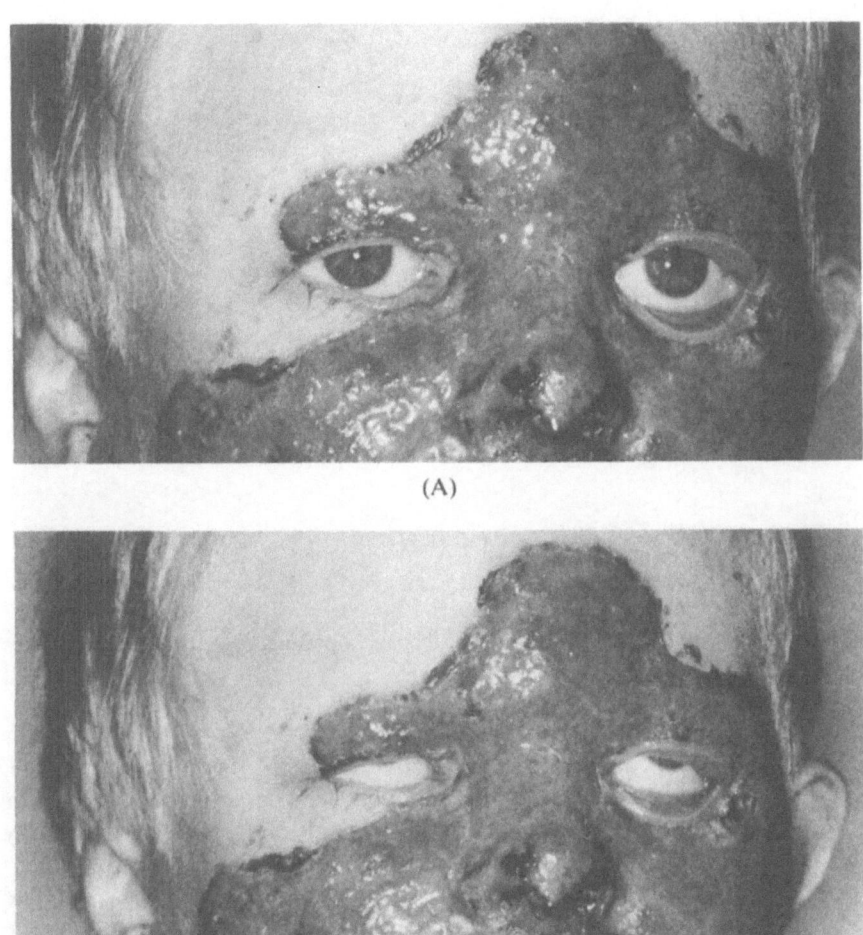

(A)

(B)

FIGURE 12.1. Ectropion and lagophthalmos in a boy with junctional EB. A: Scarring and contracture of the lower eyelids severely limits the mobility of the lids. The left eye is more severely affected than the right eye. B: The eyes cannot be closed, even with forceful contraction of the orbicularis muscles. The corneas rotate up under the upper lids (Bell's phenomenon), but the lid fissures remain open.

Dystrophic EB

Patients with recessive dystrophic EB generally suffer frequent corneal abrasions, particularly during infancy and early childhood.[2,6] Each cycle of abrasion and healing adds only a small increment, but the damage to the cornea is cumulative, and clouding of the corneal stroma may progress to the point of

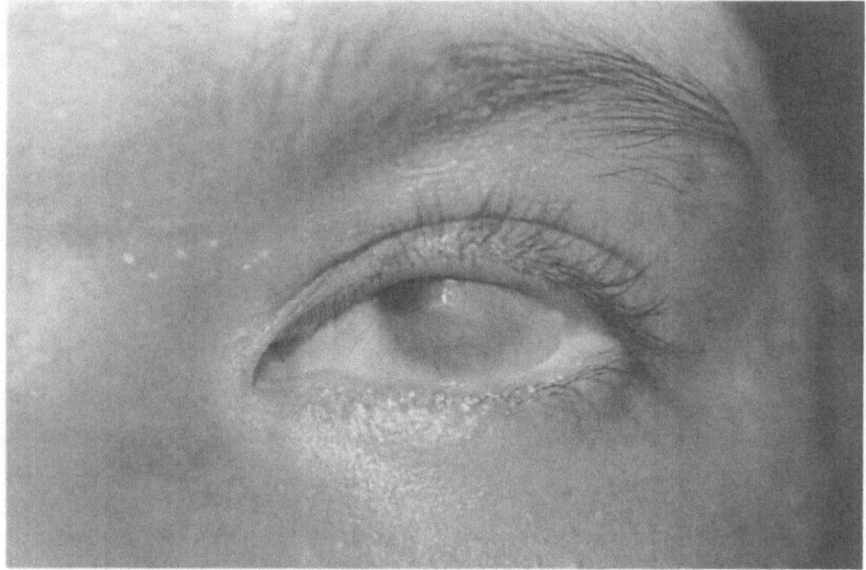

FIGURE 12.2. Symblepharon formation with corneal pannus obscuring the visual axes in a girl with recessive dystrophic EB.

serious visual compromise. The conjunctiva is also at risk in these patients, and they occasionally develop adhesions between the palpebral and bulbar conjunctiva. These may be fairly benign if small and peripheral, but may severely compromise ocular motility, or even prevent the eyelids from opening, if severe. The adhesions may grow onto the surface of the cornea, where they may serve to facilitate the development of a neovascular pannus over the corneal surface. If the pannus covers the visual axis, vision is severely impaired (Fig. 12.2). Systrophic EB patients are also susceptible to cicatricial ectropion and lagophthalmos after repeated formation of blisters on the eyelids.

Few descriptions of ocular findings in patients with dominant dystrophic EB have been reported. As a rule, the findings are similar to those in patients with recessive dystrophic disease, but is generally not as severe.

Intraocular Findings

There have been few reports of intraocular abnormalities in EB patients. In general, intraocular structures are affected only through secondary complications of damage to the ocular surface. In particular, the crystalline lens, although embryologically a purely ectodermal structure, does not seem to be involved in the EB disease process.

Therapy

The mainstay of therapy for the many EB patients with irritation of the ocular surface is the provision of supplementary moisture to supplement the deficient tear film, and compensate for poor lid function. Eyedrops suitable for use as artificial tears are available under many brand names. These may be instilled as frequently as necessary to prevent discomfort. Some patients prefer thicker, more viscous preparations, whereas others may prefer hypotonic drops, which may serve to dilute the concentrated tears found in eyes with poor lid function or reduced tear secretion. Unpreserved formulations may be helpful for patients with sensitivities to preservatives. During sleep, the corneas are frequently protected by Bell's phenomenon, in which the eyeballs spontaneously roll upward under the upper lid, even if the lids are not fully closed. In the absence of an adequate Bell's phenomenon, bland ophthalmic ointments may prove helpful for use at night in severe cases of lagophthalmos. Drying is typically most severe during the winter months, when indoor humidity is very low. An ultrasonic humidifier placed strategically at the bedside, in the playroom, or in the workplace may substantially mitigate the problem.

Corneal abrasions are a recurring problem for many EB patients. Preverbal infants will suddenly cry and tear, often inconsolably, and the abraded eye may become injected. It is important for parents to recognize the problem and obtain definitive treatment promptly after *each* abrasion, in order to minimize progressive scarring of the cornea. The initial examination is often greatly facilitated by instilling a topical anesthetic in the eye. The abrasion can then be highlighted by instilling a drop of fluorescein into the tear film—the abrasion will appear bright yellow under illumination with a blue penlight. If an abrasion is found, a prophylactic antibiotic should be instilled. If the abrasion is large, healing will be facilitated by a pressure-patch dressing. Of course, this must be fashioned using a wrapped head-roll bandage, as taping eye pads to the skin is contraindicated in EB patients. If the patient is photophobic, a cycloplegic eyedrop should also be instilled in the injured eye. If possible, the eye should be examined daily until the corneal epithelial defect has closed completely.

Cicatricial damage to the eyelids is treated supportively with ocular lubricants for as long as possible. If the exposure becomes severe, chronic epithelial defects of the corneal surface will be observed, perhaps most predominant in a horizontal band corresponding to the lid fissure. When ocular discomfort or visual compromise becomes intolerable, it becomes necessary to attempt to restore the normal relationship of the eyelids to the globe surgically. This procedure is best delegated to an experienced ophthalmic plastic surgeon. It is generally necessary to release the contracture of the external lid skin by autograft transplants from an area of uninvolved skin. If no source is available near the eyes, retroauricular skin is a traditional source, but this area is itself frequently damaged in EB. The autografts generally survive well, but genuine improvement of lid position or motility is inconsistently achieved.[7]

Adhesions between the lid and globe (symblepharon) are frequently well tolerated if they are small, and if they do not substantially limit motility of lid or globe. If the restriction becomes severe, surgical lysis may greatly enhance visual or cosmetic function. The procedure may be performed under general or local (retrobulbar) anesthesia. In order to prevent reformation of the adhesions, it may be helpful to place a conformer in the conjunctival sac, along with liberal use of steroid ointment. If the anatomy of the adhesion is fairly simple, it may be possible to completely approximate the cut edges of the conjunctiva with interrupted absorbable sutures, in order to provide an intact epithelial surface as a guard against recurrence of the adhesions.

In severe cases, a vascularized pannus will destroy the optical clarity of the cornea. This membrane can frequently be removed by careful lamellar dissection, with substantial visual improvement.

Refractive errors require special attention in EB patients. Small refractive errors do not require treatment. Larger errors should be corrected, generally with spectacles. A close alliance with a concerned optician is mandatory in order to provide spectacles with large bearing surfaces and an accurate fit, so as not to unduly stress the skin of the nose, temples, or ears. Hard contact lenses are likely to cause frequent corneal abrasions in EB patients, and are therefore contraindicated. In the milder forms of EB, it may be possible to fit a patient with soft contact lenses, provided the patient retains sufficient manual dexterity to manipulate the lenses.

In the most severe cases, generally in dystrophic disease, corneal scars may reduce visual function to bare light perception. In desperate cases, it may be reasonable to consider corneal transplantation, particularly if lid function and tear secretion are relatively intact. Experience in such cases is limited, and the prognosis remains guarded.

References

1. Lin AN and Carter DM, Epidermolysis bullosa: when the skin falls apart. *J Pediatr*. 1989;114:349–355.
2. Gans LA, Eye lesions of epidermolysis bullosa. *Arch Dermatol*. 1988;124:762–764.
3. Aurora AL, Madhavan M, Rao S. Ocular changes in epidermolysis bullosa letalis. *Am J Ophthalmol*. 1975;79:464–470.
4. Granek H, Baden HP. Corneal involvement in epidermolysis bullosa simplex. *Arch Ophthalmol*. 1980;98:469–472.
5. Tabas M, Gibbons 5, and Bauer EA. The mechanobullous diseases. *Dermatol Clin*. 1987;5:123–136.
6. McDonnell PJ, Spalton DJ. The ocular signs and complications of epidermolysis bullosa. *J R Soc Med*. 1988;81:576–578.
7. Hill JC, Rodrigue D. Cicatricial ectropion in epidermolysis bullosa and in congenital icthyosis: its plastic repair. *Can J Ophthalmol*. 1971;6:89–97.

13
Hematologic Problems in Epidermolysis Bullosa

PATRICIA J. GIARDINA and ANDREW N. LIN

The major hematologic problem encountered in epidermolysis bullosa (EB) is anemia. It is multifactorial in origin, and its severity varies with the type of EB. In some cases, the anemia associated with EB can be refractory to therapy. Other hematologic disorders reported in EB include coagulation abnormalities in a small number of patients, and immunological alterations.

Anemia in EB Patients

Anemia in EB patients is multifactorial in origin. Patients may have difficulty maintaining adequate nutritional intake because of painful oral blisters, carious teeth, and in some patients esophageal strictures. As a result, their diet is often deficient in iron, trace metals, and proteins, all of which contribute to the development of anemia. Also, chronic loss of blood and proteins from nonhealing skin and mucosal erosions and the frequent presence of skin infections are additional causes of anemia.

Anemia in EB patients is usually chronic, and patients often present with pallor, fatigue, or increased susceptibility to infections. Because the anemia usually develops gradually, the patient is hemodynamically stable, even with hemoglobin levels as low as 5 to 6 g/dl. However, acute blood loss can occur with esophageal perforation and these patients may present in shock.

As with many other manifestations of EB, the severity of anemia depends on the type of EB. Patients with EB simplex are usually not anemic because the extent of blistering is mild, oral mucosal involvement is infrequent, and cutaneous blood loss is minimal. An exception is severe infantile EB simplex (Dowling-Meara EB simplex), where blistering during infancy can be extensive and patients may be so anemic that transfusion is required.[1] Most patients with the Hallopeau-Siemens type of recessive dystrophic EB have extensive cutaneous blistering, and anemia can often be severe. In the generalized gravis type of junctional EB of Herlitz-Pearson (also called "EB letalis"), severe anemia is often seen, and the hemoglobin in one 12-year-old patient was 2.3 g/dl.[2]

The anemia seen in EB patients is usually microcytic and hypochromic, and is related to iron deficiency. However, anemia of chronic disease (ACD) caused by chronic inflamation associated with skin and mucosal infection may play a contributory role in patients with extensive cutaneous blistering.

Iron Deficiency in EB

Iron deficiency may result from inadequate dietary intake of iron-containing foods or iron salts, and possibly decreased absorptive capacity of the gastrointestinal tract. However, chronic loss of blood through open cutaneous wounds is no doubt the most significant cause. Fine et al. reported low serum iron levels in at least 25% of patients with junctional and recessive dystrophic forms of EB.[3] Loss of serum transferrin and its bound iron from cutaneous wounds may further account for the chronicity of iron deficiency seen in EB patients.[2]

Absent stainable bone marrow iron has been reported in two patients with junctional EB of Herlitz-Pearson.[2] Additional findings in those patients included low normal values for erythrocyte survival, increased plasma iron turnover, increased turnover of albumin, and accelerated plasma iron clearance. Despite "reasonably good" gastrointestinal iron absorption in both these patients, red cell incorporation of radioactive ^{59}Fe was slightly less than normal, findings more typical of anemia of chronic disease than iron deficiency.[2]

Some patients with recessive dystrophic EB have esophageal webs. Such an association may represent coexistence of EB and the Paterson-Brown Kelly syndrome, in which iron deficiency anemia is a prominent feature.[4]

Correction of iron deficiency in EB patients is not always easily accomplished. Patients with esophageal strictures often have difficulty swallowing pills, and will require oral liquid preparations. Unfortunately, most liquid iron preparations have an alcohol base that may be irritating to the gastric mucosa. In addition, different preparations have varying concentrations of elemental iron, and dosage must be carefully calculated. The usual techniques to enhance gastrointestinal absorption of iron supplemnents, such as administration on an "empty" stomach or with juices high in ascorbic acid, may not be practical for the EB patient with gastrointestinal complications. The patient with severe esophageal strictures may have difficulty swallowing even liquid preparations. Oral iron supplements can also worsen existing constipation in the EB patient.

Continuing blood loss through cutaneous wounds may result in persistent iron deficiency despite oral iron supplements if the rate of loss exceeds the rate of absorption or if the anemia is also related to chronic infections. Patients with the Herlitz form of junctional EB can experience persistent iron deficiency despite oral iron supplementation.[3] In those patients in whom serum iron fails to respond to oral iron therapy, parenteral iron should be considered. Because many EB patients with severe anemia are markedly emaciated with decreased muscle mass, intravenous iron therapy would be preferable to intramuscular therapy. The risks of anaphylaxis associated with intravenous iron dextran therapy, however, must be kept in mind and thoroughly explained to patients and their families. Premedication with antihistamines and/or corticosteroids should minimize this risk.[5]

In those patients with extremely low hemoglobin levels in whom hemodynamic compromise is present or imminent, transfusion with packed red blood cells should be considered. Currently, screening of blood products for the detection of donor exposure to hepatitis A, B, and C as well as human immunodeficiency virus (HIV) and human lymphotropic virus (HTLV I) is available in most American blood banks. However, risk of exposure to untected viruses still exists and must be cautiously weighed against the risks of withholding transfusion therapy.

Erythropoietin (EPO) is a glycoprotein produced primarily by the kidney and is the principal factor regulating red blood cell production. Clinical trials have shown that EPO is an effective treatment for anemia associated with end-stage renal disease; such efficacy, however, depends on mobilization of iron stores to sustain red blood cell production.[6] In rheumatoid arthritis, EPO levels are inappropriately low for the degree of anemia detected, and the increment in EPO for a particular hemoglobin level in these patients is less than in patients with uncomplicated iron deficiency. Administration of EPO to rheumatoid arthritis patients has been associated with a rise in hemoglobin level, suggesting that low serum EPO levels may be an indicator of a relative deficiency.[7] Investigators are currently studying the effect of EPO on chronic anemia of inflammatory disease, and these results may provide clues about its possible efficacy in EB.

Anemia of Chronic Disease in EB

Because EB patients experience frequent episodes of purulent infections involving open cutaneous wounds, it is likely that anemia of chronic inflammation and/or infection is an important component of the persistent anemia in many EB patients. The anemia of chronic inflammation and infection is also due to a disturbance in iron metabolism and is characterized by hypoferremia despite iron stores that range from adequate to increased. Anemia of chronic disease (ACD) is most often normocytic (mean cell volume greater than 80 μm^3) and normochromic (mean corpuscular hemoglobin greater than 30 pg); however, it is sometimes hyprochromic and sometimes microcytic. In patients with chronic infections, a reduced mean corpuscular hemoglobin concentration is found in 28% to 50% of patients and in 50% to 100% in those with rheumatoid arthritis.[8]

ACD is usually mild with hematocrits rarely falling below 30%, with subnormal values of serum iron concentration and transferrin saturation in association with evidence of normal or increased iron stores. Transferrin saturations are generally between 5% and 16% as compared with 0% to 16% in iron deficiency, and serum ferritin concentration is usually increased; the latter finding is often most useful in distinguishing ACD from iron deficiency. Decreased serum transferrin level is frequent in ACD but it is neither sensitive nor specific enough to be useful in excluding iron deficiency. Free erythrocyte protoporphyrin values are increased in ACD since the supply of iron to the marrow results in reduced marrow sideroblast iron.

In ACD an impaired flow of iron from tissues to plasma appears to be the major explanation of hypoferremia. It is thought to be related to the defective release of iron from reticuloendothelial cells, particularly from macrophages, but also from hepatocytes and intestinal epithelium. An altered state of iron metabolism also occurs in ACD and is related to defective incorporation of iron into red blood cells.[9,10] It is postulated that liberation of lactoferrin from neutrophils or induction of apoferritin synthesis is the cause of altered iron metabolism. In ACD a modest reduction of red blood cell survival without an adequate compensatory increase in the rate of red cell production also occurs.[8] The reduced survival is probably related to an increased phagocytic activity by activated macrophages. Bone marrow responsiveness is also impaired, probably related to the restricted supply of iron; however, an additional defect in erythropoietin production may also play a part.

It is now recognized that bacterial endotoxins, certain lymphokines, and phagocyte challenges all play some role in the biosynthesis and release of interleukin-1 (IL-1) or leukocyte endogenous mediator (LEM). It is postulated that long-term production of LEM and its release is the common pathogenetic factor in illnesses associated with ACD.

Coagulation Disorders

Several reports have documented coagulation abnormalities in EB patients. Tio[11] quoted European studies showing that certain EB patients have "a shortened whole blood clotting time," and noted shortened clotting times in EB patients and some of their relatives.[11,12] In a separate report, spontaneous episodes of purpura were noted in one of two brothers with dystrophic EB.[13] Hruby and Esterly reported low levels of Hageman factor (factor XII) in two patients with junctional EB.[2] Gedde-Dahl Jr. et al.,[14] however, quoted Schnyder et al.[15] who found "no general coagulation abnormality in 33 Swiss patients comprising 21 of the dominant simplex type, 3 with dominant and 9 with recessive dystrophic type of EB," and showed that no consistent abnormality in parameters of hemostasis was present in 16 Norwegian families with various types of hereditary EB. Furthermore, Fischer and Lodin[16] studied 10 EB patients and failed to confirm "previous reports of shortened blood clotting time," and they did not show any disturbance in the mechanism of coagulation. Two patients with hereditary EB showed normal values for ^{131}I-labeled fibrinogen turnover, and normal values in coagulation analysis.[17] Because the number of reports documenting coagulation abnormalities are small, their clinical significance remains unclear. In general, coagulation abnormalities are not a constant feature of EB.

Immunological Disorders

In EB patients it is well recognized that host defense is compromised through malnutrition and the loss of blood and protein, placing the patient at constant risk of infection.

Altered immunocompetence and depression of host resistance with increased rates of infection and depressed wound healing have been previously reported to occur in states of severe malnutrition.[18]

In a preliminary study Cunningham-Rundles et al[19] demonstrated that mild zinc deficiency in EB patients is negatively associated with major loss of immune response. EB patients with lower serum zinc levels had significantly less immune responses to phytohemagglutin (PHA) than patients with higher zinc levels ($p < .01$). Interestingly, four patients studied with recessive dystrophic EB all had serum zinc levels below 80 μg/dl and none responded in vitro to S. aureus.[19]

Although intake of dietary zinc in EB patients has been reported to be only two thirds of the Recommended Dietary Allowance,[20] extensive trials of dietary zinc supplementation have not been thoroughly investigated.[21]

Natural killer (NK) cell activity has also been reported to be reduced in patients with malnutrition.[22] This activity is important in host defenses against virus, cancer cells, and certain bacteria. Tyring et al. studied NK cell activity in 34 EB patients and noted that the reduction of NK activity was related to the severity of the skin involvement, with recessive dystrophic EB patients having the lowest NK activity.[23] Compared to controls, patients with severe forms of EB had decreased total number of T cells with greater decreases in helper cells, decreased NK cells, and decreased number of T cell interleukin 2 receptors.[24]

Acknowledgments. Supported in part by a General Clinical Research Center grant (M01-RR00102) from the National Institutes of Health to The Rockefeller University Hospital; by a training grant (AR07525) from the National Institutes of Health to the Laboratory for Investigative Dermatology; by contracts AR62269 and AR62270 from the National Institutes of Health to the Laboratory for Investigative Dermatology; by a grant from the Dystrophic Epidermolysis Bullosa Research Association (D.E.B.R.A.) of America, Inc.; and with general support from the Pew Trusts.

References

1. Buchbinder L, Lucky AW, Ballard E, et al. Severe infantile epidermolysis bullosa simplex, Dowling-Meara type. *Arch Dermatol.* 1986;122:190–198.

2. Hruby MA, Esterly NB. Anemia in epidermolysis bullosa letalis. *Am J Dis Child* 1973;125:696–699.
3. Fine J-D, Tamura T, Johnson L. Blood vitamin and trace metal levels in epidermolysis bullosa. *Arch Dermatol.* 1989;125:374–379.
4. Marsden RA, Gowar FJS, MacDonald AF, Main RA. Epidermolysis bullosa of the esophagus with esophageal web formation. *Thorax.* 1974;29:287–295.
5. Auerbach M, Witt D, Toler W, Fierstein M, Lerner RG, Ballard H. Clinical use of the total dose intravenous infusion of iron dextran. *J Lab Clin Med.* 1988;111:566–570.
6. Eschbach JW, Egrie JC, Downing MR, Browne JK, Adamson JW Correction of the anemia of end-stage renal disease with recombinant human erythropoietin: results of a combined phase I and II clinical trial. *N Engl J Med.* 1987;316:73–78.
7. Hochberg MC, Arnold CM, Hogans BB, Spivak JL. Serum immunoreactive erythropoietin in rheumatoid arthritis: impaired response to anemia. *Arthritis Rheum.* 1988;31:1318–1321.
8. Cartwright GE. The anemia of chronic disorders. *Semin Hematol.* 1966;3:351–375.
9. Freireich EJ, Miller A, Emerson CP, Ross JF. The effect of inflammation on the utilization of erythrocyte and transferrin bound radioiron for red cell production. *Blood.* 1957;12:972–983.
10. Finch CA, Deubelbeiss K, Cook JD, et al. Ferrokinetics in man. *Medicine.* 1970;49:17–53.
11. Tio TH. Blood coagulation and genetic observations in epidermolysis bullosa hereditaria (EBH). *Pediatr Indonesia.* 1965;5:499–508.
12. Tio TH, Waardenburg PJ, Vermeulen HJ. Blood coagulation in epidermolysis bullosa hereditaria. *Arch Dermatol.* 1963;88:24–31.
13. Goltz RW, Good RA. Benign hyperglobulinemia purpura: relation to Mikulicz's disese, sicca syndrome, and epidermolysis bullosa dystrophica. *Arch Dermatol.* 1961;83:26–39.
14. Gedde-Dahl Jr T, Niewiarowska M, Sotrmorken H. Parameters of hemostasis in epidermolysis bullosa: absence of significant deviations from normal. *Acta Derm Venereol (Stockh).* 1966;46:436–442.
15. Schnyder UW, Jung EG, Salamon T. Zur Klassifizierung, Histogenetik, Gerinnungsphysiologie und Therapie der hereditaren Epidermolysen. *Arch Klin Exp Derm.* 1964;220:38.
16. Fischer T, Lodin A. Biochemical studies in epidermolysis bullosa. *Acta Derm Venereol (Stockh).* 1966;46:324–337.
17. Blomback B, Carlson LA, Franzen S, Zetterqvist E. Turnover of 131-I-labelled fibrinogen in man: studies in normal subjects, in congenital coagulation factor deficiency states, in liver cirrhosis, in polycythemia vera and in epidermolysis bullosa. *Acta Med Scand.* 1966;179:557–574.
18. Law DK, Dudrick SJ, Abdou NI. Immunocompetence of patients with protein-calorie malnutrition: the effects of nutritional repletion. *Ann Intern Med.* 1973;79:545–550
19. Cunningham-Rundles S, Bockman RS, Lin AN, Giardina PV, Hilgartner MW. Physiological and pharmacological effects of zinc on immune response. *Ann NY Acad. Sci.* 1990;587:113–122.
20. Gruskay DM. Nutritional management in the child with epidermolysis bullosa. *Arch Dermatol.* 1988;124:760–761.

21. Weismann K. Dystrophic epidermolysis bullosa treated unsuccesfully with oral zinc (letter). *Arch Dermatol Res.* 1985;277:404–405.
22. Auer IO, Ziemer E, Sommer H. Immune status in Crohn's disease: V. Decreased in vitro natural killer cell activity in peripheral blood. *Clin Exp Immunol.* 1980; 42:41–49.
23. Tyring SK, Chopra V, Johnson L, Fine J-D. Natural killer cell activity is reduced in patients with severe forms of inherited epidermolysis bullosa. *Arch Dermatol.* 1989;125:797–800.
24. Chopra V, Tyring SK, Johnson L, Fine J-D. Peripheral blood mononuclear cell subsets in patients with severe inherited forms of epidermolysis bullosa. *Arch Dermatol.* 1992;128:201–209.

14
Dental Aspects of Epidermolysis Bullosa

John J. Putnam and George. W. Sferra, Jr.

Because the skin and teeth are both ectodermal in origin, it is not surprising they are similarly affected in many pathologic processes. This is well illustrated in epidermolysis bullosa (EB), a heterogeneous group of genetic disorders in which blistering of the skin and mucosa occur as a result of minor trauma.[1-4] In many patients, chewing and eating may cause formation of painful oral blisters that severely compromise nutritional intake. In addition, primary dental abnormalities such as enamel defects predispose patients to caries development. In severely affected patients crippling deformities of the hands make it almost impossible to maintain adequate oral hygeine. In this chapter, we review the unique spectrum of intraoral problems faced by EB patients and discuss management guidelines.

Classification of EB

Because EB is a heterogeneous group of diseases, the nature and severity of intraoral involvement depends on the type of EB. Based on the precise ultrastructural level at which blisters occur, EB is classified into three major types. EB simplex is characterized by intraepithelial blisters and is transmitted as an autosomal dominant trait. Junctional EB is an autosomal recessive condition characterized by blister formation at the level of lamina lucida, an electron-lucent zone located between the basal cell plasma membrane and the lamina densa. The dystrophic type is further classified into dominant or recessive forms, both of which are characterized by blister formation below the lamina densa. Further subclassification based primarily on clinical features has resulted in approximately 16 subtypes[1-4] and is discussed in detail elsewhere in this volume. For the purpose of reviewing intraoral pathology, it is sufficient to confine our classification to one of the three major types.

Anatomy and Embryology of the Tooth

The tooth consists of three distinct types of tissue. Enamel is a layer of hard, acellular, crystalline material that covers the crown, or exposed portion of the tooth. Most discussion of "dentition" in fact refers to the enamel. Just beneath the enamel is the dentin, a tubular structure consisting of specialized cells (odontoblasts) and intercellular substance that together make up the bulk of the tooth. Covering the root of the tooth is a mineralized dental tissue called cementum, which along with collagen fibers form the attachment apparatus of the tooth to the surrounding structures.

Histodifferentiaton of the tooth begins when the ectodermal lining of the embryonic oral cavity begins to proliferate over the area where the dental arches will form. At approximately 6 weeks of fetal life, buds begin to develop from this lining. Each tooth bud consists of an enamel organ of ectodermal origin, plus a dental papilla and a dental sac both derived from the mesenchyme.[5]

The cells of the enamel organ are connected to one another by desmosomes.[6-8] Approximately 10 weeks after initiation of tooth bud formation, the ectodermal portion of the bud resembles a bell whose mouth opens away from the primitive oral cavity, the so-called bell stage. Cells lining the inner aspect of this epithelial bell are derived from the basal cell layer of the oral epithelium, and are called the inner enamel epithelium. They are separated from the connective tissue of the dental papilla by a basement membrane. Before differentiation of these cells, hemidesmosomes are visible.[8,9] Subjacent to the basement membrane is a zone containing argyrophilic fibers and the cytoplasmic processes of the mesenchymal cells of the dental papilla. Cells of the inner enamel epithelium differentiate into ameloblasts. This triggers differentiation of adjacent mesenchymal cells into odontoblasts. The odontoblasts immediately begin to produce dentin, which in turn stimulates the ameloblasts to initiate enamel formation.[10,11]

The skin and oral mucosa are both ectodermal in origin and share structural similarities. They both consist of stratified squamous epithelium and a subjacent layer of connective tissue with a rete ridge configuration. In the oral mucosa the connective tissue component is called the lamina propria and is analogous to the dermis or corium of the skin. Oral epithelium over the gingiva and hard palate is keratinized, but remains nonkeratinized over the inside of the cheek, faucal and sublingual areas. Keratinized portions consist of multiple layers analogous to the basal, spinous, granular, and cornified layers of the skin. Also, hemidesmosomal attachments are visible between basal cells and the underlying lamina propria, and desmosomes are present between basal cells.[12,13] In addition, the lamina propria is dense and is firmly bound down to the underlying periosteum. In contrast, the lamina propria in nonkeratinized portions of the oral mucsoa is thin and loose and may be highly elastic.[13]

Spectrum of Intraoral Pathology seen in EB Patients

EB Simplex

Primary malformation of the teeth has not been observed in EB simplex,[1,3,4,14-16] and the teeth appear normal.[1,4,15,16] Likewise, the oral mucosa appears normal except for the occasional blister, which often heals within several days. As in the skin, mucosal bullae heal without scar formation.[1,4,15,16] There is neither ankyloglossia nor is there adhesion of the mucobuccal fold. Patients tolerate soft tissue manipulation, although mucosal blistenng is always a possibility.

Junctional EB

Enamel dysplasia is commonly seen in junctional EB.[2,4,17,18] This is due to a deranged relationship between the ameloblasts of the epithelial enamel organ and the odontoblasts of the dental papilla.[19-21] It appears that ameloblasts develop normally until dentin is laid down. A small amount of enamel matrix is deposited but premature squamous metaplasia of the ameloblasts follows. The timing of this event occurs at a similar point in the development of all involved teeth.[21]

Histologic studies of unerupted teeth obtained at autopsy from patients with junctional EB reveal not only severe reduction of enamel formation, but also the presence of globules, which appear throughout the residual stellate reticulum and enamel organ. These globules stain similar to enamel with hematoxylin and eosin. Dentin formation, however, is unaffected.[4,18-21] These findings were corroborated in a study using tetracycline staining to measure the growth rate of enamel and dentin in teeth taken from patients with junctional EB. The rate of enamel formation was greatly reduced but the dentin formation was unaffected. Globules were again noted and tetracycline staining of the calcified globules was again similar to that of enamel.[22]

Vacuolization occurs at the basal end of the ameloblasts and is due to a split between the ameloblasts and the odontoblasts.[19,21,22] This is analogous with cutaneous blistering, which occurs at the level of the lamina lucida.[2,23,24]

Clinical examination of these patients will show that oral bullae form readily and may be numerous, but healing generally occurs without scarring.[1,2,4] Studies of bullae found in the oral mucosa of junctional EB patients indicate the level of separation to be identical to that of bullae found in skin.[12] The teeth show definite enamel dysplasia and will appear denuded of enamnel[2,4,17,18] (Fig. 14.1). Ankyloglossia does not occur, and the mucobuccal fold shows neither adherence nor obliteration. Severe perioral erosions can be seen on the face.

Dystrophic EB

In dystrophic EB intraoral blistering often leads to severe mucosal scarring, making examination and treatment of the teeth almost impossible for the dentist and patient.[2,4,14-16,25-27] Routine oral hygiene is greatly compromised. Frequent and severe lesions are noted in all areas of the oral mucosa. The scarring that quickly ensues soon results in the adhesion of the adjacent

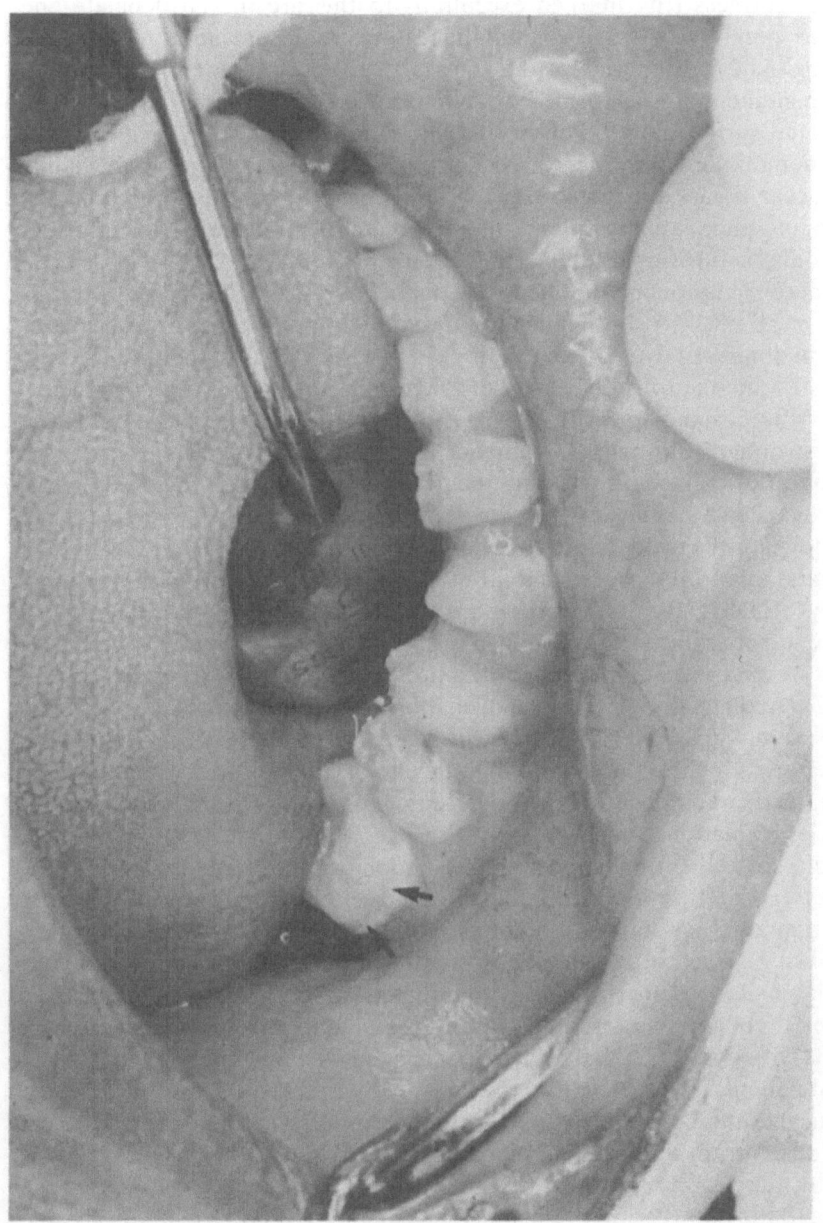

FIGURE 14.1. Junctional EB. Note enamel dysplasia of anterior and posterior teeth. Such dysplasia typically involves the entire dentition. Enamel is absent on crown of tooth above cementoenamel junction (*arrows*). Note also ragged occlusal surfaces and incisal edges with abnormal "wear facets."

mucosal surfaces (the marked exceptions to this are the hard palate and attached gingiva). The labial and buccal vestibule are soon obliterated. Ankyloglossia is observed as the tongue fuses to the floor of the mouth. Permanent indentations formed by an impression of the mandibular teeth on the lingual surface may be observed. Microstomia eventually ensues as the labial commissure becomes fused and the general mobility of the labial and buccal tissues decreases. Blisters and scarring can also occur in the esophagus, and patients often suffer esophageal strictures, which further compromises nutritional intake (Fig. 14.2).

Numerous authors have stated that enamel dysplasia occurs in dystrophic EB,[2,14,17,19,26,28–30] but clinically normal dental structures have been observed in dominant dystrophic EB,[1,2,4,17,28,31] in which cutaneous blistering appears to be due to a deficiency of anchoring fibrils which may be defective.[32,33] Decayed or possibly dysplastic teeth have been described in recessive dystrophic EB in which cutaneous blistering appears to result from the dissolution of collagen fibers and anchoring fibrils through increased fibroblast collagenase activity.[2,34] However, it is still unclear whether the severe breakdown of the teeth, which is commonly observed, is due to the defects in the dental structures or the inability of patients to perform even the most cursory oral hygiene.[1,4] Furthermore, in recessive dystrophic EB-inversa where cutaneous blisters are confined to specific regions of the body, the teeth appear normal although decayed despite the fact that the dermal defect is caused by collagenolysis indistinguishable from that seen where teeth are more severely involved.[2,35] It must be remembered that soft starchy foods are preferred by these patients to minimize the trauma of eating and deglutination, further complicating oral cleansing and creating a preferred medium for caries formation.

Studies of cementum in teeth taken from patients with dystrophic EB reveal large defects in both cellular and acellular cementum.[36] Cellular cementum displays increased thickness, large lacuna, or large, irregular, cavernlike defects not resembling normal lacuna. Acellular cementum contains large dark defects that are attributed to the presence of necrotic Sharpey's (collagen) fibers. Radiographic examination reveals cementum of patients with dystrophic EB to be hypocalcified when compared with that of normal patients.[36]

Clinical examinations of patients with dystrophic forms of EB often reveal numerous intraoral blisters and mucosal scarring.[1,4,14–16,25–27,37] This leads to ankyloglossia and adherence of the buccal and alveolar mucosa leading to the obliteration of the mucobuccal fold. Depending on the specific type of dystrophic EB, the teeth have been described as dysplastic, but they are almost always severely carious. This occurs because of extremely poor oral hygiene and destructively soft diets. Oral tissues such as the mucosa and gingiva appear angry red and swollen. In addition, the basically immovable tongue and mucobuccal fold are unable to perform their usual supportive

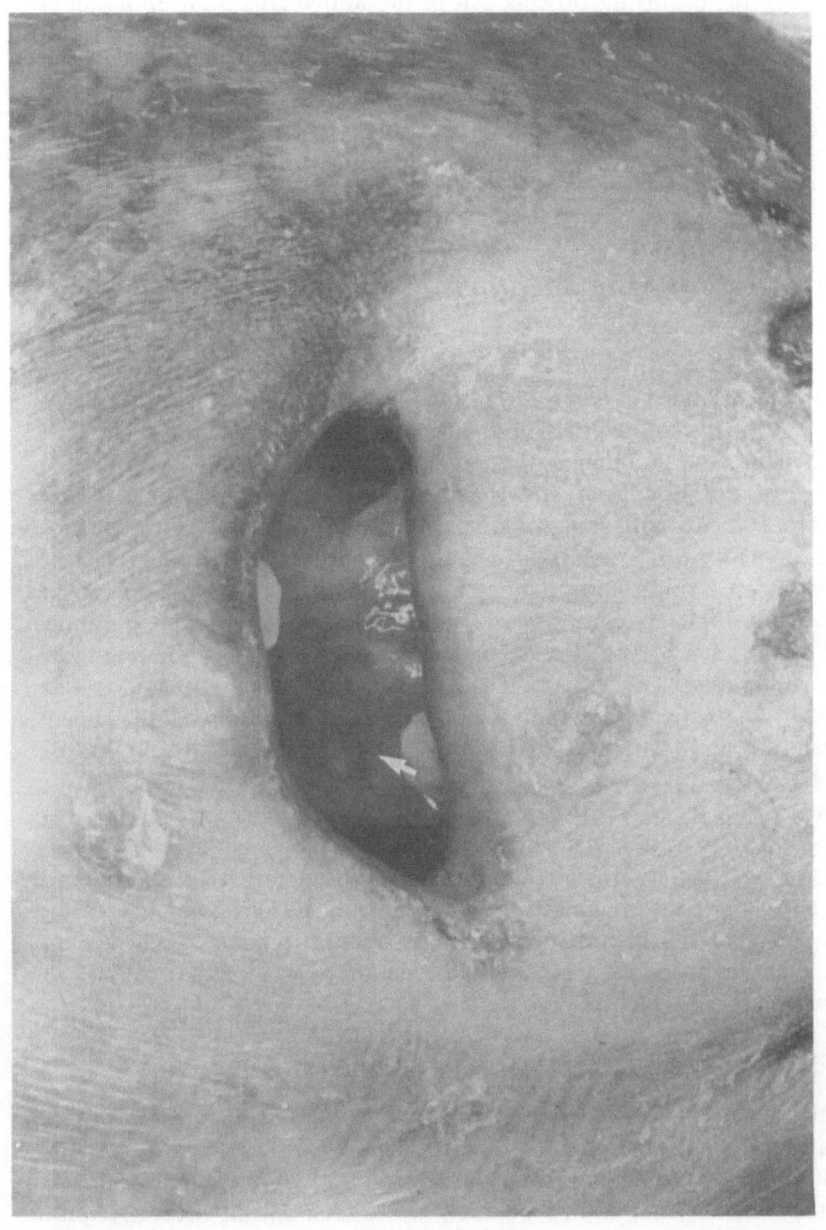

FIGURE 14.2. Recessive dystrophic EB. Mouth is fully opened and tongue is maximally extended, illustrating severe microstomia and ankyloglossia due to recurrent scarring of intraoral mucosa. Erosions are present on ventral surface of tongue (*arrow*).

functions in the cleansing process. All of the above create an optimum environment for the progression of rampant caries.

Decreased salivary flow rate, either due to obstructive scarring of the salivary ducts or inherent structural abnormalities of the salivary glands, has been suggested as a possible cause of rampant caries in patients with dystrophic Eb. However, studies have shown no demonstrable decrease in salivary flow rate or function in these patients.[38]

Other Intraoral Manifestations

Caries

In general, the pattern of caries formation in patients with EB simplex follows that of the general populace. These patients are subject to and react to the same environmental influences that affect normal individuals.

It is with the junctional and the dystrophic types that the real problems arise. Patients with junctional EB are likely to have defectively formed enamel to begin with, which in turn can predispose to rampant dental caries. In dystrophic EB this is compounded by the results of severe mucosal blisters and scarring. First, hygiene suffers seriously as the tongue and the mucobuccal fold of the lips and cheeks becomes adherent. Second, the oral tissues are so vulnerable to trauma that simple brushing is painful and is often avoided by the patient. Brushing is not only painful but also contributes to the blistering and scarring that the tongue and mucobuccal fold undergo (Fig. 14.3).

Patients with recessive dystrophic EB often experience severe cutaneous scarring, so that mitten deformities of the hands often develop by early childhood, making it virtually impossible to hold any type of device to clean the teeth. Thus, at an early age these patients develop huge carious lesions. As with the skin lesions, however, dental pain is rarely a major feature whether from pulp exposures or dental abscesses that follow. The exact reason for this lack of pain remains unknown.

Orthodontic

EB patients are subject to all the usual developmental problems that result in disparate arch size in relation to each other that any individual might experience. In addition, however, the large carious lesions present in the posterior teeth cause the teeth to change their position in the arch and in effect precipitate the same problems that the premature loss of deciduous teeth would. EB patients are not good candidates for intraoral placement of orthodontic bands, brackets, wires, or even the most simple removable devices. Such devices would result in additional blistering and scarring. With close monitoring orthodontic treatment could be initiated for the EB simplex patient.

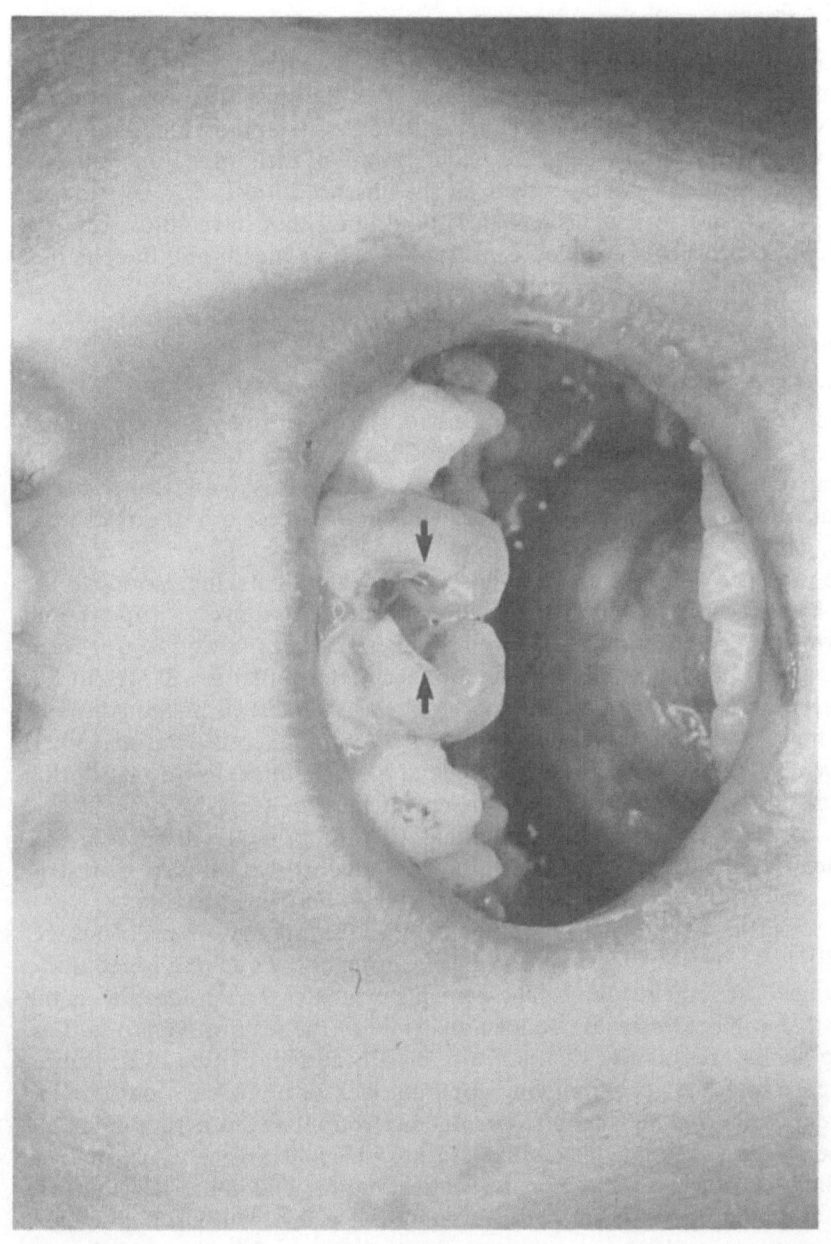

FIGURE 14.3. Recessive dystrophic EB. Marked destruction of medial surfaces of maxillary central incisors (*arrows*) due to severe caries. These teeth do not show enamel dysplasia. Destruction shown is due entirely to caries (see text).

Social Aspects

EB patients must contend with the disfigurement that the blistering and scarring have on the face itself as well as with the unsightly appearance of grossly carious anterior teeth, missing anterior teeth, and malposed anterior teeth. On probing, EB patients are acutely aware of their appearance and the visual effect caused by carious teeth or the absence of teeth.[4,39] By the time they have reached their teens and early adulthood they have adjusted to the functional aspects of a crippled dentition. A main concern and the one that they can do little or nothing about is their appearance.

Restorative

Search of the literature turns up little on this subject other than that restorative procedures were performed with the use of silver amalgam, stainless steel crowns, and bonding.[4,14,15,30] There are no contraindications to restorative procedures.[4,30,39] Microstomia, ankyloglossia, and adherence of the mucobuccal fold resulting in decidedly limited access is the restricting factor. The soft tissues are also painful to touch.

The presence of EB does not by itself imply any contraindications to the use of local anesthesia.[4,14,16,27,39,40] Restorative procedures can and should be performed on EB patients. There are differences in reaction to treatment according to the type of EB. In general, EB simplex patients will present few problems for the restorative dentist.[1,4,14,16] As with all EB patients the soft tissue must be treated carefully and delicately. Special consideration should be given to gentle retraction. Wherever possible, finger positions during instrumentation should be on hard tissues such as the teeth.

The teeth of patients with junctional EB are generally dysplastic and denuded of enamel.[4,18-21] If they are to be touched with fingers or instruments, they will be sensitive and local anesthesia may be necessary.

It is with the patient with dystrophic EB that the most severe problems will arise.[4,14-16,25-27,37,40] Some form of blistering and sloughing is certain to follow restorative procedures. The dentist's estimate of such sequelae is the factor that will determine the scope and extent of the restorative procedures. To the dentist, restorative dentistry for the EB patient can be a frustrating experience with the accompanying apparent lack of home care and ensuing recurrent caries. Dentists tend to become perfectionists but here is definitely not the place to exercise this quality. Rather, this is the place to use innovative skills employing all of the newer techniques and materials that are constantly coming to the market, to name but a few dentinal and enamel bonding agents, sealants, and the glass ionomers. Careful and gentle handling and manipulation of the soft tissue, as noted before, is paramount to all restorative procedures.

Prevention

This area cannot be stressed too often or too emphatically. Everyone must get involved—patient, parents, nutritionist, social worker, physician, and dentist. It cannot begin too early and there should be no let-up. Deciduous teeth and some permanent teeth will calcify in utero. If fluoride is not added to the local water supply it should be given to the EB infant in the form of vitamin supplements. EB infants should be seen by the dentist, preferably a pedodontist, as soon as possible. Sealants should be placed in posterior teeth where indicated and again as soon as possible. The dentist must be told in advance of the first appointment that he will be dealing with an EB patient and the exact classification of EB. Parents must be counseled as to preventive measures and must be instructed as to the actual brushing procedure itself. When the child is old enough and responsible enough not to swallow the medication inadvertently, topical application of fluoride should be initiated. The use of antiplaque agents, fluoride rinses, and fluoride toothpastes should also be instituted at an early age, due consideration being given to the age of the patient and his ability not to swallow the medication. The preventive effort is a total effort and will need constant reinforcement.

Dental Education

EB is certainly an uncommon condition and will never be a prominent part of a dental practice. However, it should be covered as part of the student curriculum in dental schools. Students must be aware that this is not a communicable disease, that they as dentists are at no risk when treating these patients, that patients can be helped if but to a limited extent, and that there will be sequelae to any treatment and how important it is to get these patients into a regular, monitored preventive program.

From the beginning, EB patients themselves should be made aware of the problems that can and will occur with their teeth and oral structures. They must realize that theirs is the most important role in the preventive process; that they are the ones with the most to lose. EB as we know it is a difficult entity at best to cope with in daily life. The more cooperation between all parties, the better will be the resolution. Thus, at some point, an in-depth consultation should occur among patient, parents, and dental practitioner in order to consider carefully all the facets and the probable course of this condition.

EB is a rare disorder that can be intimidating to the patient and dental practitioner confronted with it for the first time. Through education, coverage in the dental curriculum, and the use of standard reference books, such intimidation hopefully will disappear.

References

1. Gorlin RJ. Epidermolysis bullosa. *Oral Surg.* 1971;32:760–766.
2. Gedde-Dahl Jr T, Anton-Lamprecht I. Epidermolysis bullosa. In: Emery AEH, Rimion DL, eds. *Principles and Practice of Medical Genetics.* Edinburgh: Churchill-Livingstone; 1983:672-687.

3. Lin AN, Carter DM. Epidermolysis bullosa: when the skin falls apart. *J Pediatr.* 1989;114:349–355.

4. Crawford EG, Burkes Jr EJ, Briggaman RA. Hereditary epidermolysis bullosa: oral manifestations and dental therapy. *Oral Surg.* 1976;42:490–500.

5. Sharawy M, Bhussrt RB. Development and growth of teeth. In: Bhaskar SN, eds. *Orban's Oral Histology and Embryology.* St. Louis: CV Mosby; 1986:24–36.

6. Mathiessen ME, Molloary K. Cell junctions of the human enamel organ. *Z Zellforsch Mikrosk Anat.* 1973;146:69–81.

7. Pannese E. Observation on the ultrastructure of the enamel organ III. Internal and external enamel epithelium. *J Ultrastruct Res.* 1962;6:186–204.

8. Reith EJ. The stages of amelogenesis as observed in molar teeth of young rats. *J Ultrastruct Res.* 1970;30:111–151.

9. Preis FG. Epidermolysis bullosa simplex: a case in which tooth re-implantation was unsuccessful. *Birth Defects: Original Article Series.* 1971;VII:276.

10. Noble HW. Electron microscopy of human developing dentin. *Arch Oral Biol.* 1962;7:395–399.

11. Sharawy M, Jaeger JA. Enamel. In: Bhaskar SN, eds. *Orban's Oral Histology and Embryology.* St. Louis: CV Mosby; 1986:71–100.

12. Arwill T, Bergenholtz A, Thilander H. Epidermolysis bullosa hereditaria. V: The ultrastructure of oral mucsoa and skin in four cases of the letalis form. *Acta Pathol Microbiol Scand.* 1968;74:311–324.

13. Stern IB. Oral mucous membrane. In: Bhaskar SN, eds. *Orban's Oral Histology and Embryology.* St. Louis: CV Mosby; 1986:253–293.

14. Boyer EH, Owens RH. Epidermolysis bullosa: a rare disease of dental interest. *Oral Surg Oral Med Oral Pathol.* 1961;14:1170–1177.

15. Howden EF, Oldenburg TR. Epidermolysis bullosa dystrophica: report of two cases. *J Am Dental Assoc.* 1972;85:1113–1118.

16. Gormley JW, Schow CE. Epidermolysis bullosa and associated problems in surgical treatment. *J Oral Surg.* 1976;34:45–52.

17. Cooper, TW, Bauer EA. Epidermolysis bullosa: a review. *Pediatr Dermatol.* 1984;1:181–188.

18. Koshiba H, Kimura O., Nakata M. A clinical and histologic observation of enamel hypoplasia in a case of epidermolysis bullosa hereditaria. *Oral Surg.* 1977;43:585–590.

19. Arwill T, Bergenholtz A, Olsson 0. Epidermolysis bullosa hereditaria. III. A histologica study of changes in teeth in the polydysplastic dystrophic and lethal forrns. *Oral Surg Oral Med Oral Pathol.* 1965;19:723–744.

20. Brain EB, Wigglesworth JS. Developing teeth in epidermolysis bullosa hereditaria letalis: a histological study. *Br Dental J.* 1968;124:255–260.

21. Gardner DG, Hudson CD. The disturbances in odontogenesis in epidermolysis bullosa hereditaria letalis. *Oral Surg.* 1975;40:483–493.

22. Arwill T, Bergenholtz A. Epidermolysis bullosa hereditaria. VIII. Growth rate of the dentin in deciduous teeth in epidermolysis bullosa revealed by tetracycline lines. *Arch Oral Biol.* 1968;13:819–822.

23. Pearson RW. Studies of the pathogenesis of epidermolysis bullosa. *J Invest Dermatol.* 1962;39:551–575.

24. Hashimoto I, Gedde-Dahl Jr T, Schnyder UW, Anton-Lamprecht I. Ultrastructural studies in epidermolysis bullosa hereditaria IV. Recessive dystrophic types with junctional blistering (Infantile or Herlitz-Pearson type and adult type). *Arch Dermatol Res.* 1976;257:17–32.

25. Haas CD. Epidermolysis bullosa dystrophica: report of a case. *Oral Surg Oral Med Oral Pathol.* 1968;26:291–295.
26. Gisanti JS. Oral nodular excrescences in epidermolysis bullosa. *Oral Surg.* 1975; 40:385–390.
27. Morgan WC. Dental and anesthetic management of epidermolysis bullosa: a new approach. *Oral Surg.* 1975;40:732–735.
28. Haber RM, Hana W, Ramsay CA, Boxall LBH. Hereditary epidermolysis bullosa. *J Am Acad Dermatol.* 1985;13:252–278.
29. Fine J-D. Epidermolysis bullosa: clinical aspects, pathology, and recent advances in research. *Int J Dermatol.* 1986;25:143–157.
30. Wright JT. Epidermolysis bullosa: dental and anesthetic management of two cases. *Oral Surg Oral Med Oral Pathol.* 1984;57:155–157.
31. Tabas M, Gibbons S, Bauer EA. The mechanobullous diseases. *Dermatol Clin.* 1987;5:123–136.
32. Hashimoto I, Anton-Lamprecht I, Gedde-Dahl Jr T, Schnyder UW. Ultrastructural studies in epidermolysis bullosa hereditaria. I. Dominant dystrophic type of Pasini. *Arch Dermatol Res.* 1975;252:167–178.
33. Hashimoto I, Gedde-Dahl Jr T, Schnyder UW, Anton-Lamprecht I. Ultrastructural studies in epidermolysis bullosa hereditaria. II. Dominant dystrophic type of Cockayne and Touraine. *Arch Dermatol Res.* 1976;255:285–295.
34. Valle K-J, Bauer EA. Enhanced biosynthesis of human skin collagenase in fibroblast cultures from recessive dystrophic epidermolysis bullosa. *J Clin Invest.* 1980; 66:176.
35. Hashimoto I, Schnyder UW, Anton-Lamprecht I, Gedde-Dahl Jr T, Ward S. Ultrastructural studies in epidermolysis bullosa hereditaria III. Recessive dystrophic types with dermolytic blistering (Hallopeau-Siemens types and inverse type). *Arch Dermatol Res.* 1976;256:137-150.
36. Hitchin AD. The defects of cementum in epidermolysis bullosa dystrophica. *Br Dental J.* 1973;135:437–442.
37. Block MS, Gross BD. Epidermolysis bullosa dystrophica recessive: oral surgery and anesthetic considerations. *J. Oral Maxillofacial Surg.* 1982;40:753–758.
38. Wright JT, et al. Salivary gland function of persons with hereditary epidermolysis bullosa. *Oral Surg Oral Med Oral Pathol.* 1991;71:553–554.
39. Putnam JJ, Sferra G, Lin AN, Carter DM. Junctional epidermolysis bullosa: report of a case with treatment considerations. Submitted.
40. Winstock D. Oral aspects of epidermolysis bullosa. *Br J Dermatol.* 1962;74:431–438.

15
Otorhinolaryngologic Aspects of Epidermolysis Bullosa

Andrew N. Lin, Shelley R. Berson, and Robert F. Ward

Although epidermolysis bullosa (EB) affects mainly the keratinizing stratified squamous epithelium of the skin, virtually any mucosal surface can be involved.[1] This is well illustrated by cases in which blisters occur in the larynx. Except for the true vocal cords and parts of the epiglottis, the larynx is covered with pseudo-stratified columnar epithelium containing goblet cells. And yet, blister formation has been noted in almost all parts of the larynx, sometimes with serious consequences. In general, it appears that the supraglottic region including the epiglottis, arytenoids, and aryepiglottic folds are most often affected. Respiratory arrest due to obstructing laryngeal blisters can occur with alarming suddenness, and death has been reported. Any patient with respiratory symptoms requires careful laryngeal assessment to formulate an individualized treatment plan. Fortunately, laryngeal involvement is rare, and a search of the English literature revealed only 10 cases, including one we had managed ourselves.[2] We are aware of an additional case managed by others (Scott Schaeffer, M.D., personal communication). In this chapter, we review these cases and discuss guidelines in problem recognition and management.

Laryngeal Involvement

Clinical features of these 11 cases are summarized in Table 15.1. Seven of these patients had junctional EB[2-6,6a] (Scott Schaeffer, M.D., personal communication), whereas two others had dystrophic EB.[7,8] One case had "probable dystrophic EB"[9] and the type was not specified in another patient.[10] In one additional patient with Dowling-Meara EB simplex, "severe hoarseness" was noted, but no clinical details were given.[11]

In most cases, onset of respiratory symptoms occurred very early in life, ranging from the time of birth to childhood. Most patients presented with hoarseness or stridor. Laryngoscopy revealed abnormal findings in all 11 patients, uncovering lesions in virtually all parts of the larynx. These include blisters, ulcerations, mucosal inflammation, and scarring (Fig. 15.1).

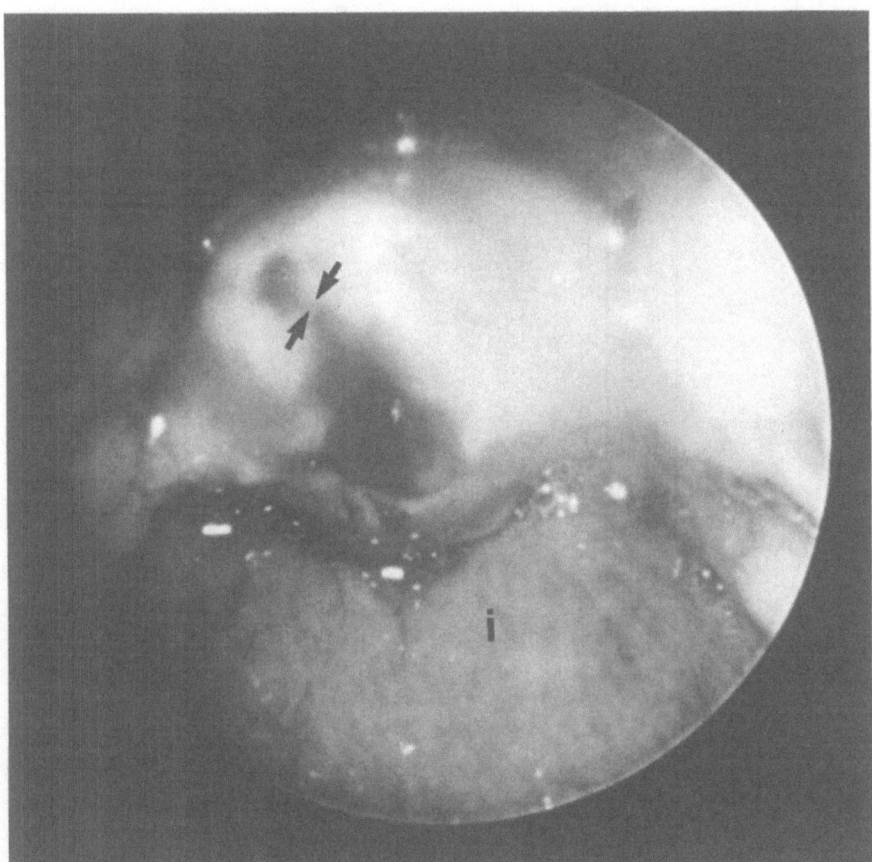

FIGURE 15.1. Photograph taken at direct laryngoscopy, showing supraglottic narrowing (*arrows*) caused by recurrent blistering and scarring in a 27-month-old patient with junctional EB ("i," introitus to esophagus).

Blistering and stenosis could also extend into the trachea[6,7]; however, it appears that tracheal involvement has been in the subglotttic region and not in the distal trachea. In one patient with letalis junctional EB,[5,6a] airway compromise was thought to be due mainly to cyst formation in the aryepiglottic folds. These cysts were believed to result from obstruction of seromucinous glands by squamous metaplastic epithelium, a mechanism distinct from the way cutaneous blisters resulted from mechanical trauma. Squamous metaplasia of laryngeal mucosa with invasion of yeast forms was noted in one other patient with letalis junctional EB, but respiratory distress was not mentioned.[12]

X-ray films of the neck revealed abnormal findings in three of five patients in whom it was done, showing a narrowed trachea and sublottic space. In the

TABLE 15.1. Laryngeal involvement reported in 11 EB Patients.

Author	Age/sex	Type of EB	Initial symptom (age of onset)	Laryngoscopy findings	X-ray findings	Treatment	Outcome
Berson et al.[2]	29 months-male	JEB letalis	Stridor, cyanosis, feeding difficulty (1 month)	Supraglottic stenosis Normal vocal cords	Normal	Tracheotomy	Doing well
Glossop et al.[5], Davies and Atherton[6a]	29 months-male	JEB letalis	Mild stridor (15 months)	Narrow supraglottis, Cyst aryepiglottic fold Mucosal inflammation	Narrow trachea	Dilatation of larynx	GI bleed, death
Kenna and Stool[3]	11 months-male	Benign JEB	Stridor (at birth)	Ulcer of supraglottis, Postcricoid bulla, Web	Narrow sub-glottic space	Tracheotomy	Recurrent symptoms Unsuccessful decannulation
Paller et al.[4]	14 years-female	Benign JEB	Hoarseness (infancy)	Thick, scarred vocal cords Tracheal stenosis	Not reported	Tracheotomy Vocal cord stripping	Improved
Paller et al.[4]	25 years-male	Benign JEB	Hoarseness (childhood)	"Blisters and scars"	Not reported	Vocal rest	Resolution of symptoms
Gonzalez and Roth[6]	2 months-male	JEB	Hoarse cry, stridor (29 days)	Bullae in epiglottis, glottis, trachea	Not reported	Tracheotomy	Death from hemoptysis

Author	Age/sex	Type of EB	Initial symptom (age of onset)	Laryngoscopy findings	X-ray findings	Treatment	Outcome
(Scott Schaeffer, M.D.,) personal communication	3 years-male	JEB	Stridor (16 months)	Left vocal cord paralysis Laryngeal web	Normal	Laser Tracheotomy	Doing well
Thompson et al.[7]	3 weeks-male	Dystrophic	Stridor, retractions (3 weeks)	Narrow glottis Interarytenoid and tracheal vesicles	Not reported	Tracheotomy	Resolution of symptoms Decannulation
Ramadass and Thangavelu[8]	5 years-male	Dystrophic	Noisy breathing Voice change (5 years)	Cicatricial stenosis at anterior commissure and interarytenoid region Irregular margin of vocal cords	Normal neck films	Observation	"Under observation"
Shackelford et al.[9]	6 months-male	"Probable dystrophic"	Stridor (4 months)	Edematous supraglottis Edematous subglottic region with inflammatory membrane Normal vocal cord	Subglottic narrowing	Suction	Death from hemoptysis
Cohen et al.[10]	8 years-male	Not specified	"Loss of vocal power" (6 months)	Subglottic edema Web at cordal level	Not reported	Tracheotomy	Stenotic larynx in spite of web incision and stenting

patient with a normal x-ray examination of the neck,[8] indirect as well as direct laryngoscopy revealed cicatricial stenosis at the anterior commissure and interarytenoid region. The lateral and anteroposterior neck films appear to be particularly valuable in demonstrating subglottic involvement. The region of the larynx is not well visualized by this radiologic evaluation.

Outcome varied greatly, even among the seven patients who underwent tracheotomy. Among this group, two were successfully decannulated within 18 days[7] and after 6 months.[4] In another patient, marked blister formation occurred around the tracheotomy tube, and repeated attempts at decannulation within 12 months were unsuccessful.[3] Another patient experienced repeated laryngeal blockage during the 12 years after tracheotomy, and required multiple incisions of web and scar tissues.[10] Two patients were "doing well"[2] (Scott Schaeffer, M.D., personal communication), but another died of postoperative sepsis after tracheotomy.[6]

Other ENT Complications

External auditory canal stricture resulted in conductive hearing loss in a 24-year-old woman with "EB simplex."[13] Favorable results followed scar excision, bony canal enlargement, and split-thickness skin graft. Electron microscopic evidence in support of EB simplex was not presented. Two of her siblings also had EB, but neither parent was affected, suggesting her condition was inherited as an autosomal recessive trait. Because EB simplex is generally inherited as an autosomal dominant disorder, it is unclear on what basis that patient was felt to have EB simplex.

One 4-year-old boy with junctional EB developed gradual stenosis of the nares and collapse of the anterior nose caused by extensive facial erosions.[14] Conventional skin grafting and nasal dilatation resulted in no improvement. He was subsequently treated with an experimental technique using cultured autologous keratinocyte grafts, with complete healing of facial erosions and surgical reconstruction of nasal tissues.[15]

Conclusions

Laryngeal involvement is a rare but serious complication that appears to occur primarily in junctional EB, but has also been noted in other types. Onset is generally early in life. Any patient presenting with stridor and/or hoarseness requires prompt assessment of the airway. X-ray films of the neck may be helpful in documenting airway narrowing, and laryngoscopy often reveals blisters and scarring in virtually any part of the larynx and upper airway. However, invasive procedures may further damage the mucosa and should be performed with extreme care. Because the number of reported patients with laryngeal involvement is small, it is unclear if prophylactic tracheotomy should be performed in patients presenting with severe respiratory distress. Until further experience develops through management of additional patients, treatment should be individualized to maximize airway preservation and minimize the risk of further mucosal damage.

Acknowledgments. Supported in part by a General Clinical Research Center grant (M01-RR00102) from the National Institutes of Health to The Rockefeller University Hospital; by a training grant (AR07525) from the National Institutes of Health to the Laboratory for Investigative Dermatology; by contracts AR62269 and AR62270 from the National Institutes of Health to the Laboratory for Investigative Dermatology; by a grant from the Dystrophic Epidermolysis Bullosa Research Association (D.E.B.R.A.) of America, Inc.; and with general support from the Pew Trusts.

References

1. Holbrook KA. Extracutaneous epithelial involvement in inherited epidermolysis bullosa. *Arch Dermatol.* 1988;124:726–731.
2. Berson S, Lin AN, Ward RW, Carter DM. Junctional epidermolysis bullosa of the larynx: report of a case and literature review. *Ann Otol Rhinol Laryngol.* (in press).
3. Kenna MA, Stool SE. Junctional epidermolysis bullosa of the larynx. *Pediatrics.* 1986;78:172–174.
4. Paller AS, Fine J-D, Kaplan S, Pearson RW. The generalized atrophic benign form of junctional epidermolysis bullosa: experience with four patients in the United States. *Arch Dermatol.* 1986;122:704–710.
5. Glossop LP, Michaels L, Bailey CM. Epidermolysis bullosa letalis in the larynx causing acute respiratory failure: a case presentation and review of the literature. *Int J Pediatr Otorhinolaryngol.* 1984;7:281–288.
6. Gonzalez C, Roth R. Laryngotracheal involvement in epidermolysis bullosa. *Int J Pediatr Otorhinolaryngol.* 1989;17:305–311.
6a. Davies H, Atherton DJ. Acute laryngeal obstruction in junctional epidermolysis bullosa. *Pediatric Dermatol.* 1987;4:98–101.
7. Thompson JW, Ahmed AR, Dudley JP. Epidermolysis bullosa dystrophica of the larynx and trachea: acute airway obstruction. *Ann Otol.* 1980;89:428–429.
8. Ramadass T, Thangavelu TA. Epidermolysis bullosa and its E.N.T. manifestations: two case reports. *J Laryngol Otol.* 1978;92:44–46.
9. Shackelford GD, Bauer EA, Graviss ER, McAllister WH. Upper airway and external genital involvement in epidermolysis bullosa dystrophica. *Radiology.* 1982;143:429–432.
10. Cohen SR, Landing BH, Isaacs H. Epidermolysis bullosa associated with laryngeal stenosis. *Ann Otol Rhinol Laryngol.* 1978;87(Suppl 52, part 2):25–28.
11. Buchbinder L, Lucky AW, Ballard E, et al. Severe infantile epidermolysis bullosa simplex, Dowling-Meara type. *Arch Dermatol.* 1986;122:190–198.
12. Pearson RW, Potter B, Strauss F. Epidermolysis bullosa hereditaria letalis: clini-

cal and histologic manifestations and course of the disease. *Arch Dermatol.* 1974; 109:349–355.
13. Thawley SE, Black MJ, Dudek SE, Spector GJ. External auditory canal stricture secondary to epidermolysis bullosa. *Arch Otolaryngol.* 1977;103:55–57.
14. Kaluza C, Kennedy BJ, Harman L. Head and neck complications of epidermolysis bullosa. *Laryngoscope.* 1985;95:599–600.
15. Carter DM, Lin AN, Varghese MC, Caldwell D, Pratt L, Eisinger M. Treatment of junctional epidermolysis bullosa with epidermal autografts. *J Am Acad Dermatol.* 1987;17:246–259.

16
Rheumatologic Aspects of Epidermolysis Bullosa

Thomas J.A. Lehman

Although epidermolysis bullosa (EB) is not routinely considered a rheumatologic disorder, many of its manifestations parallel those found in patients with collagen vascular disease. Awareness of these parallels prompted consideration of two important issues, which I will address in this chapter. The first is whether the rheumatologic concept of chronic inflammatory disease provides a useful model for consideration in the pathogenesis of EB and its complications. The second is how the experience of rheumatologists in working to maintain function and prevent deformity may be brought to bear for the benefit of EB patients.

Mild variants of EB such as EB simplex are rarely associated with significant systemic manifestations or functional limitation and will not be considered here. In contrast, the junctional and recessive dystrophic forms of EB may be associated with marked disability. The greatest disability is associated with the Hallopeau-Siemens recessive dystrophic form of disease. The blistering skin lesions of these patients are associated with severe flexion contractures, weakness, as well as anemia and other manifestations of a chronic inflammatory response. The well described mittenlike scarring of the hands and feet results in marked disability.

Although much has been written about the histopathology of the skin in EB, little has been reported about other manifestations of inflammation in these children. The anemia in patients with recessive dystrophic EB has been routinely ascribed to chronic blood loss, but there is evidence to suggest that it is the anemia of chronic disease.[1] Our own studies have indicated that the anemia is accompanied by markedly elevated erythrocyte sedimentation rates, hypergammaglobulinemia, thrombocytosis, and elevated total protein levels, a constellation of findings that suggest that these children have a true chronic inflammatory state much like that seen in rheumatic diseases of childhood.

The resorption of the distal tufts of the terminal digital phalanges is a characteristic that recessive dystrophic EB shares with progressive systemic sclerosis (scleroderma). In EB this has been ascribed to autoamputation secondary to the tightness of the skin.[2] A similar pathogenesis was suspected for the distal tuft resorption that occurs in scleroderma, but subsequent investigation revealed it to be the result of small blood vessel compromise.[3] In scleroderma this vascular disease is accompanied by small vessel disease in the kidneys, which leads to glomerular sclerosis.[4] Severe glomerular sclerosis was noted in the autopsy reports of two patients with recessive dystrophic EB that have come to our attention, but this association has not been described in the literature.

Large numbers of EB patients for systematic study are not routinely available. EB and progressive systemic sclerosis are both diseases of connective tissue. Both have prominent cutaneous involvement, and both are well recognized to involve the esophagus. Although a significant vascular component has been recognized in scleroderma, a vascular component of EB has not been described. The observations I have described here are indications that the recessive dystrophic form of EB may be a multisystem disease with a chronic inflammatory response. If this is true, then our concepts of the overall nature of the disease and its therapy may need revision. These comments come from the initial rheumatologic evaluation of patients followed at the Rockefeller University Hospital. The observations are preliminary, but suggest that children with dystrophic EB and perhaps junctional EB may have chronic inflammatory disease manifestations that extend to multiple organ systems. If this is true, then appropriate use of antiinflammatory medications may prove beneficial in the care of these children.

Further progress in the evaluation of the rheumatic disease model of chronic inflammation in children with EB awaits additional information. The national EB registry which has been established for the accumulation of data (including autopsy reports) is a major step forward in gathering the necessary information.[5]

We are currently engaged in a prospective study of acute phase reactants in the sera of EB patients, clinical evaluation for manifestations of internal organ involvement, and careful examination of autopsy findings (where available) to determine whether the evidence of chronic inflammation is indeed ascribable to repeated low grade skin infections, or a manifestation of a systemic and perhaps vascular component to this disease.

Rehabilitative Management

Because children with EB are seen only infrequently even in large medical centers, there is a tendency to avoid aggressive intervention out of fear that it may increase blistering. If the child with recessive dystrophic disease is chronically bandaged and discouraged from physical activity for fear of blistering, weakness, limitation of motion, and joint contractures invariably result in severe disability and often confinement to a wheel chair. Appropriate splinting to prevent flexion contractures using both upper and lower extremity "night resting splints," and appropriate daytime splinting can prevent the development of flexion contractures and allow the child to maintain functional mobility. The flexion contractures of the wrists and ankles that are frequently illustrated in textbook pictures of this condition and that severely limit functional utility are preventable.

Children with junctional forms of EB with recurrent blistering of the feet may also become disabled. The recurrent blistering often leads to an abnormal gait pattern. In some patients recurrent blistering of the heel may lead to plantar flexion contractures and heel cord shortening whereas in others blistering over the metatarsal heads may result in either internal or external tibial version so severe as to ultimately require surgical correction. These abnormalities can be prevented by careful observation of the child's early gait development and provision of appropriate orthotics to prevent the development of deformity. A detailed discussion of the appropriate rehabilitative procedures and techniques is provided in Chapter 20.

It is important that as our ability to prevent infection and manage the systemic manifestations of EB improves the prognosis for long-term survival in these patients, appropriate consideration is given to improving their functional outcome as well.

References

1. Hruby MA, Esterly NB. Anemia in epidermolysis bullosa letalis. *Am J Dis Child.* 1973;125:696–699.
2. Alpert M. Roentgen manifestations of epidermolysis bullosa. *Am J Roentgenol.* 1957;78:66–72.
3. Rodnan GP, LeRoy EC. The vascular hypothesis in scleroderma. In: Black CM, Myers AR, eds. *Current Topics in Rheumatology: Systemic Sclerosis (Scleroderma).* New York: Gower Medical Publishing Co; 1985:239–241.
4. Rodnan GP, Schreiner GE, Black RL. Renal involvement in progressive systemic sclerosis (generalized scleroderma). *Am J Med.* 1957;23:445–462.
5. Carter DM. Announcement of the national epidermolysis bullosa registry. *J Invest Dermatol.* 1987;89:120.

V
Special Management Considerations

17
Reconstructive Surgery for Patients with Epidermolysis Bullosa

KENNETH O. ROTHAUS and MICHAEL J. PAGNANI

Epidermolysis bullosa (EB) is a group of hereditary disorders of skin characterized by the formation of blisters following minor trauma.[1] In severe cases, scarring occurs at sites of healing blisters. Repeated cycles of blistering and scarring may lead to crippling and disfiguring deformities of the hands, feet, and face especially in the dystrophic form of EB.

Management in the Operating Room

Special precautions and techniques must be used in the anesthetic and intraoperative management of patients with EB. The use of adhesive substances for securing intravenous lines, electrocardiographic leads, pulse oximeter sensors, etc. is contraindicated as blistering or loss of underlying epidermis will occur with their removal.

Intravenous lines are secured in place with a single silk suture and then wrapped with gauze rolls. Electrocardiogram leads are similarly held in place with gauze rolls. The disposable form of pulse oximeter terminals are generally employed. Their adhesive ends are cut off and they may be easily secured with a large office paper clip. Bipolar cauteries only or those not requiring an adhesive ground are used. The blood pressure cuffs and operating table should be well padded to prevent any shearing forces.

The anesthetic techniques used in the care of these patients has previously been described[2-4] and is reviewed in chapter 18 of this text. In our patients, regional anesthesia or local anesthesia with intravenous sedation is generally employed. As general anesthesia with endotracheal intubation is associated with a higher risk of complications, when general anesthesia is necessary a well-padded face mask with xeroform gauze placed against the skin of the face is generally employed.

Scrubbing of the skin is to be avoided at all costs as a shearing injury will result. Antiseptic solution is therefore poured or patted over the operative site.

Harvesting of Skin Grafts

As previously noted, the skin of the patient with EB is extremely sensitive to shearing forces. The use of air-driven or electrical dermatomes are therefore contraindicated in this group of patients. In our practice, split-thickness skin grafts are harvested using a goulian knife, although any type of hand dermatome is suitable for use. Full-thickness skin grafts are generally harvested from the inguinal crease using a #15 blade. The donor site is then primarily closed using absorbable sutures of vicryl and subcuticular polydioxanone synthetic absorbable suture (PDS). Steristrips are never used to close a wound.

The donor sites are generally treated as one would routinely treat any split-thickness skin graft donor site; however, a donor site dressing with any type of adhesive cannot be employed. There is some feeling that the donor sites in this group of patients is slower to reepithelialize, although, this may just represent their vulnerability to minor trauma.

Management of Deformities of the Head and Neck

Involvement of the head and neck can occur with as devastating and crippling a deformity as commonly seen with the extremities in patients diagnosed as having EB. No area is spared, with patients not only suffering cosmetic deformities but also significant functional deficits as well. Ectropion of the upper and lower eyelids, loss of the nares with scar contracture and total obstruction of the primary valve of the nose (nostril), and scar contracture of the oral commissure are among the deficits seen and treated around the face in our patients at Rockefeller University Hospital. Flexion contractures of the neck, similar to those seen in burn patients, also can be seen.

Although surgical management requires meticulous and stringent attention toward the particular needs of the patient with EB, the principles and procedures used for the surgical correction of each problem do not substantially differ from those applied for correction of similar problems in patients not afflicted with EB but suffering from similar problems as a result of burns, tumors, or prior surgery.

Eyelid ectropion is best treated with release of the contracture, recreation of the defect, and reconstruction with a full-thickness skin graft. Routine plastic surgical principles and techniques apply to the choice of donor site, harvesting of the graft, and closure of the donor site, as well as for immobilization of the full-thickness skin graft and eyelids.

Alar reconstruction can be performed with composite grafts harvested from the ear. For extensive alar deficits, multiple grafts may be required for each alar. These grafts may be layered one on top of the other in a staged fashion as long as each one is less than 0.5 cm in width and sufficient time is allowed between procedures to insure revascularization of the preceding graft.

Scar contractures of the oral commissure are similar in anatomy and physiology to those seen with electrical burns of the mouth. As with burn reconstruction of the oral commissure, mucosal flaps may be used to reconstruct these patients. Similarly, skin grafts or rotation of myocutaneous flaps may be used to treat flexion contractures of the neck.

Surgical Management of the Upper and Lower Extremities

Although sequelae of EB may affect the more proximal portion of the upper and lower extremities, the hands, wrist, feet, and ankles are most commonly involved and are usually the most severely affected. In severe cases, characteristic mitten like deformities result in significant functional disabilities.

Progressive loss of hand web spaces occurs as epidermal bridging extends across adjacent digits (pseudo-syndactyly). Eventually a bridging scar creeps distally to encase the entire hand in a glovelike envelope. Formation of this "epidermal cocoon" is accompanied by the development of metacarpophalangeal, interphalangeal, and wrist flexion contractures. In addition, marked adduction of the thumb occurs with loss of the first web space. Joint subluxation may be noted. Nails are often absent. Resorption of the distal phalanges is often noted radiographically. Soft tissue calcification of the distal digits has also been reported. Loss of independent finger motion, pinch, and prehension makes fine motor manipulation difficult and interferes with the simple tasks of daily life.

Similar involvement of the foot and ankle, with syndactyly and flexion contractures of the toes, contractures of the ankle, and even joint dislocation have been noted. Foot involvement may preclude shoe fitting and normal ambulation.

Initial management of the upper and lower extremities should obviously be directed toward prevention of the factors leading to epidermal injury, proper care of open wounds, and prevention of the sequelae of injury and subsequent scar formation. The use of custom splints and maintenance of full range of motion is important in attempting to prevent the development of the syndactyly, scar contractures, and flexion deformities.

Operative intervention is indicated to improve hand and foot function in patients with severe deformities of the extremities. An aggressive approach may be indicated in that better function can be achieved postoperatively in younger patients. Correction of long-standing deformities in the older patient is extremely difficult. Surgical correction of the hand is indicated in any patient with a pseudo-syndactyly extending up to the proximal interphalangeal joint, an adduction contracture of the thumb, a flexion contracture of the pinky finger, and a flexion contracture of the metacarpophalangeal joint greater than 30° or any degree of involvement of the proximal interphalangeal joint. Inability to fit proper footwear and difficulty with ambulation are indications for surgery on the foot, toe, and ankle.

Although previous reports state the need for skin grafts and K-wire fixation,[5-3] our experience is that this is not usually the case. As this syndactyly represents more of an epidermal bridging than a true fusion, one is often able to find a dermis-to-dermis interface that separates easily and that reepithelializes relatively rapidly in the post-operative period. In patients with long-standing flexion contractures of the proximal phalangeal joint, skin grafts may be needed because of shortening of the soft tissues. Postoperatively the patient's wounds are dressed with a nonadherent dressing and moist gauze sponges and placed in a custom splint. The first dressing change is performed after 48 to 72 hr. In the younger patient this may have to be performed in the operating room under anesthesia. Subsequent dressing changes are performed every 48 hr and can easily be done at home. Early splinting and range of motion exercises are important to maintain the achieved surgical results. Custom gloves are sometimes employed to prevent the recurrence of the syndactyly.

Recurrence is inevitable. Close follow-up and early reoperation for recurrence appears to prevent changes that are permanent in nature. Similar techniques for surgery on the foot and ankle in this group of patients is employed.

Treatment of Cutaneous Tumors and Malignancies

As in any patient with a malignancy of the skin, wide resection is the primary treatment of choice. Squamous cell carcinoma is a frequent finding in this group of patients often involving the lower extremity.[14-18] In our patients afflicted with squamous cell carcinoma, wide resection and reconstruction with a split-thickness skin graft remain the treatment of choice. The most difficult problem in the treatment of these patients is determination intraoperatively of tumor margins. The scarring of the surrounding skin and fragility of the tissues make clinical and frozen section determination of tumor margins difficult at best. It is often found, therefore, on permanent sections that one margin may have tumor.

References

1. Lin AN, Carter DM. Epidermolysis bullosa: when the skin falls apart. *J Pediatr.* 1989;114:349–355.
2. Kelly RE, Koff HE, Rothaus KO, Carter DM, Artusio JF. Brachial plexus anesthesia in eight patients with recessive dystrophic epidermolysis bullosa. *Anesth Analg.* 1987;66:1318–1320.
3. Kaplan R, Strauch B. Regional anesthesia in a child with epidermolysis bullosa. *Anesthesiology.* 1987;67:262–264.
4. Speilman FJ, Mann ES. Subarachnoid and epidural anesthesia for patients with epidermolysis bullosa. *Can Anaesth Soc J.* 1984;31:549–551.

5. Greider JL, Flatt AE. Surgical restoration of the hand in epidermolysis bullosa. *Arch Dermatol.* 1988;124:765–767.
6. Greider Jr JL, Flatt AE. Care of the hand in recessive epidermolysis bullosa. *Plast Reconstr Surg.* 1983;72:222–227.
7. Horner RL, Wiedel JD, Brailliar F. Involvement of the hand in epidermolysis bullosa. *J Bone Joint Surg.* 1971;53-A:1347–1355.
8. Cuono C, Finseth F. Epidermolysis bullosa: current concepts and management of the advanced hand deformity. *Plast Reconstr Sung.* 1978;62:280–285.
9. Pers M. Skin grafting in a case of epidermolysis bullosa. *Acta Chir Scand.* 1965; 129:333–339.
10. Rees TD, Swinyard CA. Rehabilitative digital surgery in epidermolysis bullosa. *Plast Reconstr Surg.* 1967;40:169–174.
11. Zarem HA, Pearson RW, Leaf N. Surgical management of hand deformities in recessive dystrophic epidermolysis bullosa. *Br J Plast Surg.* 1974;27:176–181.
12. Swinyard CA, Swenson JR, Rees TD. Rehabilitation of hand deformities in epidermolysis bullosa. *Arch Phys Med Rehab.* 1968;49:138–144.
13. Gough MJ, Page RE. Surgical correction of the hand in epidermolysis bullosa dystrophica. *Hand.* 1979;11:55–58.
14. Yoshioka K, Kono T, Kitajima J, et al. Squamous cell carcinoma developing in epidermolysis bullosa dystrophica. *Int J Dermatol.* 1991;30:718–721.
15. Lentz SR, Raish RJ, Orlowski EP, Marion JM. Squamous cell carcinoma in epidermolysis bullosa: treatment with systemic chemotherapy. *Cancer.* 1990;66: 1276–1278.
16. Carapeto FJ, Pastor JA, Martin J, Agurruza J. Recessive dystrophic epidermolysis bullosa and multiple squamous cell carcinoma. *Dermatologica.* 1982;165: 39–46.
17. Reed WB, College Jr J, Francis MJO, et al. Epidermolysis bullosa dystrophica with epidermal neoplasm. *Arch Dermatol.* 1974;110:894–902.
18. Wechsler JL, Krugh FJ, Domonkos AN, Scheen SR, Davidson CL. Polydysplastic epidermolysis bullosa and development of epidermal neoplasms. *Arch Dermatol.* 1970;102:374–380.

18
Anesthesia for the Epidermolysis Bullosa Patient

ROBERT E. KELLY

The more than 16 forms of epidermolysis bullosa (EB) have been categorized by genetic, clinical, and histologic criteria. Recessive dystrophic epidermolysis bullosa (RDEB), characterized by mucous membrane involvement, is the form of special interest to the anesthesiologist. The successful anesthetic for the RDEB patient is one with minimal contact to skin or mucous membranes,[1] as minor trauma during the course of airway management may cause damage to epithelial surfaces. Perfecting such an anesthetic technique has confounded anesthesiologists for decades; although multiple techniques of anesthetic management have been proposed,[2-22] none has been wholly successful. Planning a safe anesthetic for the RDEB patient requires a thorough familiarity with not only the disease process, but also the various techniques available and their limitations. Armed with this knowledge, one may appropriately tailor an anesthetic to the needs of the RDEB patient and the operative procedure.

Preoperative Visit

Every well constructed anesthetic plan begins with the preoperative visit. Most afflicted patients requiring surgery are in the pediatric age group and a visit with the child and his parents is especially helpful. Specifics of the anesthetic plan, including preoperative medications and transport to the operating suite, should be explained in appropriate detail; an informed patient of any age will be more cooperative in the perioperative period, reducing the likelihood of combative behavior that could lead to the creation of bullae.

The assessment of the patient with RDEB begins with a careful history. These patients are often developmentally delayed and one must appreciate the child's capabilities and limitations, as activity level will provide useful information regarding muscle function and tone. Corticosteroid use is common in these patients[2] and one should determine if steroid dependency has occurred. Prior surgical history and any associated complications should be explored in depth.

The physical examination will typically reveal a patient who is malnourished and has muscle wasting. The limbs should be examined for flexion contractures with particular attention to proper positioning and protection during the operative procedure. Pseudo-syndactaly is often present and reflects prior trauma with scar formation.[3] Oral examination is especially important in these patients as poor dentition is common; the patient and parents must be warned of the possibility of dental damage during instrumentation of the airway. Ankyloglossia, when present, should also be noted.[4]

The laboratory evaluation of the RDEB patient must be extensive. Electrolyte imbalance, iron deficiency anemia, protein wasting, and amyloidosis with associated impairment of renal function are the most frequent abnormalities encountered.[3] There has been debate in the literature concerning an association of RDEB with porphyria; if there is an association, it is with porphyria cutanea tarda rather than acute intermittent porphyria.[5] Most authors recommend screening of urine for porphyrins; however, one large series felt this did not provide useful information.[6]

Preoperative medication is usually not necessary after a thorough visit. An awake and alert patient is better able to cooperate and therefore is less likely to incur injury.[7]

Monitoring Techniques

Appropriate monitoring is critical to the safe administration of any anesthetic. The patient with RDEB presents a special challenge to even routine monitoring; however, this does not preclude their safe use. In general, the placement of monitors must be done with utmost caution and care for the skin to prevent friction that could lead to the creation of new bullae.

In the past, the fear of epithelial injury had led clinicians to recommend against sphygmomanometry[7-9]; however, a moist wadding placed around the arm before careful application of a blood pressure cuff permits safe and atraumatic measurement.[10] If invasive blood pressure monitoring is necessary, one may place a percutaneous arterial catheter and secure it by wrapping the site with gauze. The electrocardiogram is safely obtained by the use of needle electrodes; however, these obviously are not easily placed on an awake patient. Consequently, gel electrode pads may be used safely if the adhesive is trimmed and the pad carefully placed under the patient to maintain electrical contact.[10] Temperature should be monitored with an axillary probe; measurement of esophageal or rectal temperature can be traumatic to mucous membranes and adhesive skin temperature devices will damage epithelial surfaces. Pulse oximetry has become a standard of care and should be measured with a nonadhesive sensor. A weighted precordial stethescope should be placed on the precordium of all patients to monitor cardiac and respiratory function. Measurement of inspired oxygen concentration, end-tidal carbon dioxide, airway pressure, and minute or tidal volume bring no risk to these patients and, as standards of care, should be performed.

Anesthestic Management

General Anesthesia

An anesthesiologist's primary concern when providing a general anesthetic is maintaining the patency of the patient's airway. Unfortunately, many of the tools available to assist in this goal may lead to the formation of bullae in the RDEB population. For this reason, these patients pose a unique challenge to the anesthesiologist administering general anesthesia and this technique should be reserved for those patients who cannot be anesthetized in any other fashion.

As with any anesthetic, the induction may safely proceed after placement of the appropriate monitors. If intravenous access has been established, a short-acting barbiturate is satisfactory for induction[6]; if not, one should establish access after a breathing induction to avoid possible trauma during venipuncture in an awake child. Regardless of induction technique, mask fit can be problematic; mere application of the mask can generate frictional forces of sufficient severity to generate new bullae.[11] Thus, all areas of facial contact (with both the mask and the hand of the anesthesiologist) should be protected with soft cotton wadding laden with sterile lubricant and steroid cream.[12,13] Once the mask is applied, care must be taken to ensure that movement of the mask is kept to a minimum. Oral or nasal airway devices should be avoided as their use may result in massive bullae formation in the oral cavity. Fortunately, ankylostomia is common in these patients and frequently obviates the need for these devices.[4]

In the past, intubation of the trachea was avoided for fear of creating life-threatening laryngeal bullae; however, no cases of laryngeal bullae formation after intubation have been reported. It is now postulated that RDEB affects the stratified squamous epithelium of the oral cavity but not the pseudo-stratified ciliated columnar epithelium of the tracheobronchial tree.[12] Thus, current recommendations advocate expeditious tracheal intubation in order to minimize contact with the facemask and reduce the risk of aspiration, which is high in this population because of associated esophageal strictures.[2,14] Intubation of the RDEB patient can be difficult; scarring of the oral cavity, leading to microstomia, occurred in 51% of cases in one major series of RDEB patients reported[15] and 6% of these patients could not be intubated. Further, the poor dentition that is common in these patients often leads to dental trauma.

Before laryngoscopy is attempted, profound muscle relaxation must be established as movement at this time may lead to the creation of major oropharyngeal bullae.[1,7] Succinylcholine has been used successfully in these patients[4,6,13] despite early fears of hyperkalemia due to their typically large, dystrophic muscle mass.[5,7,14] The short-acting nondepolarizing muscle relaxants may be used as an alternative, but one must be prepared to maintain the airway for a longer period if intubation is unsuccessful.

Laryngoscopy should be performed only by an experienced anesthesiologist and utmost care taken to prevent trauma in the oral cavity. A well lubricated MacIntosh blade is better suited than the Miller blade for prevention of injury to the posterior epiglottis.[11] If one is unable to visualize the vocal cords during laryngoscopy, a "blind pass" attempt at intubation is not recommended because of the trauma that it may cause. Fiberoptic laryngoscopy for the most difficult intubations may be undertaken with great caution. Once the endotracheal tube is in place, it should be secured in the midline with umbilical tape to prevent movement or lateral force at the corner of the mouth. Adhesive tape must be rigorously avoided.[2]

After the airway has been secured, the anesthetic may proceed with any technique appropriate for the type of surgery. An inhalation technique offers the advantages of easy titration of anesthetic depth and rapid emergence from anesthesia, whereas a narcotic-based anesthetic results in profound analgesia in the postoperative period, minimizing patient thrashing. Regardless of anesthetic technique, an intermediate-acting muscle relaxant is recommended for prevention of patient movement or "bucking." Protection of the eyes is extremely important during any general anesthetic and application of a sterile lubricant is effective for the RDEB patient; taping the eyelids closed should be avoided.

At the conclusion of the anesthetic, protection of the airway remains the utmost concern for the anesthesiologist. Suctioning of the airway can lead to life-threatening bullae[16] and must be done with extreme caution, if at all. Extubation should be attempted only when the patient is able to manage his own airway in order to prevent aspiration and undesirable use of a mask or artificial airway; however, the patient must be extubated before reacting to the endotracheal tube in order to prevent "bucking" and the associated movement. Once the trachea has been successfully extubated and the airway is adequate, one may proceed to the recovery room.

Dissociative Anesthesia

Dissociative anesthesia induced with ketamine provides profound analgesia without the alterations in the CO_2 response curve that are associated with inhalational or narcotic-based anesthetic techniques. Further, airway reflexes are not ablated under ketamine anesthesia.[9,14,17,18] These effects combine to allow the patient under ketamine anesthesia to maintain his own airway, thereby minimizing the complications of airway management in the RDEB patient. As a result, the choice of ketamine as an anesthetic agent has emerged as an attractive alternative to general anesthesia for the RDEB patient's unique anesthetic needs.

Every anesthetic technique has undesirable side effects and, unfortunately, ketamine is no exception. First, ketamine causes airway hyperreactivity, and consequently is not appropriate for any surgical procedure in which there may be blood or secretions in the oropharynx. Second, ketamine induces central nervous system activation of the cardiovascular centers, which can lead to hypertension and tachycardia[10]; as a result, hemodynamics and the electrocardiogram must be monitored closely. Third, nonpurposeful patient movement and violent thrashing upon emergence are quite common and can result in formation of new bullae. Finally, although unusual in the pediatric population, nightmares and personality changes after ketamine analgesia have been reported.[23]

Despite this, ketamine remains a mainstay in the anesthetic treatment of the RDEB patient because the advantage of airway maintainence often outweighs any other side effects. As a result, ketamine is particularly useful in this population for any operative procedure that does not involve the patient's airway. Ketamine anesthesia should be used with caution, if at all, for dental procedures in the RDEB patient.

Regional Anesthesia

Regional anesthesia was initially proposed in 1966 as an alternative to general anesthesia for the RDEB patient[8]; however, clinicians initially dismissed it as unfeasable based on the fear of infection as well as that of new bullae formation secondary to the physical and chemical irritation asssociated with this technique.[2,14] It was not until 1983 that the first report of a regional anesthetic appeared in the literature,[19] and since that time there have been many case reports of the successful use of regional anesthesia in this population.[6,10,20-22] The difficulty of airway management during general anesthesia renders regional anesthesia the technique of choice whenever possible.[10]

The foundations of a successful regional anesthetic are identical to those of a general anesthetic, commencing with a thorough preoperative visit. Special emphasis should be given to the anticipated events in the operating suite, including pertinent details concerning positioning and needle placement. Upon arrival at the operating suite, appropriate monitors should be placed. One may then proceed with the anesthetic using the following modifications of standard techniques. First, asepsis should be achieved via betadine soaks, as the use of abrasive sponges will result in epithelial injury.[8] Similarly, only nonadhesive drapes should be used. Second, local infiltration of the subcutaneous tissue should be avoided, as this will result in sloughing and bullae formation.[8] Third, when performing a peripheral nerve block, the use of a nerve stimulator is indicated to ensure proper location and to minimize placement trauma.[22] Finally, intravenous adjuncts for sedation may be used judiciously before or after placement of the block; however, an awake and cooperative patient is optimal.

The appropriate regional technique will be dictated by the location of the surgical field. Spinal, epidural, and axillary plexus blockade have all been successfully employed.[10,19-22] Conversely, techniques such as ankle blocks that rely on subcutaneous infiltration of local anesthesia will likely lead to bullae formation and should be avoided. The choice of local anesthetic agent should be dictated by the operative procedure; epinephrine has been used successfully as an adjunct to peripherial nerve blocks.[10] An operating tourniquet may be used if carefully wrapped over protective gauze.[6,10] Meticulous handling of the patient, with emphasis on avoiding the shearing forces of abrasion, is critical to successful regional blockade in the RDEB patient.

Postanesthetic Recovery

Management of the RDEB patient in the postanesthetic recovery period uses the same principles as in the operative period and centers upon meticulous handling of the patient. Parents should be allowed in the recovery area whenever possible to allay patient anxiety and agitation and minimize combative emergence from the anesthetic. In addition, postoperative pain should be treated promptly and aggressively to keep patient movement to a minimum. Oxygen, if needed, should be delivered by hood, as facemasks and nasal cannulae may be associated with unnecessary trauma.[11] Finally, the use of restraints is contraindicated in this population. Using these modifications to the normal postanesthetic rocovery period, the RDEB patient should emerge from the recovery room without significant injury.

References

1. Pratilas V, Biezunski A. Epidermolysis bullosa manifested and treated during anesthesia. *Anesthesiology.* 1975;43:581–583.
2. Reddy ARR, Wong DHW. Epidermolysis bullosa: a review of anaesthetic problems and case reports. *Can Anaesth Soc J.* 1972;19:536–547.
3. Milne B, Rosales JK. Anaesthesia for correction of oesophageal stricture in a patient with recessive epidermolysis bullosa dystrophica: a case report. *Can Anaesth Soc J.* 1980;27:169–171.
4. Young DA, Hartwick PB. Anaesthesia for epidermolysis bullosa dystrophica. *Anaesthesia.* 1968;23:264–267.
5. Smith GB, Shribman AJ. Anaesthesia and severe skin disease. *Anaesthesia.* 1984; 39:443–455.
6. Boughton R, Crawford MR, Vonwiller JB. Epidermolysis bullosa—a review of 15 years' experience, including experience with combined general and regional anaesthetic techniques. *Anaesth Intens Care* 1988;16:260–264.
7. Tomlinson AA. Recessive dystrophic epidermolysis bullosa. *Anaesthesia.* 1983; 38:485–491.
8. Mark LC, Marx GF, Arkins RE, et al. Anesthesia in epidermolysis bullosa. *NY State J Med.* 1966;66:511–512.
9. Hamann RA, Cohen PJ. Anesthetic management of a patient with epidermolysis bullosa dystrophica. *Anesthesiology.* 1971;34:389–391.
10. Kelly RE, Koff HD, Rothaus KO, et al. Brachial plexus anesthesia in eight patients with recessive dystrophic epidermolysis bullosa. *Anesth Analg.* 1987;66: 1318–1320.

11. Petty WC, Gunther RC. Anesthesia for nonfacial surgery in polydysplastic epidermolysis bullosa (dystrophic). *Anesth Analg.* 1970;49:246–250.
12. Berryhill RE, Benumof JL, Saidman LJ, et al. Anesthetic management of emergency cesarean section in a patient with epidermolysis bullosa dystrophica polydysplastica. *Anesth Analg.* 1978;57:281–283.
13. Hubbert CH, Adams JG. Anesthetic management of patients with epidermolysis bullosa. *South Med J.* 1977;70:1375–1377.
14. Lee C, Nagel EL. Anesthetic management of a patient with recessive epidermolysis bullosa dystrophica. *Anesthesiology.* 1975;43:122–124.
15. James I, Wark H. Airway management during anesthesia in patients with epidermolysis bullosa dystrophica. *Anesthesiology.* 1982;56:323–326.
16. Block MS, Gross BD. Epidermolysis bullosa dystrophica recessive: oral surgery and anesthetic considerations. *J Oral Maxillofac Surg.* 1982;40:753–758.
17. LoVerme SR, Oropollo AT. Ketamine anesthesia in dermatolytic bullous dermatosis (epidermolysis bullosa). *Anesth Analg.* 1977;56:398–401.
18. Kelly AJ: Epidermolysis bullosa dystrophica—anesthetic management. *Anesthesiology* 1971;35:659.
19. Rowlingson JC, Rosenbaum SM. Successful regional anesthesia in a patient with epidermolysis bullosa. *Reg Anesth.* 1983;8:81–83.
20. Spielman FJ, Mann ES. Subarachnoid and epidural anaesthesia for patients with epidermolysis bullosa. *Can Anaesth Soc J.* 1984;31:549–551.
21. Broster T, Placek R, Eggers GWN. Epidermolysis bullosa: anesthetic management for cesarean section. *Anesth Analg.* 1987;66:341–343.
22. Kaplan R, Strauch B. Regional anesthesia in a child with epidermolysis bullosa. *Anesthesiology.* 1987;67:262–264.
23. Meyers EF, Charles P. Prolonged adverse reactions to ketamine in children. *Anesthesiology.* 1978;49:39.

19
Prenatal Diagnosis and Genetic Screening for Epidermolysis Bullosa

Virginia P. Sybert and Karen A. Holbrook

Prenatal Diagnosis

Prenatal diagnosis of embryonic and fetal abnormalities is a multidisciplinary field of medicine whose techniques have been applied to an increasing number of inherited and sporadic disorders and malformations. Prenatal diagnosis for epidermolysis bullosa (EB) by fetoscopy was first reported in 1980.[1] Since that initial report, numerous successful diagnoses and exclusions of EB in pregnancies at risk have been published.

The methods available for the detection of in utero abnormalities include maternal serum alpha-fetoprotein (AFP) screening, chorionic villus sampling (CVS), amniocentesis for amniotic fluid analysis and cell culture, fetoscopy for fetal visualization, blood sampling and skin biopsy, ultrasonography, and fetal radiographs. To date, electron microscopic examination of fetal skin samples obtained by fetoscopy has been the only reliable technique used for EB. As the metabolic and genetic causes for these disorders are established, less invasive and perhaps more accurate means may become possible.

Maternal Serum AFP Screening

Although both fetal cells and fetal metabolic products cross the placenta into the maternal circulation, the proportion of fetal to maternal cells $(1:1000)$[2] is so low that culturing of fetal cells obtained from maternal blood samples for metabolic and/or chromosomal analysis is not yet possible. It has been possible to measure certain metabolic products, primarily AFP, in maternal serum for the purpose of prenatal diagnosis. AFP is a fetal product that is made in the liver and the gastrointestinal tract, excreted into the urine and then into the anmiotic fluid, from which it diffuses into the maternal circulation. AFP levels in maternal serum rise from the 10th week gestational age until early in the third trimester, when they begin to fall.[3-5]

Any abnormal membrane or serosa-covered defect of the normal epidermis (e.g., omphalocele, myelomeningocele, anencephaly) results in increased transudation of AFP into the amniotic fluid and thus into maternal serum.

Routine maternal serum AFP screening is now offered to all pregnant women at about 16 to 17 weeks of gestation for the purpose of detecting open neural tube defects. Levels of AFP elevated 2.5 times the mean are reasonably sensitive for detecting such defects. The test is not specific; fetal demise, multiple pregnancy, and even normal fetuses may cause elevated levels. Accurate dating of the pregnancy is important for interpretation of AFP levels.

Abnormally high levels of maternal serum AFP have been reported in one pregnancy in which the fetus had EB simplex.[6] The authors suggested that extensive blistering and denudation of skin resulted in increased diffusion of AFP from the fetal surface. This method could not be depended on reliably to detect or exclude the possibility of EB in a pregnancy at risk as an affected fetus might not have sufficiently large areas of denuded skin to result in increased maternal serum AFP levels.

Other fetal metabolic products can also be measured in maternal serum, and have been used for prenatal diagnosis of other genetic conditions. As the biochemical bases of the EB become known, this noninvasive method of screening pregnant women at risk may become more useful.

Ultrasonography

Ultrasound examination of the fetus is a noninvasive method of fetal visualization. It is used for the in utero diagnosis of fetal malformations and as an adjunct to fetoscopy, anmiocentesis, and chorionic villus sampling.[7-9] The technique relies on the different acoustical densities of fetal tissues, placenta, and amniotic fluid to ultrasonic pulses applied to the mother's abdomen. The differential echoes produced are displayed on a cathode ray tube. Realtime ultrasonography gives excellent resolution and allows visualization of fetal movement. Routine ultrasound examinations provide information about gestational age (based on femur length and biparietal diameter), location of the placenta and insertion of the umbilical cord, fetal viability, multiple pregnancy, amount of amniotic fluid, and may detect some structural malformations. Level II ultrasound examinations are used for the detection of neural tube defects, and other major, and some minor, structural malformations such as abdominal wall defects, cardiac abnormalities, limb deficiencies, skeletal dysplasias, and renal malformations.[7,9-11]

Some animal studies and in vitro laboratory data have caused concern about the long-term safety of ultrasonography.[12-14] Follow-up evaluations of children exposed to ultrasound in utero have not demonstrated untoward effects.[15-17] Ultrasonography has become routine in obstetric practice for dating of pregnancies; its use for definitive prenatal diagnosis requires significant expertise and remains the domain of tertiary care perinatal units.

Chorionic Villus Sampling

CVS first came into vogue in the late 1960s,[18] but was discarded because of an unacceptably high rate of pregnancy loss. In the mid-1970s, Chinese investigators began to use the technique for sex determination[19]; it was further refined in the U.S.S.R.,[20] the U.K.,[21] and Italy.[22] The rate of pregnancy loss at experienced centers has dropped to 3% to 5%. It is much higher in less experienced hands. More than 41,000 pregnancies have undergone CVS and entered in a multinational ongoing registry.[23] Transcervical aspiration of the developing chorionic villi can be accomplished between the 8th and 11th weeks of pregnancy. The villi develop from the trophoblast of the blastocyst and rapidly proliferate during the early stages of embryogenesis. They provide a source of embryonic tissue for rapid and direct chromosomal and DNA analysis. Villous cells can also be cultured for karyotyping and for biochemical studies.[24]

Any genetic condition for which the gene defect is known, closely linked DNA polymorphisms are available, or in which the biochemical basis is understood and expressed in villous cells can be prenatally diagnosed using this method. CVS offers the dual advantages of first-trimester diagnosis and a shorter time than amniocentesis between sampling and results from cultured cells, allowing for early termination of affected fetuses. The major disadvantage is the relatively high rate of pregnancy loss—about tenfold greater than that of amniocentesis. Although this higher rate of loss may be in some part due to the higher frequency of spontaneous abortion in the first trimester than second trimester, it is nonetheless prudent to limit CVS to pregnancies at high risk for specific abnormalities and to restrict its use to those centers conducting well monitored clinical trials.

To date, CVS is not a technique that has played a role in the prenatal diagnosis of EB. With the exception of EBS-1 (EBS-Ogna)[25] and EBS-Köbner,[26] linkage studies have not proven successful in finding closely linked DNA polymorphisms that might make prenatal diagnosis by restriction fragment length polymorphism (RFLP) analysis of villous cells' DNA possible.[27-30] It is reasonable to assume that CVS will become useful as more is discovered about the underlying biochemical mechanisms of the inherited disorders of blistering and as the gene for each condition is mapped and the DNA sequences determined.

Amniocentesis

First used for the in utero treatment of erythroblastosis fetalis,[31] amniocentesis has become the major method of prenatal diagnosis. It is performed between the 15th and 20th weeks of gestation, and gives access to fetal cells and fetal metabolic products that are excreted into the amniotic fluid. After the fetus and placental position have been determined by ultrasound examination (some centers do the procedure with concurrent ultrasonography), approximately 20 ml (5–10% total volume) of amniotic fluid are aspirated by sterile transabdominal percutaneous needle puncture of the amniotic cavity. Amniocentesis is a relatively low-risk procedure with a 0.5% rate of pregnancy loss [32,33]; in addition to pregnancy loss, Rh sensitization, fetal puncture, and uterine cramping may occur.[34]

The amniotic fluid can be assayed for AFP (see discussion of maternal AFP screening) and other fetal secretions or excretions. Amniotic fluid acetylcholinesterase (AChE) levels can be measured and have been used to increase the specificity of AFP levels in detecting open neural tube defects.[35-37] Elevated AFP and AChE levels have been reported in a pregnancy of a fetus with recessive dystrophic EB.[38] The diagnosis was confirmed by fetal skin biopsy, which demonstrated a split below the basement membrane and absence of anchoring fibrils. AFP levels were similarly elevated in the amniotic fluid from a fetus with extensive aplasia cutis congenita.[39] Just as with maternal serum AFP levels, prenatal diagnosis of EB by assaying levels of these substances would only detect those fetuses with significant loss of skin surface.

DNA can be harvested from uncultured amniotic fluid cells for RFLP analysis using restriction endonucleases.[40] Electron microscopic examination of amniotic fluid cells is also possible and has been used in the prenatal diagnosis of bullous congenital ichthyosiform erythroderma.[41,42] Cultured amniotic fluid cells can be karyotyped, assayed for specific biochemical defects, and used for DNA analysis. As amniotic fluid cells, which are derived from several fetal sources,[8,43,44] appear to express collagenase, it may be possible to do prenatal diagnosis in those families with recessive dystrophic EB of the Hallopeau-Siemens type (RDEB-H-S) in which abnormal collagenase or abnormal collagenase activity has been demonstrated.[45,46]

Although amniocentesis for prenatal diagnosis is a relatively safe procedure, it is not without disadvantages. The risk of pregnancy loss, puncture of the fetus (Fig. 19.1), and other obstetric complications is approximately 0.5%. As it is performed during the second trimester and culturing of cells requires at least 1 to 2 weeks, elective termination of affected fetuses requires either saline or prostaglandin induction of labor, which has greater maternal morbidity as well as greater psychological burden. An increased incidence of clubfoot and respiratory distress has been noted in liveborn infants of pregnancies that have undergone amniocentesis.[32,34] Studies in animals have suggested that lung development may be compromised if chronic leakage of amniotic fluid occurs.[47] Nevertheless, amniocentesis appears to be a relatively low-risk procedure and remains the primary tool for prenatal diagnosis of most disorders.

Fetoscopy

Fetoscopy is a procedure that allows direct visualization of the fetus and provides access for fetal biopsy and blood sampling.[8,48-60] It was first performed in the 1950s[61] but did not become generally useful until the 1970s when endoscopes that were small enough to provide transabdominal entry into the womb with a relatively low risk of pregnancy loss were manufactured. Visualization of the fetus is most easily done between the 15th and 18th menstrual weeks (13th–16th GA) because the fetus is small and the amniotic

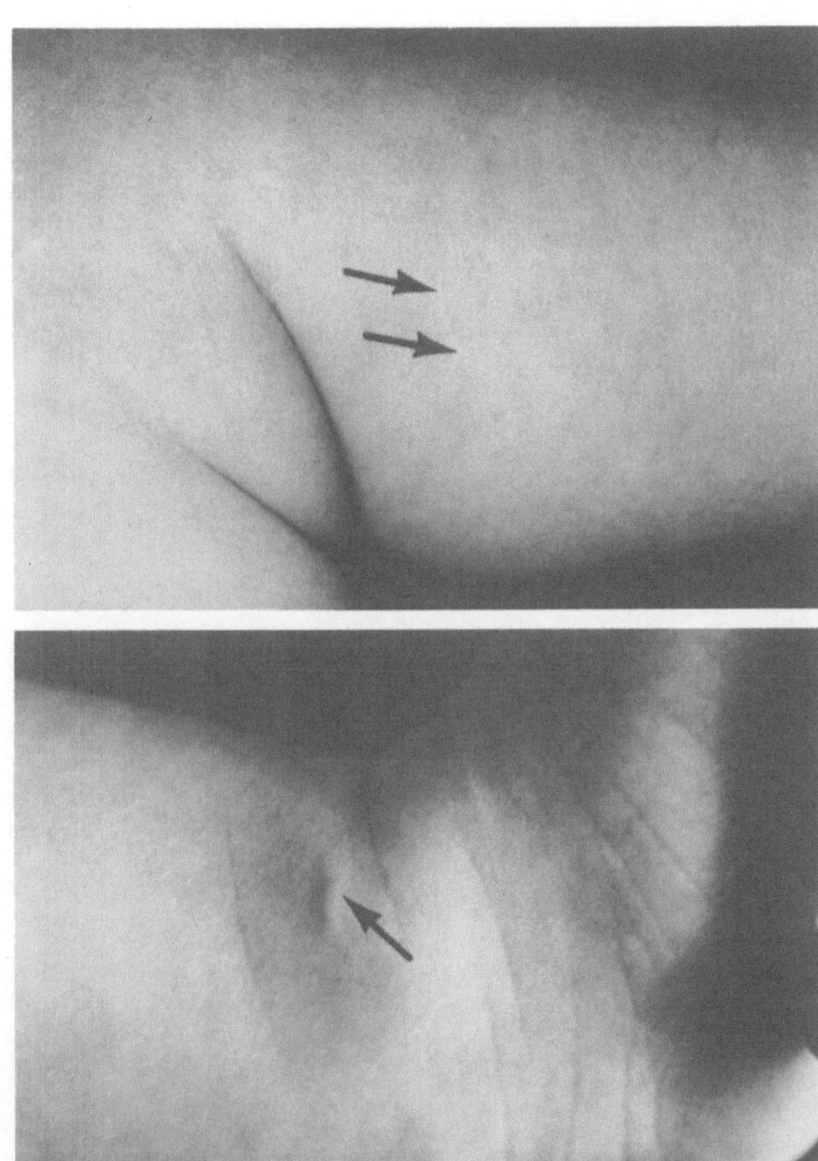

FIGURE 19.1. Elevated scar on the ankle and hairline scar on the medial surface of the leg at birth that remain from a skin biopsy obtained in utero (photographs obtained courtesy of Tracy B. Perry, Montreal).

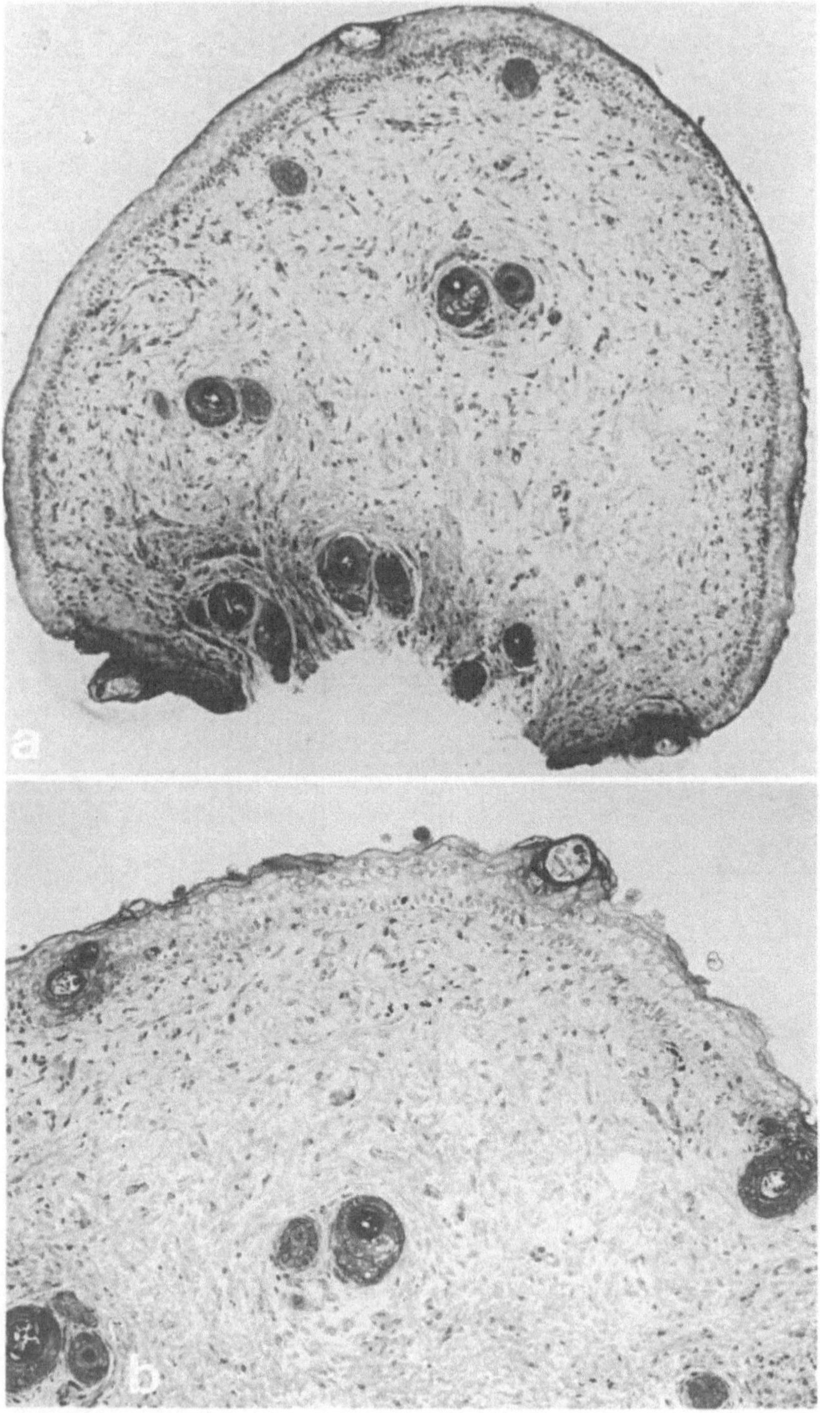

(A)

(B)

fluid has not yet become cloudy. Fetoscopy for the purpose of fetal blood sampling is performed between the 18th and 21st menstrual weeks (16th–19th GA) because of the larger umbilical vessels and greater blood volume in the older fetus. Skin biopsy for prenatal diagnosis is also performed at the later gestational ages.

After maternal sedation to decrease fetal movement, and ascertainment of placental position and umbilical cord insertion by ultrasound, a cannula with a trocar is inserted under sterile conditions into the amniotic cavity. The trocar is withdrawn and a rigid fiberoptic fetoscope with a visual field of 2 to 4 mm^2 is passed through the cannula. The restricted range of vision precludes seeing the fetus in entirety, but fetal parts can be visualized as the fetus moves and presents them. A 25–27 gauge needle can be passed down a side channel in the fetoscope to aspirate fetal blood from the umbilical vessels near the site of placental insertion. Fetal skin biopsies of 1 to 2 mm^2 (Fig. 19.2) can be obtained by using small, cup-shaped biopsy forceps. When the procedure is performed "blind" (i.e., the fetoscope is withdrawn and the biopsy forceps passed down the cannula), fetal membranes rather than fetal skin may be biopsied in error.[62,63] When the biopsy forceps are passed down a sidearm on the fetoscope so that samples can be obtained under visualization, the biopsies are more likely to be useful, but a larger fetoscope is required and the pregnancy may be put at greater risk for loss. Extremely small biopsy forceps have been developed to overcome this disadvantage, but they are more difficult to make and more likely to break. Needle biopsy under ultrasound guidance has also been used. Three or more biopsies are usually taken from the back, buttocks, chest, or abdomen. The scalp may be biopsied for certain disorders. These biopsy sites usually heal quickly and are difficult to find when the newborn is examined (Fig. 19.1). Fetal liver biopsy has also been successfully obtained for prenatal diagnosis.

In experienced hands, fetoscopy carries about a 5% risk of pregnancy loss when blood or skin is obtained. The rate of loss is less for fetal visualization alone. Maternal bleeding, maternal bladder or bowel injury, infection, chronic leakage of amniotic fluid, and prematurity can also ensue.[41,64,65] Fetoscopy is currently performed in a limited number of centers and should not be performed outside of accomplished units as the risks increase significantly with inexperience.

Fetoscopy with fetal skin biopsy has been the primary method of prenatal

---

◁ FIGURE 19.2. **A**: Section through a skin biopsy from a normal fetus sampled at 17 weeks estimated gestational age. There is sufficient tissue in one specimen to evaluate the morphology of the epidermis, dermal–epidermal junction, dermis, and hair follicles. **B**: Enlarged view of a portion of the biopsy sample showing detail of their epidermis and follicles in cross-section. Note that the hair follicles are keratinized and the sebaceous glands are formed and synthesizing sebum; the interfollicular epidermis still retains periderm on the surface. **A**, × 95; **B**, × 152.

diagnosis for EB and inherited skin diseases in general. Examination of fetal skin by transmission electron microscopy (TEM) has been, until recently, the only reliable method of diagnosis, and its reliability directly depends on the expertise of the laboratory personnel who process the specimens and the individual who interprets the results.[66] EB letalis (Herlitz) has been successfully diagnosed or excluded using the ultrastructural criterion of hypoplastic or absent hemidesmosomes[1,67-70] (Fig. 19.3), as has EB atrophicans inversa.[67] Heterogeneity exists within junctional EB, and at least one affected adult individual has been reported to have normal hemidesmosomes.[71] The

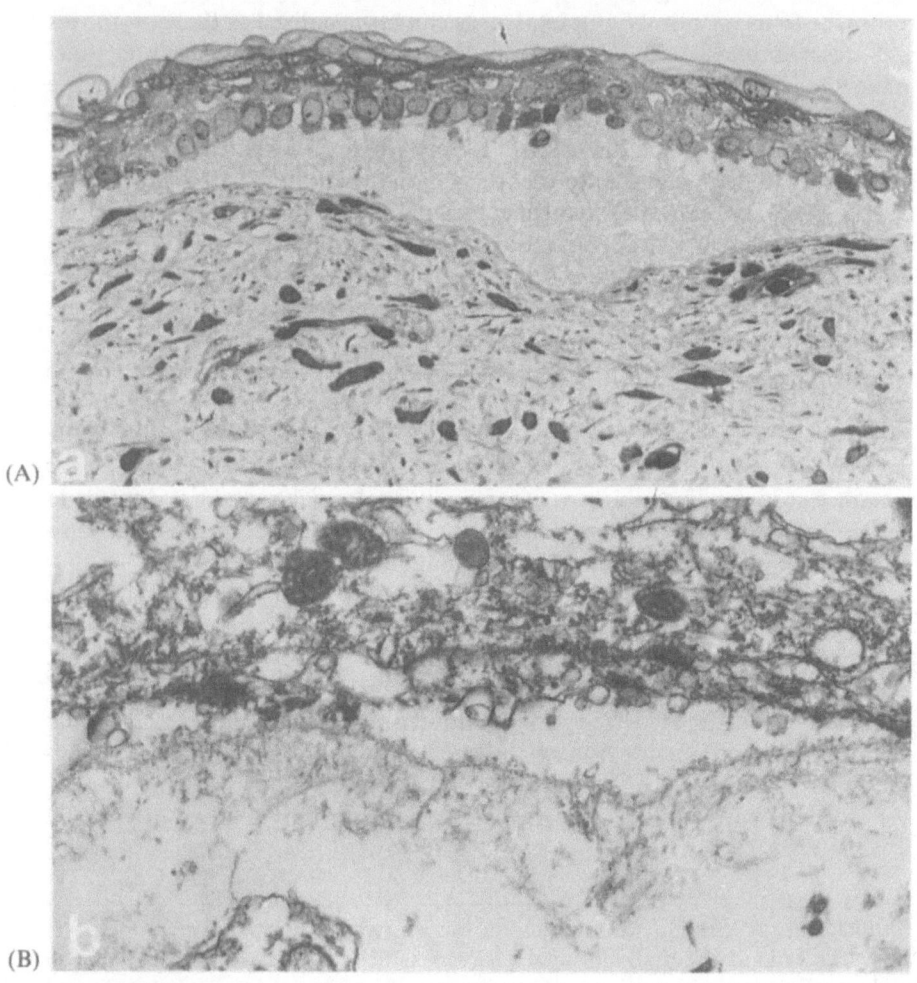

(A)

(B)

FIGURE 19.3. Portion of a skin biopsy from a fetus affected with junctional epidermolysis bullosa (A). Note that the plane of separation above the basal lamina (in the lamina lucida) is evident in both the light (A) and the electron micrographs (B). A, × 340; B, × 11,400.

skin of an affected fetus is typically detached from the dermis as a consequence of the biopsy procedure, making it possible for an experienced individual to identify the defect with the dissecting microscope. Nonetheless, electron microscopy must be done to confirm the presence of diagnostic ultrastructural features. Every effort should be made to establish the ultrastructural findings in the liveborn affected relative(s) before examination of skin biopsy samples from the fetus at risk.

RDEB-H-S has been excluded or diagnosed prenatally using the ultrastructural criteria of reduced or absent anchoring fibrils[67,68,72,73] (Fig. 19.4). In this form, as in all the other types of EB diagnosed prenatally, the level of the separation of the epidermis from the dermis is also used as a criterion. As in EB letalis, blister formation occurs almost uniformly as a consequence of the biopsy procedure, making this disorder one of the most reliable to diagnosis in utero.

Prenatal exclusion of two autosomal dominant dystrophic forms of EB, the albopapuloidea Pasini and Cockayne-Touraine variants, has also been reported. Exclusion of both was based on the presence of normal anchoring fibrils,[74] and in the latter case, on the absence of clefting and the normal binding of specific monoclonal antibodies to antigens of the dermal–epidermal junction.[75]

Heagerty and colleagues[76] have reported the successful prenatal diagnosis of RDEB-H-S and the successful exclusion of junctional EB using the monoclonal antibody LH 7:2 and the polyclonal antibody AA3, respectively, for indirect immunofluorescence evaluation of fetal skin biopsies. LH 7:2 binds to epidermal basement membrane and is expressed as early as 10 weeks gestation. Its binding is severely reduced or absent in patients with RDEB-H-S.[77] However, this same antigen has been shown to be unreliable in staining biopsies from a fetus at risk for dominant dystrophic EB.[75] AA3 binds to normal epidermal basement membrane, and shows reduced binding in patients with the lethal form of junctional EB.[78] Fine and colleagues[79] have shown absence of expression of both GB3 and 19-DEJ-1 (a monoclonal antibody that binds specifically to the midlamina lucida of the dermal–epidermal junction, in close association with hemidesmosomes) in three fetuses with junctional EB. A fourth, at risk, fetus showed normal binding and, at delivery, was clinically normal. In all studied instances the diagnoses were confirmed by TEM. The immunofluorescence studies required 4 h to perform, rather than the days required for TEM evaluation of tissue, a significant advantage for prenatal diagnosis. If chorionic villous cells express these antigens it may be possible to perform prenatal diagnosis for these two forms of EB much earlier in pregnancy. Monoclonal antibodies against other antigens may prove useful for prenatal diagnosis in the future.[78]

Among the simplex forms of EB, only Dowling-Meara has been identified in utero using fetal skin biopsy samples. Blister formation occurred within the basal layer, and clumped keratin filaments associated with desmosomes were identified in disrupted and intact basal cells (unpublished findings).

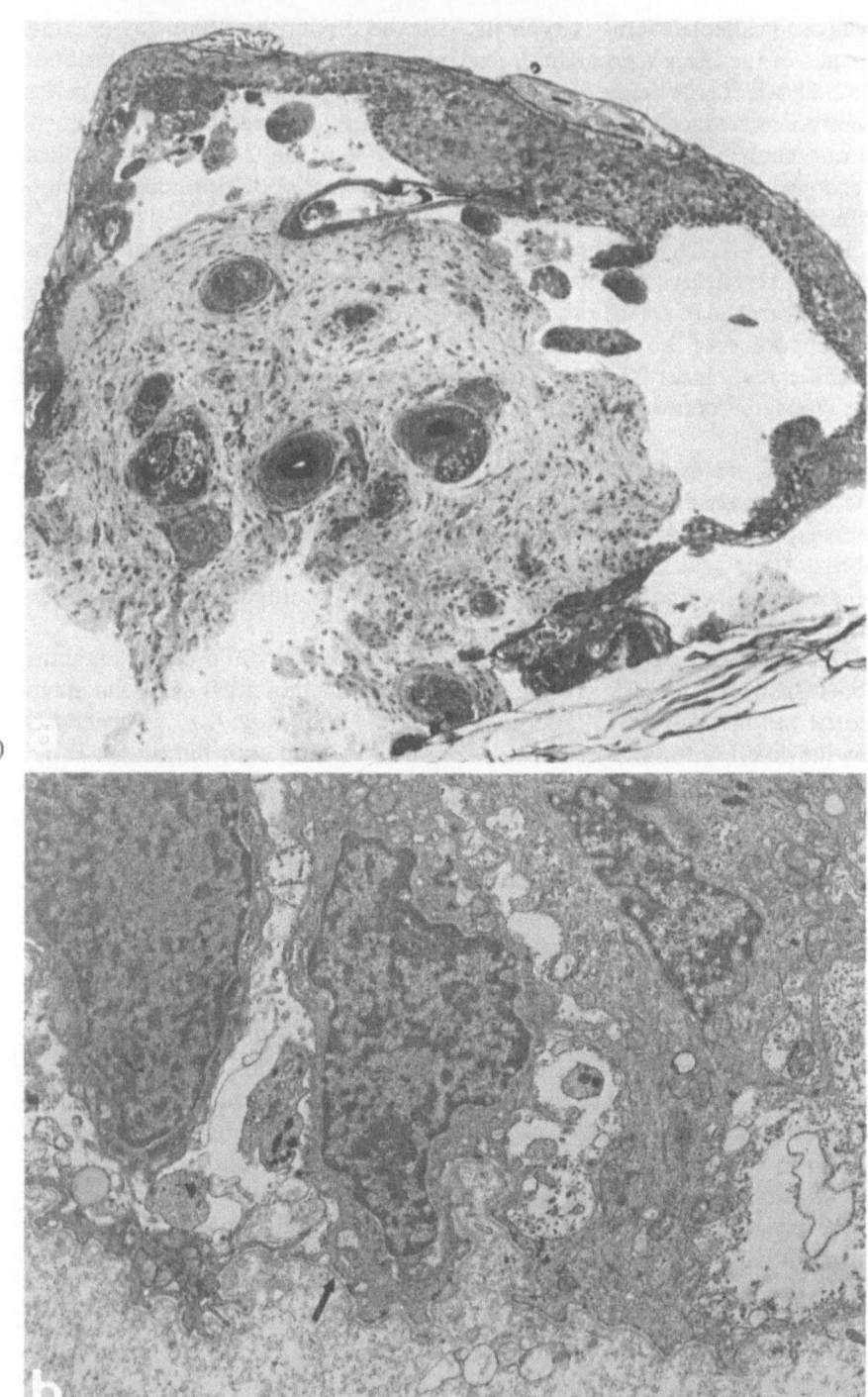

(A)

(B)

The goal of prenatal diagnosis is to obtain as much information as possible in the least deleterious way to allow parents to make fully informed decisions about reproductive options. At this time, TEM evaluation of fetal skin samples remains the accurate and reliable mainstay of prenatal diagnosis for EB. The advent of recombinant DNA RFLPs will hopefully allow for earlier (first trimester) and accurate prenatal detection of these genetic disorders of blistering.

Genetic Counseling

Genetic counseling refers to the process in which patients and families are evaluated and informed regarding the inherited disorder for which they are either at risk or with which they are affected. The process includes establishing the correct diagnosis, discussion of the natural history of the condition, treatment of complications, referral for management and community resources, and provision of information regarding recurrence risks and prenatal diagnosis. Genetic counseling is a nondirective process. Families and patients need to be given the information to allow them to arrive at their own decisions based on their needs, beliefs, and value systems.

Accurate diagnosis is a prerequisite for genetic counseling. Different forms of EB are inherited differently and carry differing prognoses and recurrence risks (genetic heterogeneity). Even where the diagnosis seems secure based on clinical and pedigree data (e.g., a family in which many members in multiple generations are affected with blistering limited to the palms and soles is likely to have Weber-Cockayne, an autosomal dominant EB simplex), biopsy confirmation of the diagnosis is important. There may be genetic heterogeneity even within apparently similar conditions and it is important to establish the ultrastructural findings in a specific famlly so that accurate prenatal diagnosis can be offered.

The natural history of the disorder is extremely important information to transmit to patients. Parents of a newborn infant with autosomal dominant EBS-herpetiformis (Dowling-Meara) need to know that the disorder improves over time and that adults may have relatively little difficulty with the disease, in contrast to severe recessive dystrophic EB. Variability of expression is common in genetic conditions. Treatment for genetic conditions may be specific (e.g., phenytoin in some forms of RDEB) or symptomatic (unroofing of blisters, avoidance of trauma, antibiotics, etc). Families need to

---

◁ FIGURE 19.4. A: Skin biopsy sample from a fetus affected with recessive dystrophic epidermolysis bullosa. Note the obvious separation of the epidermis from the dermis that is characteristic of skin biopsies from affected individuals. B: The ultrastructure of the separated epidermis confirms that the cleavage plane is beneath on the dermal side of the basal lamina (*arrows*). The flocculent material beneath the basal lamina is blister fluid. A, × 140; B, × 7600.

know when referral to a tertiary or specialty clinic is necessary, and what their family physician can be expected to manage when EB occurs in a family.

Discussion of the recurrence risks includes the actual likelihood of transmission, the likelihood of manifestation (penetrance), and the variability of expression. The family history or pedigree should be obtained and documented in the medical record. In some autosomal dominant conditions, an individual can inherit the gene for the disorder and yet not show any signs of it. This is referred to as "nonpenetrance." To our knowledge, penetrance for the autosomal dominant forms of EB is 100%, so this is not an issue in counseling for EB.

Variability of expression is common in genetic conditions. Individuals with the same genetic disorder differ in the severity with which they manifest the condition. A person who has a dominant form of EB may not realize that his/her children, who are at 50% risk to inherit the same gene, may be more or less severely involved. Individuals with one form of EB may incorrectly believe that their offspring are at risk for other, more severe types and need to be reassured. A common misconception about genetic disease is the idea that disorders worsen in subsequent generations (anticipation). This is not true; severity of expression can vary greatly, but does not attenuate or increase with vertical (generational) transmission. Decisions about reproduction are often based more on the likely severity of the disorder than on the magnitude of the recurrence risk.

For the autosomal recessive forms of EB, it is assumed that both parents of a clinically affected individual are heterozygote carriers for the abnormal allele and have a 25% recurrence risk in each pregnancy, irrespective of the sex or birth order of the conceptus. Unaffected siblings of an individual with autosomal recessive EB have a 2 out of 3 likelihood of being carriers for the abnormal gene but a low risk to have affected children unless they marry a relative. The carrier frequency in the general population for rare recessive disorders is estimated at 1 in 50 to 1 in 100; therefore, the likelihood that a sibling would have an affected child is $\frac{2}{3}$ (sib's carrier risk) $\times \frac{1}{100}$ (carrier frequency) $\times \frac{1}{4}$ (risk of having affected child born to two carriers) $= \frac{1}{600}$. Although this risk is higher than that of the general population, it is low in comparison with the 1 out of 20 to 1 out of 30 risk that every pregnancy carries of resulting in a child with a significant birth defect. Aunts and uncles of children with autosomal recessive forms of EB have a 50% chance of being carriers, and similar risk calculations can be made for them. Persons who themselves have an autosomal recessive form of EB also have a low risk to have affected children; although they will transmit the gene to all of their offspring, unless the other parent is also a carrier, none of the children will have the disorder. For all intents and purposes, the only persons at risk for recurrences of autosomal recessive EB are the parents of the affected child, and these couples should be offered prenatal diagnosis if it is available. Other options include artificial insemination and ovum transfer, which reduce the couple's risk to that of aunts and uncles of the proband. For all other relatives, unless they marry a blood relation, the risk of prenatal diagnostic procedures is far greater than the risk for a pregnancy to be affected.

For autosomal dominant forms of EB, recurrence risks depend on whether the proband represents a new or spontaneous mutation for the condition or if a parent is affected. In both situations, every child born to an affected individual has a 50:50 chance to inherit the normal allele or the abnormal allele, irrespective of sex or birth order. Although expression (severity) may vary, penetrance is 100%. Therefore, an individual who was at risk to inherit autosomal dominant EB who shows no sign of the disorder can be assumed to have inherited the normal gene and to have no risk to pass EB on to his/her children. Genes do not skip generations. If a child with autosomal dominant EB is born to unaffected parents, the assumption is made that the disorder has resulted from a new or spontaneous mutation that occurred in one of the gametes that resulted in the child. Although the child's offspring will be at 50% risk to inherit EB, the parents do not have an increased risk in subsequent pregnancies, as the mutation is assumed to have been a one-time event. Gonadal mosaicism (a mutation involving a significant proportion of the sperm or eggs of an individual) has been implicated for some autosomal dominant disorders that have recurred in offspring of healthy parents, but this is a rare event and parents can be reassured that recurrence is unlikely.

There is only one form of EB that is known to be X-linked: this is the rare Mendes da Costa form of EB simplex that is associated with a variety of other abnormalities. In X-linked conditions, carrier mothers have a 25% risk with each pregnancy to have an affected child (1 out of 2 to transmit the gene × 1 out of 2 to have a male) and a 25% risk to have a carrier (1 out of 2 to transmit × 1 out of 2 to have a female). New mutations can occur for X-linked disorders; in this situation there is no increased recurrence risk. Males with Mendes da Costa do not reproduce. If they were able to do so, all of their daughters would be carriers, having inherited the paternal X chromosome, and none of their sons would be affected, as they would inherit the Y chromosome. An acquired late-onset form of dystrophic EB, EB acquisita, does not appear to have a genetic component.

In summary, the process of genetic counseling is one of education. All relevant aspects of the disorder need to be addressed and it may require more than one session. It is the practice of most genetics clinics to send families follow-up letters, reiterating the information presented during the clinic visit. This provides the family with written documentation that they can review, forward on to other medical caretakers, and share with other family members. Last, referral to support organizations such as D.E.B.R.A. (Dystrophic Epidermolysis Bullosa Research Association) is an integral part of the counseling process.

Acknowledgments. This work was supported in part by NIH Grants GM 15253, AM 17664-01, AR 21557, HD 17664, NIH contract NO1 ARG2272, and a grant from D.E.B.R.A.

References

1. Rodeck CH, Eady RAJ, Gosden CM. Prenatal diagnosis of epidermolysis bullosa letalis. *Lancet.* 1980;1:949–952.
2. Schroder JM, Herzenberg LA. Fetal cells in the maternal circulation: prenatal diagnosis by cell sorting using a fluorescence-activated cell sorter (FACS). In: Milunsky A, ed. *Genetic Disorders and the Fetus.* New York: Plenum; 1979:541–555.
3. UK Collaborative Study on Alpha-Fetoprotein in Relation to Neural Tube Defects. Maternal serum alpha-fetoprotein measurement in antenatal screening for anencephaly and spina bifida early in pregnancy. *Lancet.* 1977;1:1323–1332.
4. Adams MJ Jr, Windham GC, James LM, et al. Clinical interpretation of maternal serum alpha-fetoprotein concentrations. *Am J Obstet Gynecol.* 1984;148:241–254.
5. Crandall BF, Robertson RD, Lebherz TB, et al. Maternal serum alpha-fetoprotein screening for the detection of neural tube defects: report of a pilot program. *West J Med.* 1983;138:524–530.
6. Yacoub T, Campbell CA, Gordon YB, et al. Maternal serum and amniotic fluid concentrations of alphafetoprotein in epidermolysis bullosa simplex. *Br Med J.* 1978;2:307.
7. Campbell S, Pearce JM. Ultrasound visualization of congenital malformations. *Br Med Bull.* 1983;39:322–331.
8. Perry TB. Clinical procedures for prenatal diagnosis of inherited skin disease: amniocentesis, ultrasound, fetoscopy and fetal skin biopsy and blood sampling, chorionic villus sampling. *Semin Dermatol.* 1984;3:155–166.
9. Vandenberghe K, De Wolf F, Fryns JP, et al. Antenatal ultrasound diagnosis of fetal malformations: possibilities, limitations and dilemmas. *Eur J Obstet Gynecol Reprod Biol.* 1984;18:279–297.
10. Blackwell R. New developments in equipment. *Clin Obstet Gynaecol.* 1983;10:371–394.
11. Epstein CJ, Cox DR, Schonberg SA, et al. Recent developments in the prenatal diagnosis of genetic diseases and birth defects. *Annu Rev Genet.* 1983;17:49–83.
12. Liebskind D, Basea R, Elequin F, et al. Diagnostic ultrasound: effects on the DNA and growth patterns of human cells. *Radiology.* 1979;131:177–184.
13. Liebskind D, Basea R, Mender F, et al. Sister chromatid exchanges in human lymphocytes after exposure to diagnostic ultrasound. *Science.* 1975;205:1273–1275.
14. Stratmeyer ME. Research in ultrasound bioeffects. A public health overview. *Birth Fam J.* 1980;7:92–100.
15. Bolsen B. Question of risk still hovers over routine prenatal use of ultrasound. *JAMA.* 1982;247:2195–2197.
16. Kinnier-Wilson LM, Waterhouse JAH. Obstetric ultrasound and childhood malignancies. *Lancet.* 1984;2:998–999.
17. Stark CR, Orleans M, Haverkamp AD, et al. Short- and long-term risks after exposure to diagnostic ultrasound in utero. *Obstet Gynecol.* 1984;63:194–200.
18. Hahnemann N, Mohr J. Genetic diagnosis in the embryo by means of biopsy from extraembryonic membranes. *Bull Eur Soc Hum Genet.* 1968;2:23–29.
19. Tietung Hospital, Department of Obstetrics and Gynecology. Fetal sex prediction

by sex chromatin of chorionic villi cells during early pregnancy. *Chin Med J.* 1975;1:117–126.
20. Kazy Z, Rozovsky IS, Bakharev VA. Chorion biopsy in early pregnancy: a method of early prenatal diagnosis for inherited disorders. *Prenat Diagn.* 1982; 2:39–115.
21. Ward RHT, Modell R, Petrou M, et al. A method of chorionic villus sampling in the first trimester of pregnancy under real time ultrasonic guidance. *Br Med J [Clin Res].* 1983;286:1542–1544.
22. Simoni G, Brambati B, Danesino C, et al. Efficient direct chromosome analyses and enzyme determinations from chorionic villi samples in the first trimester of pregnancy. *Hum Genet.* 1983;63:349–357.
23. Jackson LG. CVS Newsletter. Philadelphia, Jefferson Medical College. 1984 (ongoing).
24. Rodeck CH, Morsman JM. First-trimester chorion biopsy. *Br Med Bull.* 1983;39:338–342.
25. Olaisen B, Gedde-Dahl T Jr. GPT-Epidermolysis bullosa simplex (EBS Ogna) linkage in man. *Hum Hered.* 1973;23:189–196.
26. Humphries MM, Sheils D, Lawler M, et al. Epidermolysis bullosa: evidence for linkage to genetic markers on chromosome 1 in a family with the autosomal dominant simplex form. *Genomics.* 1990;7:377–81.
27. Mulley JC, Turner T, Nicholls C, et al. Genetic linkage analysis of epidermolysis bullosa dystrophica, Cockayne-Touraine type. *Clin Genet.* 1985;28:31–35.
28. Gedde-Dahl T, Jr. *Epidermolysis Bullosa, a Clinical, Genetic and Epidemiological Study.* Oslo: Universitetsforlaget/Baltimore: The Johns Hopkins Press; 1971.
29. Joensen HD, Hansen HE, Henningsen K, et al. A study of the linkage relations of epidermolysis bullosa dystrophica. *Hum Hered.* 1979;29:221–225.
30. Gedde-Dahl T Jr. Classification of epidermolysis bullosa. In: Herzberg JJ, Korting GW, eds. *Padiatrische Dermatologie.* Stuttgart/New York: F.K. Schattauer Verlag; 1978.
31. Liley A. Intrauterine transfusion of fetus in hemolytic clisease. *Br Med J.* 1963;2:1107–1109.
32. MRC (Medical Research Council). Working party on amniocentesis. *Br J Obstet Gynaecol.* 1985;85(Suppl):2.
33. National Institute of Child Health and Human Development National Registry for Amniocentesis Study Group. Mid-trimester amniocentesis for prenatal diagnosis: Safety and accuracy. *JAMA.* 1976;236:1471–1476.
34. Turnbull AC, Mackenzie IZ. Second trimester amniocentesis and termination of pregnancy. *Br Med Bull.* 1983;39:315–321.
35. Aitken DA, Morrison NM, Ferguson-Smiths MA. Predictive value of amniotic acetylcholinesterase analysis in the diagnosis of fetal abnormality in 3700 pregnancies. *Prenat Diagn.* 1984;4:329–340.
36. Brock DHJ, Hayward C. Gel electrophoresis of amniotic fluid acetylcholinesterase as an aid to the prenatal diagnosis of fetal defects. *Clin Chim Acta.* 1980;108:135–141.
37. Report of the collaborative acetylcholinesterase study. Amniotic fluid acetylcholinesterase electrophoresis as a secondary test in the diagnosis of anencephaly and open spina bifida in early pregnancy. *Lancet.* 1981;2:321–324.
38. Leschot NJ, Treffers PE, Becker-Bloemkolk MJ, et al. Severe congenital skin defects in a newborn. *Eur J Obstet Gynecol Reprod Biol.* 1980;10:381–388.

39. Bick DP, Balkite EA, Baumgarten A, et al. The association of congenital skin disorders with acetylcholinesterase in amniotic fluid. *Prenat Diagn.* 1987;7:543–549.

40. Humphries SE, Williamson R. Application of recombinant DNA technology to prenatal detection of inherited defects. *Br Med Bull.* 1983;39:343–357.

41. Eady RAJ, Gunner DB, Doria-Lamba-Carbone L, et al. Prenatal diagnosis of bullous ichthyosiform erythroderma: detection of tonofilament clumps in fetal epidermal and amniotic fluid cells. *J Med Genet.* 1986;23:46–51.

42. Holbrook KA, Dale BA, Sybert VP, et al. Epidermolytic hyperkeratosis: ultrastructure and biochemistry of skin and amniotic fluid cells from two affected fetuses and a newborn infant. *J Invest Dermatol.* 1983;80:222–227.

43. Holbrook KA. The biology of human fetal skin at ages related to prenatal diagnosis. *Pediatr Dermatol.* 1983;1:97–111.

44. Holbrook KA, Hoff MS. Structure of the developing human embryonic and fetal skin. *Semin Dermatol.* 1984;3:185–202.

45. Bauer EA. Recessive dystrophic epidermolysis bullosa: evidence for an altered collagenase in fibroblast cultures. *Proc Natl Acad Sci USA.* 1977;74:4646–4650.

46. Bauer EA, Ludman MD, Goldberg JD, et al. Antenatal diagnosis of recessive dystrophic epidermolysis bullosa: collagenase expression in cultured fibroblasts as a biochemical marker. *J Invest Dermatol.* 1986;87:597–601.

47. Hislop A, Fairweather DVI. Amniocentesis and lung growth: an animal experiment with clinical implications. *Lancet.* 1982;2:1271–1272.

48. De Vore GR, Mahoney MJ, Hobbins JC. Fetoscopy: an update. *Clin Gynecol Obstet.* 1980;23:481–498.

49. Filkins K, Benzie RJ. Fetoscopy. *Clin Obstet Gynecol.* 1983;26:339–345.

50. Golbus MS for the International Fetoscopy Group. Special report: the status of fetoscopy and fetal tissue sampling. *Prenat Diagn.* 1984;4:79–81.

51. Hopkins EL, Carey J. Amniocentesis and fetoscopy. In: Scott RB, ed. *Advances in the Pathophysiology, Diagnosis and Treatment of Sickle Cell Disease.* New York: Alan R Liss; 1982:27–45.

52. Mahoney MJ. Fetoscopy. *Pediatr Ann.* 1981;10:61–68.

53. Mahoney MJ. Fetoscopy and genetic disease. *Birth Defects.* 1981;17:9–16.

54. Perry TB. Fetoscopy. In: Marois M, ed. *Prevention of Physical and Mental Congenital Defects. Part B: Epidemiology, Early Detection and Therapy, and Environmental Factors.* New York: Alan R Liss; 1984:207–212.

55. Rauskolb R. Fetoscopy. *J Perinat Med.* 1983;11:223–231.

56. Rodeck CH. Prenatal diagnosis by fetoscopy and chorion biopsy. *Aust NZ J Obstet Gynaecol.* 1984;24:86–90.

57. Rodeck CH, Nicolaides KH. Fetoscopy and fetal tissue sampling. *Br Med Bull.* 1983;39:332–337.

58. Rodeck CH, Nicolaides KH. The use of fetoscopy for prenatal diagnosis and treatment. *Semin Perinatol.* 1983;7:118–124.

59. Schwartz DB, Zweibel WJ, Donovan D, et al. Fetoscopic visualization in second-trimester pregnancies. *Am J Obstet Gynecol.* 1983;145:51–55.

60. Usajiw G. Prenatal diagnosis with fetoscopy. *N Engl J Med.* 1977;297:949–950.

61. Westin B. Hysteroscopy in early pregnancy. *Lancet.* 1954;2:872.

62. Lofberg L, Gustavii B. "Blind" versus direct vision technique for fetal skin sampling in cases for prenatal diagnosis. *Clin Genet.* 1984;24:37–41.

63. Lofberg L, Gustavii B. Technical difficulties in fetal skin sampling. *Acta Obstet Gynecol Scand.* 1982;61:505–507.
64. Anton-Lamprecht I, Arnold M-L, Holbrook KA. Methodology in sampling of fetal skin and pitfalls in the interpretation of fetal skin biopsy specimens. *Semin Dermatol.* 1984;3:203–215.
65. Rocker I, Laurence KM. Defect in fetal membranes after fetoscopy. *Lancet.* 1978;2:716.
66. Anton-Lamprecht I, Schnyder UW. Ultrastructure of inborn errors of keratinization. VI. Inherited ichthyosis—a model system for heterogeneities in keratinization disturbances. *Arch Dermatol Forsch.* 1974;250:207–227.
67. Anton-Lamprecht I. Prenatal diagnosis of epidermolysis bullosa hereditaria: a review. *Semin Dermatol.* 1984;3:229–240.
68. Anton-Lamprecht I. Prenatal diagnosis of genetic disorders of the skin by means of electron microscopy. *Hum Genet.* 1981;59:392–405.
69. Blanchet-Bardon CI, Souteyrand P, Mimoz C, et al. Epidermolyse bulleuse lethale—diagnostic d'exclusion antenatal. *Presse Med.* 1984;13:680–681.
70. Lofberg L, Anton-Lamprecht I, Michaelsson G, et al. Prenatal exclusion of Herlitz syndrome by electron microscopy of fetal skin biopsies obtained at fetoscopy. *Acta Derm Venereol (Stockh).* 1983;63:185–189.
71. Tidman MJ, Eady RAJ. Hemidesmosome heterogeneity in junctional epidermolysis bullosa revealed by morphometric analysis. *J Invest Dermatol.* 1986;86:51–56.
72. Anton-Lamprecht I. Genetically induced abnormalities of epidermal differentiation and ultrastructure in ichthyoses and epidermolyses: pathogenesis, heterogeneity, fetal manifestation, and prenatal diagnosis. *J Invest Dermatol.* 1983;81:149s–156s.
73. Anton-Lamprecht I, Jovanovic V, Arnold M-L, et al. Prenatal diagnosis of epidermolysis bullosa dystrophica Hallopeau-Siemens with electron microscopy of fetal skin. *Lancet.* 1981;2:1077–1079.
74. Blanchet-Bardon C, Dumez Y, Nazzaro V, et al. Le diagnostic antenatal des epidermolyses bulleuses hereditaires . *Ann Derm Venereol.* 1987;114:525–539.
75. Fine J-D, Robin AJ, Eady MB, et al. Prenatal diagnosis of dominant and recessive dystrophic epidermolysis bullosa: application and limitations in the use of KF-1 and LH 7:2 monoclonal antibodies and immunofluorescence mapping technique. *J Invest Dermatol.* 1988;91:465–471 .
76. Heagerty AH, Kennedy AR, Gunner DB, et al. Rapid prenatal diagnosis and exclusion of epidermolysis bullosa using novel antibody probes. *J Invest Dermatol.* 1986;86:603–605.
77. Heagerty AHM, Kennedy AR, Leigh IM, et al. LH 7:2 monoclonal antibody defines a common dermo-epidermal junction defect in recessive forms of dystrophic epidermolysis bullosa (abstr). *J Invest Dermatol.* 1985;84:448.
78. Kennedy AR, Heagerty AHM, Ortonne J-P, et al. Abnormal binding of an anti-amnion antibody to epidermal basement membrane provides a new diagnostic probe for junctional epidermolysis bullosa. *Br J Dermatol.* 1985;113:651–659.
79. Fine JD, Holbrook KA, Elias S, et al. Applicability of 19-DEJ-1 monoclonal antibody for the prenatal diagnosis or exclusion of junctional epidermolysis bullosa. *Prenat Diagn.* 1990;10:219–229.

20
Physical Rehabilitation of Epidermolysis Bullosa Patients

REBECCA L. LIPNICK and BARBARA S. STANERSON

A major frustration of the occupational or physical therapist asked to treat a patient with epidermolysis bullosa (EB) is the lack of information in the literature regarding rehabilitation for these individuals. Except for a few references to splinting after surgical releases in hands and feet,[1-4] there is no mention of therapy. It is unclear if this is because the therapies have not traditionally been a part of the treatment provided for EB, or if therapists have not published the results of their experiences with this population.

Before the establishment of research centers for EB, it was uncommon for a therapist to see more than one individual with the condition. Therefore, it was difficult for a therapist to draw conclusions from results observed, or to establish effective treatment approaches. At the Washington University Medical Center (WUMC), all patients with the diagnosis of EB of any type are referred to physical and occupational therapy for evaluation and treatment. The authors of this chapter have had the opportunity to follow numerous patients with EB and to participate as members of a multidisciplinary team in the care of these individuals. A description of the program that was developed at Irene Walter Johnson (IWJ) Rehabilitation Institute at Washington University Medical Center follows.

Occupational Therapy Evaluation

The purpose of the occupational therapy evaluation is to determine:

1. level of function in fine motor and life skills, including need for adaptive equipment or techniques,
2. active and passive range of motion of the upper extremities and,
3. web space measurements (recessive dystrophic only).

Fine motor skills are assessed in patients from birth to age 6 years using the Peabody Fine Motor Developmental Scale. Patients age 6+ to 14 years are assessed using the Bruininks-Oseretsky Test of Motor Proficiency, if they are physically capable of performing the test items. Either the long or short form of this test may be used. These evaluations are standardized and can be used for test/retest measurements. The tests are widely available to occupational therapists, and if used consistently by other therapists, could contribute to a data base of developmental information on the EB population. It is interesting to note that even individuals with seemingly benign cases of simplex and dominant dystrophic EB have been noted to score below the norm on some test items—particularly those involving balance and upper limb speed and dexterity. No standardized test is used consistently to evaluate fine motor function in EB patients over the age of 14 years. Manipulation tests such as the Purdue Peg Board or the Minnesota Rate of Manipulation Test have been used.

Self-care skills appropriate to the patient's age are assessed using patient/family interview as well as direct observation. A feeding assessment is indicated if oral intake is deemed inadequate for growth, tissue healing, and nutritional support. Intraoral blistering should be noted, as well as difficulties coordinating suck/swallow/breathing. In assessing feeding, consideration should be given to behavioral/manipulative elements that may require a behavior modification program. Work and/or academic skills should be assessed. A thorough assessment of an adolescent or adult might include technology, work tolerance, and a driving readiness evaluation. Assessment with adaptive equipment is recommended for patients with physical limitations. It is important to remember that the devices themselves may need adaptation to enable the patient to hold and manipulate them without risk of skin trauma.

Active and passive range of motion are assessed using standard goniometric measures. Although deformities and loss of range of motion are characteristic of recessive dystrophic EB, *all* individuals with EB are susceptible to soft tissue limitations if inappropriate positioning exists or active movement is limited. Therefore, splints may be indicated for persons who do not have a dystrophic disorder.

Web space measurements of both hands and feet should be monitored in all individuals with recessive dystrophic EB. The following method has been developed to allow for accurate sequential measurements. The ulnar styloid and radial head are palpated and an imaginary line constructed connecting them. The length of the long finger is measured from this line along the third metacarpal to the end of the long finger. Web spaces are measured from the imaginary line on the wrist, between the digits, to the end of the web space (Fig. 20.1). All measurements should be to the nearest millimeter. Over time, the sequential difference in long finger length will indicate how much of the change in web space measurements can be attributed to normal growth. An increase in web space measurement greater than the increase in long finger length indicates a progression of finger webbing. A change in web space measurement less than the change in long finger length indicates improvement of web space integrity.

The same technique can be applied to measuring toe web spaces. The

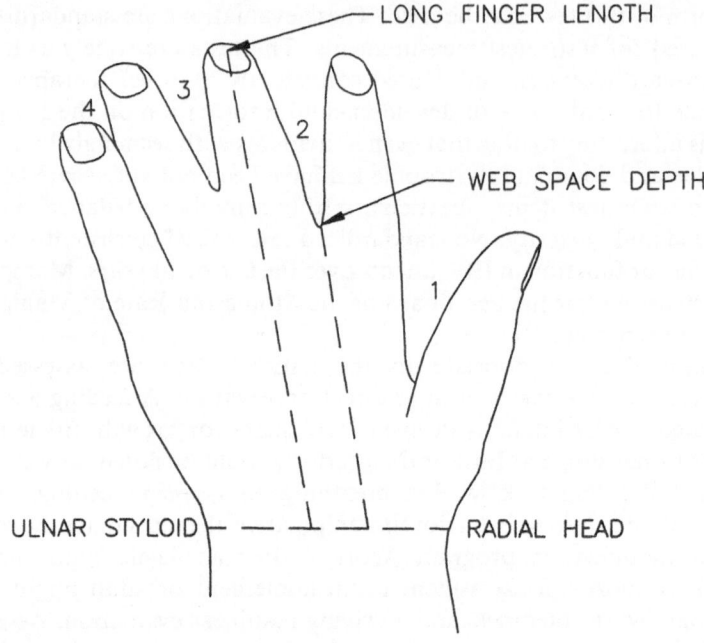

FIGURE 20.1. Diagram illustrating assessment of web space measurement.

imaginary line is drawn from medial to lateral malleolus and the length of the great toe is monitored.

Occupational Therapy Treatment

Splinting, other than after surgical releases, has not been mentioned in the literature. It may be that prophylactic or corrective splinting was deemed ineffective, as the scarring process itself cannot be prevented. At WUMC, we have drawn on information learned from burn treatment regarding scar management[5-7] and employ routine splinting for recessive dystrophic EB. We have data on five patients who have worn splints for at least 18 months and all have preserved or even improved web space integrity. The splints are also used after surgical release.

Web space splinting is achieved using Otoform, a moldable silicone-based putty available from Aquaplast Corporation. The material is molded on the patient's hand from the palmar surface, through the web spaces, to the dorsum (Fig. 20.2). In an infant or very small child, the splint can consist of a single place extending through all four web spaces. For older children, the center of a strip of Otoform is placed on the palmar aspect of the index finger and the two ends are brought to the dorsum through the web spaces

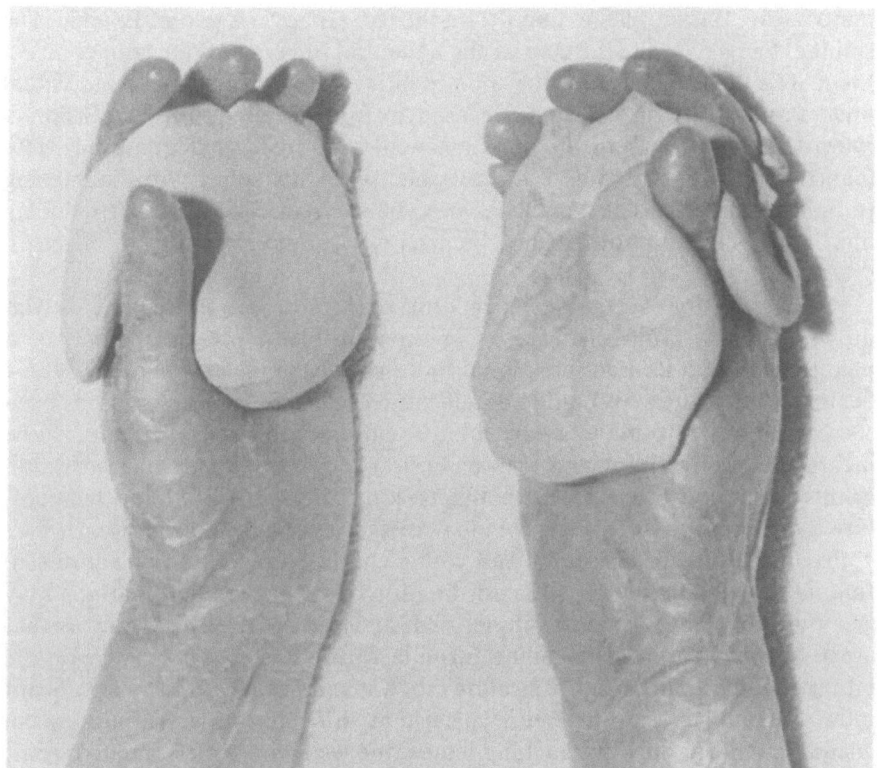

FIGURE 20.2. Web space splinting using Otoform, a silicone-based putty.

on either side of the index finger. A second strip is formed around the ring finger, thus separating the fingers at each web space. Adults usually require individual pieces through each web space. Sufficient material is placed in the web spaces to separate the fingers and allow pressure to be applied through the splinting material to the web space. Splints are secured with a strip of fabric slipped over the individual fingers and pulled firmly into each web space to provide pressure, and held at the wrist with a strap of soft material such as Velfoam.

The web space splint is worn at night only. It is clearly explained to the patient and family that the splints will not permanently prevent web space loss and decreases in hand function, but that they may delay the process. Web space splinting has been attempted on the feet, but the results have not been as good as those with the hands.

The other component of hand deformity in recessive dystrophic EB is finger flexion contractures. Finger extension splinting is a challenge because of the risk of causing skin trauma through the fabrication and/or wearing of the splint. We have had good results using a dorsally based splint of low temperature thermoplastic that fits on the forearm over a pad of Exudry. The splint extends over the dorsum of the hand and fingers but does not contract them. The finger portion of the splint pan is cut to correspond to individual fingers and strips of Velfoam are used to pull the digits into extension— *toward, but not touching* the hard plastic dorsal splint. Adequate purchase (control) on the joints has been obtained with this splint without causing trauma to the skin. This splint has been effective in controlling or reducing mild finger flexion contractures, but has not shown a significant effect on severe contractures.

It is possible for soft tissue contractures to be present in those patients who do not have scarring disorders. Common problems are maceration of a palmar thumb in infants, positional tightness of thenar musculature, elbow flexion contractures, and ankle dorsiflexion contractures. Otoform has been successfully used to make a soft splint for thumb abduction. It can also be incorporated into elbow and knee extension splints and ankle plantarflexion splints by serving as a base that contacts skin or dressings, with low temperature thermoplastic over it to provide necessary strength and rigidity.

Feeding problems in infants and young children must often be addressed. Infants showing difficulty with coordination of suck/swallow/breathing may show improvement if a soft nipple, such as various "preemie" nipples that are available, is used. Thickening formula with rice cereal may increase the infant's ability to coordinate swallowing. Some infants who have significant intraoral involvement and show persistent difficulty with establishing an adequate seal for effective sucking have done well with a cleft palate nurser, which allows formula to be gently squeezed into the mouth. This should not be confused with the lamb's nipple, which has been used with cleft palates in the past. Cheek and jaw support can be used with these infants, but care should be taken to distribute the pressure over a wide area and to avoid slipping of the feeder's hand position and subsequent skin shearing.

Many of the feeding problems seen at WUMC have no apparent organic basis; instead, these problems seem to have a behavioral basis. In such cases, it is suggested that the occupational therapist (OT) work with a psychologist and the parents in establishing a program of behavior modification to emphasize reinforcement of appropriate eating behaviors and to identify and otherwise fulfill the needs that have been satisfied by the inappropriate behaviors and patterns.

A primary concern of the OT is that of optimizing hand function. The OT should become familiar with how hand dressings are being done and, if appropriate, suggest various methods of wrapping that will promote individual digit use rather than mittening of all fingers. Hand dressings, if used at all, should be minimized during the day to allow for active hand use. Even infants with significant hand involvement should have supervised periods without hand dressings to promote awareness and use of the hands. Passive and active range of motion of the hands and arms should be performed routinely and the family trained in how to perform them. Fine motor and manipulation activities should be encouraged and families provided with suggestions for activities that involve hand use at the patient's developmental level. Patient and family education in this area should emphasize the developmental, psychological, and *functional* gains of these activities, compared to a slightly increased incidence of blistering when dressings are reduced and hand use increased.

Developmentally appropriate functional self-care and life skills training is a vital part of an OT program. The OT can help direct the patient and family in the selection of realistic goals and activities that are important and meaningful to the patient. The flexibility and mobility exercises discussed in the physical therapy section are an important element of successful self-care training. For patients with physical limitations, adaptive equipment must be considered. The therapist must remember that even an older patient may have never seen an occupational therapist before, and that previous exposure to adapted techniques and equipment cannot be assumed.

Physical Therapy Management

The purpose of this section is to describe the problems occurring in individuals diagnosed with EB who are amenable to physical therapy intervention and the programming necessary for management of these problems. The physical therapy program developed at IWJ has been designed to address specifically the rehabilitation needs of patients with EB. The program includes a) prescription of specific exercises, sports, and leisure activities, b) a specialized hydrotherapy program, and c) education of the family and other health care professionals concerning handling and positioning of the child.

Physical Therapy Evaluation

Evaluation of the patient with EB entails assessing motor development, postural faults, gait deviations, endurance, and the need for orthoses and prostheses. The severity of involvement in each of these areas is dependent on the specific type of EB. The patient with recessive dystrophic EB presents with limitations in these areas that are profoundly evident and that are representative of the range of problems in all types of the disorder. Physical therapy management, however, is required for patients with all forms of EB.

When considering the motor development of a child with EB, standardized developmental tests commonly used are the Peabody Developmental Motor Scales and, for the older child, the Bruininks-Oseretsky Test of Motor Proficiency. One explanation for the fine and gross motor delays often observed may be the restricted environment, generally set by concerned parents, in an attempt to limit blister formation. A certain amount of blistering will occur regardless of how well the child's skin is protected from shearing forces. Therefore, drastically limiting the child's ability to move may have the more profound effect of inhibiting motor development, rather than lessening blister formation. Education of the parents who have a child with EB must begin as soon as possible to encourage them to allow the child the opportunity to explore his environment and promote motor skills.

Postural and gait analysis in patients with recessive dystrophic EB will reveal poor skeletal alignment in response to a severe loss of flexibility, beginning in the cervical spine and continuing throughout the skeletal and muscular systems. As these patients reach adulthood, common postural faults seen are a forward head and shoulders, thoracic and lumbar kyphosis, and contractures in the elbows, hips, knees, and ankles. Limited flexibility in trunk rotation and elongation is frequently observed, as is a structural scoliosis. The sedentary lifestyle of these individuals also contributes to severe deconditioning and limited endurance for any type of physical activity.

The chronic poor posture alignment of a patient with recessive dystrophic EB promotes severe muscle imbalances. As an example, there is often a shortening of the anterior shoulder-girdle musculature, most commonly the pectoralis minor. In contrast, the posterior shoulder-girdle musculature, specifically the lower trapezius, becomes weakened because of the overly lengthened position. The postural deviations in this example are not just a result of the individual's occasional, or even frequent, slouched posture when sitting, but rather a response to true development of scar tissue, lack of active movement, and faulty habitual positioning.

It is important to recognize that faulty movement patterns can be apparent in infancy. These may present as hyperextension of the upper cervical spine and prolonged contraction in the paraspinal musculature producing a sustained position of trunk extension and retraction of the scapula, accompanied by the external rotation of the shoulders. The exacerbation of open wounds during infancy and the pain associated with handling and wound care appear to be at least partially responsible for the abnormal movement patterns noted at this age.

Physical Therapy Treatment

Exercise prescription is the area in which the physical therapist's expertise can play a vital role. Based on the results of the examination, specific exercises are prescribed that will promote flexibility, strength, and endurance.

Despite fragile skin, EB patients can be treated with a wide range of physical therapy techniques. Active exercise, stretching, resistive exercises, and endurance activities are essential inclusions in the program. Lengthening shortened muscles, as in the case of the pectoralis minor, can be done passively or in conjunction with strengthening exercises for the antagonist, the lower trapezius.

Correct positioning during the exercise regimen is essential for maximum effect. Suggestions to promote conditioning must also be included in the exercise prescription. Sports or leisure activities that have limited physical contact should be recommended, such as bicycling, swimming, or walking programs.

The prescription of orthoses or prostheses should also be considered to protect the skin and increase function. The feet typically become severely deformed, characterized by webbing of the toes and clublike appearance of the foot. Ambulation becomes painful because of open wounds and unstable because the ankle is poorly supported. Marr et al. described the use of a heat-molded footwear to enable a 20-year-old woman to regain independent mobility by improving the ankle position as much as possible and relieving pressure over painful areas.[8] Amputation is also common because of squamous cell carcinoma; Jain and DeLisa fitted a patient with a simple prosthesis to allow a patient to regain her mobility after a below-knee amputation.[9] In both situations the patient was able to tolerate the equipment without further damage to the skin and to increase her independent mobility.

Another component in the comprehensive physical therapy program is hydrotherapy. This provides an ideal environment for the physical therapist to examine how the patient moves, free of clothing and bandages. Wound care is also done at the time and the physical therapist can assist and consult with nursing in the procedure (see Chapter 23).

Patient and family education is a key component of a comprehensive rehabilitation program. Family and other health care professionals should receive instructions in handling and positioning to promote more normal motor development. A patient must also become aware of how to protect and care for his body. All members of the EB treatment team assume an educational role.

Explanation of handling techniques and clothing/padding options is often provided by the physical and occupational therapists. Skin integrity is best preserved during active handling with firm pressure on as wide an area as possible. For example, a whole hand stabilizing a leg for a dressing change is less likely to cause trauma than two fingers that concentrate pressure and friction on two small points. Rather than lifting infants and small children under the axillae, we suggest an arm across their chest and a hand under their bottom. Shearling moccasins have been found to be very good footwear for the young child. Soft fabrics and long sleeves protect and cover dressings. Sweat bands become knee, elbow, and hand protectors. Once parents are presented with a few basic concepts, they invariably progress to new and improved variations of their own.

Psychosocial issues are also a concern for the physical and occupational therapist. Emotional reactions to a restricted independent lifestyle and to disfigurement as a result of scarring and amputation may be as debilitating as the physical limitations imposed by the disease process.

Longitudinal studies have not been done to describe the level of independence in functional skills and self-care these patients could achieve with aggressive rehabilitation. Research is a necessary element for determining the effectiveness of physical and occupational therapy intervention. Striving for an erect posture, full range of motion, and normal hand function may not be realistic goals for this population. Treatment must be directed at promoting active movement in the most functional and efficient manner possible to allow the patient to achieve the maximum possible degree of independence. It is important to convey to practitioners information regarding rehabilitation of EB and the impact physical and occupational therapy intervention can have in achieving and promoting an individual's maximum potential.

Acknowledgments. The authors gratefully acknowledge the contributions of Michael Mueller, M.H.S., P.T., Susan Deusinger, Ph.D., P.T., Monica Perlmutter, M.A., O.T., Lucile Paden, Ph.D., and David Lipnick in the preparation of this chapter.

References

1. Greider JL, Flatt AE. Care of the hand in recessive epidermolysis bullosa. *Plast Reconstr Surg.* 1983;72:222–227.
2. Horner RL, Wiedel JD, Bralliar F. Involvement of the hand in epidermolysis bullosa. *J Bone Joint Surg.* 1971;53-A(7):1347–1356.
3. Zarem HA, Pearson RW, Leaf N. Surgical management of hand deformities in recessive dystrophic epidermolysis bullosa. *Br J Plast Surg.* 1974;27:176–181.
4. Resnick JI, Rohtich RJ, May JW. Management of advanced foot deformities in dystrophic epidermolysis bullosa. *Plast Reconstr Surg.* 1988;82:888–891.
5. Malick M, Carr J. Manual on Management of the Burn Patient. Harmarville Rehabilitation Center, Pittsburgh PA, 1982.
6. Larson DL, Abston S, Dobrkovsky M, et al. *The Prevention and Correction of Burn Scar Contracture and Hypertrophy.* Galveston, Tex: Shriner's Burns Institute, University of Texas Medical Branch; 1973.
7. Malick MH, Carr JA. Flexible elastomer molds in burn scar control. *Am J Occup Ther.* 1980;34(9):603–608.
8. Marr ST, Hoskins M, Molley HF. Report of heat moulded footwear for a patient with epidermolysis bullosa. *Austr J Dermatol.* 1979;20(2):90–92.
9. Jain SS, DeLisa JA. Successful prosthetic fitting of a patient with epidermolysis bullosa dystrophica. *Am J Phys Med Rehab.* 1988;67(3):104–107.

21
Nutritional Management of the Epidermolysis Bullosa Patient

Donna Tesi and Andrew N. Lin

Some degree of nutritional compromise is present in virtually all patients with epidermolysis bullosa (EB). As with all clinical manifestations of EB, the extent of nutritional compromise is determined by the type of EB. It tends to be mild in EB simplex, but can be very severe in junctional and dystrophic forms. In patients with the Hallopeau-Siemens type of recessive dystrophic EB, the combination of esophageal stricture, abnormal dentition, microstomia, and crippling hand deformities results in a picture of severe, recalcitrant nutritional deprivation unparalleled in all of clinical medicine. In this chapter we review the complex etiologies leading to nutritional compromise in EB patients, and discuss management guidelines.

Nutritional Requirements for Normal Growth and Development

The Food and Nutrition Board of the National Research Council–National Academy of Sciences has established formulations of daily nutrient intakes that are considered to be adequate to meet the known nutrient needs of healthy individuals.[1] Called "recommended daily dietary allowances" (RDA), these guidelines specify the recommended daily amount of calories, proteins, vitamins, and minerals (Table 21.1). These guidelines require adjustments for patients with abnormal nutritional needs. For example, it is believed that pregnancy requires an additional daily intake of 300 kcal.[1] Similarly, the burn patient requires markedly increased nutritional intake to keep up with hemodynamic and metabolic changes.[2] Although the burn patient is not entirely comparable to the EB patient, they both face problems created by the loss of large amounts of skin.[3] In one study, resting energy expenditure in two patients with recessive dystrophic EB and one with junctional EB was measured by analyzing oxygen consumption and carbon dioxide production.[4] In all three patients, the measured values exceeded calculated estimates using three different formulae. In another study, rates of whole body protein synthesis and breakdown in four EB patients were significantly higher than

TABLE 21.1. Recommended daily energy intake and dietary protein allowances.

| Age (years) | Weight (kg) | Height (cm) | Average energy allowance (kcal) | | Protein | |
			Per day	Per kg	g/day	g/kg
0–0.5	6	60	650	108	13	2.2
0.5–1	9	71	850	98	14	1.6
1–3	13	90	1300	102	16	1.2
4–6	20	112	1800	90	24	1.1
7–10	28	132	2000	70	28	1.0
Males	45	157	2500	55	45	1.0
11–14	66	176	3000	45	59	0.9
15–18	72	177	2900	40	58	0.8
19–24	79	176	2900	37	63	0.8
25–50	77	173	2300	30	63	0.8
51+						
Females	46	157	2200	47	46	1.0
11–14	55	163	2200	40	44	0.8
15–18	58	164	2200	38	46	0.8
19–24	63	163	2200	36	50	0.8
25–50	65	160	1900	30	50	0.8
51+						

Reprinted with permission from *Recommended Dietary Allowances*, 1989 by the National Academy of Sciences. Published by National Academy Press, Washington, DC.

normal controls, and were comparable to rates found in burn patients.[5] Although the number of study patients is small, these observations support the concept that EB patients have increased nutritional requirements. Satisfying these requirements can be difficult, because EB patients present with complex gastrointestinal lesions that may severely restrict oral intake.

Nutritional Deficiencies in EB Patients

Various gastrointestinal complications limit nutrition intake in EB patients. In EB simplex, patients may have oral blisters from time to time. Although these often heal within a few days, they are usually painful and will interfere with oral intake, especially in infants and children. In the subtype of EB simplex characterized by herepetiform grouping of blisters (the Dowling-Meara subtype), intraoral blistering can be extensive.[6] In addition to oral blisters, patients with junctional and dystrophic forms of EB often present with enamel defects of the teeth and extensive caries, further compromising nutritional intake. In an attempt to decrease trauma to the oral mucosa due to chewing, patients may prefer foods that are soft in texture such as ice cream, avoiding meats and fresh vegetables, thus decreasing the nutritional value of their diet. Also, esophageal blisters are common, especially in reces-

sive dystrophic EB. These often heal with scarring, causing esophageal stenosis and dysphagia. Most patients with recessive dystrophic EB also have some
degree of contracture of the fingers, and many have complete mitten deformity of the hands, making it almost impossible to hold eating utensils.
Feeding therefore becomes a time-consuming and tedious process requiring
the help of an assistant. Coupled with enhanced caloric requirements, it is not
surprising that many patients with EB have severely compromised nutrition
intake.

Although nutritional compromise is commonly seen in EB patients, very
few studies have analyzed their nutritional profiles. In one study, plasma or
erythrocyte levels of 10 nutrients were measured in 73 patients with simplex,
junctional, and dystrophic forms of EB.[7] Normal levels of plasma folate,
thiamine, ribloflavin, and copper were seen in all patients examined. Deficient
levels of other nutrients were seen in patients with specific types of EB. Low
plasma iron levels were seen in 3 of 10 patients with junctional EB and 2 of
8 with recessive dystrophic EB. All patients with the Herlitz variant of
junctional EB had low iron levels despite administration of supplemental
iron; this was cited as support for the presence of the marked malabsorptive
state that is often assumed to be present in these patients. Erythrocyte zinc
levels were normal in most patients tested, but plasma levels were reduced in
half of patients with junctional EB and 56% of those with recessive dystrophic EB. Among the latter, a definite relationship between the overall severity
of EB activity and reduced plasma zinc levels was noted, although the precise
role of zinc in wound healing is still controversial.[8] Approximately a quarter
of patients with EB simplex had low levels of vitamin C, although none had
clinical signs of scurvy. Low levels of vitamin B_6 and B_{12} were seen in some
patients with various forms of EB.

Another study analyzed the nutrition profile of four patients with junctional EB and three with recessive dystrophic EB.[4] All patients were significantly shorter and thinner than controls matched for age and sex. Dietary
intake was assessed by 24-hr recall and 3-day food records. Six patients had
inadequate intake of zinc, magnesium, calories and vitamin D; five had
inadequate intake of vitmians B and B_6, folic acid, calcium, and iron; four
had inadequate intake of Vitamin B_{12} and thiamine; and three had inadequate intake of vitamin A, protein, phosphorus, and vitmin C.

Management of Nutritional Deficits in EB Patients

Correction of nutritional deficits in EB patients can be a difficult and frustrating experience. Many patients have chronic cutaneous wounds from which
blood and electrolytes are constantly lost, making it almost impossible to
fully correct deficiency of iron and other nutrients. Factors that limit oral
intake, such as dental caries, esophageal strictures, and oral blisters must be
dealt with as outlined elsewhere in this text.

All EB patients require consultation with a dietician to assess the extent to which nutrient intake has been compromised. By analyzing food records and patients' dietary recall, one can calculate calorie counts and determine amount of nutrients consumed. Because of intermittent presence of painful oral blisters, EB patients often develop erratic eating patterns, tending to minimize oral intake when oral blisters are present. Specific enquiries about such variations must be made in order to arrive at a dietary history representative for a given patient. In addition, underweight patients tend to overestimate the actual amount of food consumed,[9] and this must be considered to maximize the accuracy of a diet history. In addition to a diet history, blood tests should be done to detect anemia and determine levels of protein, albumin, and trace metals such as iron and zinc.

Once a diet is found to be deficient in specific nutrients, steps should be taken to remedy such deficiencies. In patients who are unable to tolerate solid foods because of dysphagia, the use of nutritional supplements should be considered (Table 21.2). The market contains supplements designed to enhance specific nutrient requirements such as calories, carbohydrates, proteins, and fats (Table 21.2). Some of these are mixed with milk or water and consumed like a milkshake, whereas others are added in small quantities to beverages as well as to soft, pureed, and even solid foods. If zinc and iron deficiency are uncovered, they should be remedied by selecting foods rich in these minerals, or the use of oral supplements administered under the care of a physician.

Many EB patients suffer from constipation. This is often due to perianal erosions that make it painful to move the bowels, leading to voluntary suppression of bowel movements, which is especially common in children. The use of iron supplements to treat anemia may also lead to constipation. A diet high in fiber and fluids plus appropriate use of laxatives will help alleviate this problem. The use of prunes, prune juice, stewed dried fruits (pears, peaches, and apricots), and bran will increase dietary fiber content. Also, adherence to a routine for bowel movements is helpful in maintaining regularity.

Several steps can be taken to encourage feeding in uncooperative children. Feedings should occur in pleasant relaxed environments in which the child feels comfortable. Individual food preferences should be respected. Portions should be appropriate for age so that the child may have the satisfaction of finishing a serving and asking for more. A regular schedule of meal and snack times should be established, and eating between these times should be discouraged.

In patients with severe dysphagia caused by esophageal strictures, the use of gastrostomy feeding should be considered. Short-term use of parenteral nutrition immediately before and after surgery has been advocated in select EB patients undergoing surgery.[10]

Progress in nutritional status is best assessed by serial anthropometric measurements. Height and weight measurements are the most useful and are

TABLE 21.2. Nutritional supplements.

Product	Major nutrient source	Caloric density	Use
Carnation Instant Breakfast, Forta	Nutritionally complete	1 kcal/ml	Mix with milk or water; drink as a shake
Ensure, Resource, Sustacal, Meritene	Nutritionally complete	1 kcal/ml	Drink like a shake; use in cake, cookie, and pudding recipes
Ensure Plus, Sustacal HC, Magnacal	Nutritionally complete	1.5–2 kcal/ml	Drink like a shake; use in cake, cookie, and pudding recipes
Osmolite, Osmolite HN, Ensure HN Isocal	Nutritionally complete	1 kcal/ml	Tube feeding
Ensure Pudding, Sustacal Pudding	Nutritionally complete	240–250 kcal/5 oz	Ready to eat
Pediasure for children 1–6 years	Nutritionally complete	1 kcal/ml	Oral or tube feeding
Enrich	Nutritionally complete, fiber	1 kcal/ml	Drink like a shake
Jevity, Ultracal	Nutritionally complete, fiber	1 kcal/ml	Tube feeding
Nutrisource Carbohydrate, Polycose, Moducal	Carbohydrate	2–3 kcal/ml	Mix with juices and food
Promod, Propac, Casec Powder, Nutrisource Protein	Protein	4 kcal/g	Mix with food
MCT Oil, Microlipid, Nutrisource MCT and LCT, Vegetable Oil	Fat	100 kcal/tbsp	Mix with food

easily obtained. However, the height may not accurately reflect the growth of a patient whose stature is significantly affected by joint contractures.

Acknowledgments. Supported in part by a General Clinical Research Center grant (01-RR00102) from the National Institutes of Health to The Rockefeller University Hospital; by a training grant (AR07525) from the National Institutes of Health to the Laboratory for Investigative Dermatology; by contracts AR62269 and AR62270 from the National Institutes of Health to the Laboratory for Investigative Dermatology; by a grant from the Dystrophic Epidermolysis Bullosa Research Association (D.E.B.R.A.) of America, Inc.; and with general support from the Pew Trusts.

References

1. Subcommittee on the Tenth Edition of the RDA's. *Recommended Dietary Allowances.* 10th ed. Washington, DC: National Academy Press; 1989.
2. Curreri PW, Richard D, Marvin J, Baxter CR. Dietary requirements of patients with major burns. *J Am Diet Assoc.* 1974;5:415–417.
3. Gamelli RL. Nutritional problems of the acute and chronic burn patient: relevance to epidermolysis bullosa. *Arch Dermatol.* 1988;124:756–759.
4. Lechner-Gruskay D, Honig PJ, Pereira G, McKinney S. Nutritional and metabolic profile of children with epidermolysis bullosa. *Pediatr Dermatol.* 1988;5:22–27.
5. Conway JM, Bauer EA, Burke JF, Bier DM. Whole body protein turnover in subjects with epidermolysis bollosa. *Fed Proc.* 1981;40:852.
6. Buchbinder L, Lucky AW, Ballard E, et al. Severe infantile epidermolysis bullosa simplex, Dowling-Meara type. *Arch Dermatol.* 1986;122:190–198.
7. Fine J-D, Tamura T, Johnson L. Blood vitamin and trace metal levels in epidermolysis bullosa. *Arch Dermatol.* 1989;125:374–379.
8. Fine J-D, Wise TG, Falchuk KH. Zinc in cutaneous diseases and dermatological therapeutics. In: Moschella SL, eds. *Dermatology Update: Reviews for Physicians.* New York: Elsevier Science Publishing; 1982; 299–312.
9. Stunkard AJ, Waxman M. Accuracy of self-reports of food intake. *J Am Diet Assoc.* 1981;79:547–551.
10. Zemtsov A, Bergfeld WF, Orlowski JP, Ostrowski DJ, Petroff N. Use of parenteral nutrition in dermolytic epidermolysis bullosa patient undergoing surgery (letter). *Pediatr Dermatol.* 1988;5:212–213.

22
Medical and Surgical Treatment of the Skin in Epidermolysis Bullosa

ANDREW N. LIN and D. MARTIN CARTER

Although no cure exists for any form of EB, many agents have been tried in the hope of uncovering therapeutic success. In this chapter we review treatments aimed specifically at decreasing cutaneous blistering. General principles of wound care as applied to the EB patient and treatments designed to improve extracutaneous complications are reviewed elsewhere in this text.

Although not curative, some agents have clearly defined roles in supportive management of EB patients. For example, systemic and topical antibiotics minimize infection and play a crucial role in maintenance of cutaneous hygiene. There is sound scientific data supporting the use of phenytoin in recessive dystrophic EB, but favorable results documented in open studies have not been fully realized in a controlled study. Because EB can be such a devastating disease, clinicians and patients sometimes reach for unproven remedies for which there is no rational basis supporting their use. In some cases, the use of specific agents have been documented in only isolated reports, and no meaningful conclusions can be drawn about their efficacy. It is instructive, however, to develop an overview of reported therapeutic interventions in order to formulate informed decisions about management of individual patients.

Systemic and Topical Antibiotics

Patients with EB are deprived of the epidermal barrier to bacterial invasion. They have chronic nonhealing wounds that are often colonized by *Staphylococcus aureus* and other pathogens. Judicious use of topical antibiotics can decrease their bacterial flora and minimize the risk of soft tissue infection. Mupirocin ointment is a topical antibiotic that is effective in eradicating *S. aureus* from EB wounds.[1-3] Chronic use, however, has been associated with emergence of resistant strains of *S. aureus*.[4,5] When cellulitis or other forms of soft tissue infection develop at the site of an EB erosion, systemic antibiotics should be used.

Phenytoin

Phenytoin inhibits collagenase, an enzyme whose activity is increased in fibroblasts obtained from patients with recessive dystrophic EB.[6-8] Favorable outcome after phenytoin therapy has been documented in open studies in patients with recessive dystrophic EB.[7,9,10] In one open study, 12 of 17 patients responded to oral phenytoin administration with decrease in blistering of more than 40%, and therapeutic response was correlated with blood phenytoin levels.[9] In another open study, 14 of 22 patients treated for periods ranging from 8 to 99 weeks showed a greater than 40% mean decrease in skin blistering.[10] However, in a multicenter double-blind controlled study, no therapeutic benefit of phenytoin over placebo was observed, although it was noted that occasional patients may respond with reduced numbers of blisters.[11] In one study, investigators showed that only 4 of 18 patients with recessive dystrophic EB showed elevated levels of collagenase in cultured skin fibroblasts, suggesting that collagenase concentration cannot be taken as a genetic trait in all patients with recessive dystrophic EB.[12] In addition, a correlation had been noted between clinical response to phenytoin therapy and in vitro inhibition of fibroblast collagenase by phenytoin.[9] It is therefore possible that recessive dystrophic EB is a heterogeneous disorder, and only a subset of these patients will repond to phenytoin.

Collagenase activity has also been noted to be increased in a small number of patients with junctional EB,[13,14] and the use of systemic phenytoin therapy has been studied in a few patients with junctional EB. Improvement in cutaneous blistering was noted in two patients with the generalized atrophic benign form,[15] but conflictng results have been noted in patients with the Herlitz variant, with both improvement[16,17] and worsening.[15,18] Further study is clearly required to define further the role of systemic phenytoin therapy in junctional EB. Collagenase and connective tissue remodeling in recessive dystrophic EB is discussed in detail elsewhere in this text (see Chapter 4).

Antiperspirants

Hyperhidrosis of the palms and soles can be a bothersome problem in EB. It has been reported in several patients with the Weber-Cockayne type of EB simplex,[19-21] in which blistering occurs predominantly in the hands and feet, and rarely in the albopapuloid (Pasini) type of dominant dystrophic EB.[22] In patients with EB simplex, topical application of 10% glutaraldehyde has been effective in controlling sweating and blistering, but irritant effects can be a limiting factor.[23] Topical application of aluminum chloride has also been effective in decreasing sweating in EB simplex of Weber-Cockayne.[24,25] In a double-blind, controlled crossover study of 20% aluminum chloride hexahydrate in 23 patients with EB simplex of Weber-Cockayne, no significant difference was observed in blister counts between the active drug and placebo, although most patients reported dryness in sites treated with the active drug.[26]

Systemic Corticosteroids

Systemic corticosteroids have been used in simplex,[27] junctional,[28-40] and dystrophic[30,41-46] forms of EB, and have been found to be effective[28-33,41-43,46] as well as ineffective[27,34-40,44,45] in improving cutaneous blistering. Oral prednisone has also been found effective in relieving symptoms of esophageal stenosis.[47] However, these findings are all based on isolated case reports, sometimes with few details about type and dosage of corticosteroid administered, duration of therapy, and criteria by which response is assessed. To control cutaneous blistering, dosage as high as 140 mg of prednisolone daily has been recommended for use in infancy and the neonatal period.[48] The efficacy of systemic corticosteroids has never been tested in double-blind controlled studies.

Systemic corticosteroids were used more widely in the past when the basic pathology underlying blister formation was poorly understood. Although the basic mechanism of blister formation in all forms of EB remains to be fully understood, there is virtually no evidence to suggest that blister formation is due primarily to an inflammatory process. Any benefit from the use of systemic corticosteroids is therefore unlikely to be due to their antiinflammatory effect. There are data suggesting that corticosteroids appear to decrease collagenase activity in cultured normal human fibroblasts,[49] providing a possible rationale for their use. On the other hand, however, it is well known that chronic use of systemic corticosteroids often leads to serious side effects, including defective wound healing and predisposition to infection, which are serious complications of EB. For these reasons, routine use of systemic corticosteroids in EB cannot be recommended at this time.

Topical Corticosteroids

Topical corticosteroids have been found to improve EB in a small number of patients,[45,50] but have also been found ineffective in others.[45] Like systemic corticosteroids, the use of topical corticosteroids has not been tested in double-blind studies, and the basis for any possible therapeutic benefit is tenuous at best.

Vitamin E

Vitamin E has been tried in EB because of its purported efficacy in treatment of leg ulcers.[51] There are case reports in which patients with simplex[52,53] and dystrophic[51,52,54-56] forms of EB improved while taking oral vitamin E.

Other reports, however, show that oral vitamin E had no effect in simplex.[27,57] junctional,[58,59] and dystrophic[60-62] forms of EB. As a result, the role of vitamin E has been debated with both proponents[63-65] and critics.[66,67] Various theories have been offered to explain its possible efficacy. These include a protective effect on membrane lipoprotein[65] and inhibition of excessive collagenase activity.[68] None of these theories has been proven to apply in EB. In one double-blind crossover study involving two sisters with dermolytic EB, oral vitamin E therapy caused marked reduction in blister formation when compared witn placebo.[68] Because only two patients were studied, it is unlikely these results achieved any statistical significance. A larger double-blind crossover study involving six patients with dominant dystrophic EB and two with recessive dystrophic EB failed to demonstrate any significant difference in effect between oral vitamin E and placebo.[69] In another double-blind crossover study, eight patients with the gravis type of recessive dystrophic EB were given oral vitamin E for 3 months as well as placeobo for a similar period.[70] No objective benefit of vitamin E over placebo was seen in blister-erosion counts, suction blister times, or ultrastructural pathology.

Antimalarials

Antimalarials have been tried in the treatment of EB because of the occasional report that blistering can be made worse by exposure to sunlight.[71,72] Since antimalarials have long been known to be effective in certain photosensitive disorders, these agents have been tried in a small number of patients with EB. Chloroquine has been reported to improve EB simplex[73] and dystrophic EB,[74] but disturbance in visual acuity has been associated with its use in EB.[72] Hydroxychloroquine has also been effective in one case.[72] The number of these case reports, however, remains small, and the use of antimalarials has never been tested in a controlled study. There have also been reports in which antimalarial drugs were not effective.[38,44]

Other than a handful of reports noted above in which blistering is worse during sun exposure, there is no evidence to support the possibility that EB is a photosensitive disorder. On the other hand, it is well known that EB blisters often worsen during hot weather, and it is likely that any worsening during sun exposure is actually a response to heat rather than reflecting photosensitivity. Given the potential for serious adverse effects such as retinal toxicity and diffuse cutaneous pigment changes, it is difficult to recommend the use of antimalarials at this stage.

Retinoids

In 1982, Bauer et al. showed that 13-*cis*- and all-*trans*-retinoic acid were effective inhibitors of collagenase production in cultured fibroblasts obtained from normal human volunteers and patients with recessive dystrophic EB.[75]

This observation led to suggestions that retinoids may be a useful therapeutic agent, because collagenase activity is increased in recessive dystrophic EB fibroblasts.[6] This possibility, however, has been studied in only a small number of patients. A pilot study showed that 13-*cis*-retinoic acid at a dose of 0.4 mg/kg/day decreased blister formation by 67% in three patients with severe recessive dystrophic EB.[76] At the higher dose of 1 to 2 mg/kg/day, all three patients developed severe cutaneous fragility with an increased number of blisters and erosions, plus severe xerosis and pruritus.[77] In another study, etretinate was ineffective in one patient with recessive dystrophic EB.[78] Etretinate, however, is less effective than isotretinoin in relative collagenase—inhibitory potency.[79]

One patient with Weber-Cockayne type of EB simplex responded favorably to isotretinoin.[80] Another patient with the Dowling-Meara type of EB simplex showed worsening of blistering on etretinate, but significant improvement occurred in appearance of palmar-plantar keratoderma.[81] The role of retinoids in the treatment of EB clearly requires further study.

Skin Grafts

Different techniques using autologous and heterologous grafts have been tried in EB patients with variable success.

One patient with recessive dystrophic EB required four operations to excise multiple squamous cell and basal cell carcinoma.[82] At each procedure, skin grafts harvested from his unaffected mother were used to cover the sites from which cancers were excised. Despite initial healing, all grafted sites eventually broke down and the patient died. Successful outcome occurred in a patient with the pretibial form of dystrophic EB, in whom skin grafts from the patient's abdomen were used to cover pretibial erosions.[83] In another patient with pretibial dystrophic EB, "homograft skin dressings" were used with "some success."[84] In another report, split-thickness skin graft harvested from a man with dystrophic EB was used successfully to reconstruct his scarred oral cavity so that dentures could be inserted.[85]

A novel approach was used to treat a 12-year-old boy with dystrophic EB who suffered second and third degree burns.[86] Attempts to harvest split skin grafts using a dermatome failed because his skin was so fragile that the grafts fragmented. A new technique was then attempted. A 2 × 6 inch area of skin was outlined with superficial scalpel incisions, a corner of this skin was elevated, and the entire skin was peeled off by rolling it onto a moistened applicator stick. Several such grafts were applied to the burn wounds, and "most of these grafts had a 90% to 100% take." Donor sites apparently reepithelialized more rapidly than areas denuded in the natural course of the disease, and it was proposed that perhaps nearly all the dermal appendages were left behind in the donor sites, allowing near-normal healing.

An experimental technique using cultured autologous keratinocytes was successful in covering disfiguring facial erosions in four children with junctional EB.[87,88] This technique was extended successfully to cover a chronic erosion involving the entire back of a 25-year-old man with recessive dystrophic EB.[5] Although this technique does not reverse the basic defects of junctional and recessive dystrophic EB, it proved useful in improving function and appearance of chronic EB erosions.

A cultured allogeneic keratinocyte graft was used successfully to treat chronic erosions in a 22-year-old woman with recessive dystrophic EB.[89] Keratinocytes were obtained from an unrelated neonatal male. In another study, cultured keratinocyte allografts were applied to donor sites in six patients with recessive dystrophic EB undergoing plastic surgery involving autologous split skin grafts.[90] Preliminary findings suggested that compared with nongrafted control sites, cultured allogeneic keratinocyte grafts may promote healing and alleviate postoperative pain.

Topical Bufexamac

Bufexamac is a nonsteroidal antiinflammatory agent that is available in topical form. It has been studied in the treatment of various inflammatory dermatoses.[91] In a double-blind controlled crossover study involving 10 EB simplex patients (9 Weber-Cockayne variant, 1 generalized variant), 5% bufexemac cream was compared with the cream-based vehicle.[92] Subjects were randomized to apply one preparation four times daily for 4 weeks, then used the other preparation for another 4 weeks. Weekly evaluation included lesion counts and assessments of cutaneous pain, healing times, and activity times before further blister formation. Two patients with Weber-Cockayne variant failed to comply with the request to maintain their usual level of daily activities during the study period, and their data were excluded for analysis. For the remaining eight patients, no significant difference was detected between the active drug and placebo. This finding is not surprising, since there is no clinical or histologic evidence to suggest that EB simplex is an inflammatory disorder.

Miscellaneous Agents

Tetracyclines

Tetracyclines have been known to inhibit mammalian collagenase, possibly through a mechanism independent of their antimicrobial activity.[93] This observation may explain the efficacy of oral minocycline in suppressing blistering in two patients with dystrophic EB.[94]

Pipamperone

Pipamperone is a neuroleptic agent belonging to the butyrophenone family. It was given to a 3-year-old girl with EB simplex herpetiformis for psychological disturbance.[57] During therapy, blistering was noted to be less severe and the blisters became smaller. The basis for such improvement was not discussed in this report, and further confirmation is obviously required before meaningful conclusions can be drawn.

Topical Silver Nitrate Solution

Two infants with EB (apparently letalis form) were treated with topical 0.5% silver nitrate solution.[95] In one patient, improvement was noted during therapy, with "healing without scars and decrease in new bullae." However, concurrent therapy included "supportive therapeutic agents such as ACTH and antibiotics." Because antibiotics can improve the skin by treating infected blisters, the role of silver nitrate in causing improvement remains unclear. "Similar results" occurred in the other patient but details were not given.

Cyclosporine

A 65-year-old woman with dominant dystrophic EB (Cockayne-Touraine variant) was given oral cyclosporine[96] because of reports that it was effective in EB acquisita.[97] She was treated with vitamin E, phenytoin, prednisolone, and erythromycin without success, but addition of cyclosporine (1 mg/kg daily) improved blistering within 2 months. Because EB acquisita and hereditary EB are different diseases, there is no reason to think an agent that is effective in one will also be useful in the other. Furthermore, the potential for renal toxicity from cyclosporine must be considered before initiating therapy. One case report is obviously insufficient data for meaningful conclusions about the role of cyclosporine in EB therapy.

Zinc

Zinc deficiency has been noted in EB patients,[98,99] especially those with junctional and recessive dystrophic types.[98] Although it is prudent to recommend oral zinc supplements to patients with zinc deficiency,[98] it is unclear if such therapy is effective in improving healing of EB blisters. In two siblings with junctional EB and low serum zinc, the use of zinc supplements had no effect.[40] In another patient with dystrophc EB, oral zinc therapy also was not effective in improving the skin.[100]

Camostat Mesylate

Camostat mesylate is a synthetic serine protease inhibitor that decreased blister formation in organ cultures of normal skin induced by blister fluid obtained from patients with recessive dystrophic EB.[101] In one study comparing 1% camostat mesylate in antibiotic ointment with antibiotic ointment alone, decreased blistering was noted in parts of the body treated with camostat mesylate–containing ointment in three of four patients with recessive dystrophic EB.[101]

PUVA

Therapy with oral psoralen and UVA light (PUVA) was found effective in five EB patients (three Dowling-Meara, one Köbner, one Cockayne-touraine type).[102] After transient exacerbation, blistering "practically ceased for about 4 to 7 months."

Hormonal Influences

A 45-year-old woman with dystrophic EB (subtype unspecified) underwent oophorohysterectomy for benign leiomyoma.[103] Within a few days skin lesions completely resolved and her skin has remained lesion-free until the time of report, for a period of 2 years. Another patient with junctional EB experienced cessation of blister formation during pregnancy.[33] Blisters recurred postpartum but were dramatically reduced by administration of oral contraceptives. Because these reports concern patients with two different types of EB, it is unclear whether hormonal influences play a role in each, or whether the changes observed were coincidental to changes in hormonal status in these patients.

Human Growth Hormone

Two brothers with dominant dystrophic EB (ages 19 and 32 months) were given intramuscular human growth hormone (0.1 U/kg 3 times weekly) for 8 weeks, with no apparent decrease in number or size of blisters.[104] No substantial effect on height or weight was noted.

"Kozak Regimen"

In the 1970s, a treatment regimen developed by a European biochemist came to the attention of physicians and patients in North America. Known as the "Kozak regimen," this consisted of topical and systemic medications, plus strict attention to diet. In one open study involving 19 patients with various types of EB,[105,106] this treatment improved cutaneous blistering in 9 of 10 hospitalized patients. However, it was felt the improvement may have been due to the intense topical treatment rather than to a specific item of the treatment program.[106] This program was further evaluated during a meeting between its developer and a panel of American physicians.[107] The panel found "no evidence for any unique therapeutic feature" in this program, and was unable to "lend any legitimacy or endorsement" to it.[107]

Acknowledgments. Supported in part by a General Clinical Research Center grant (M01-RR00102) from the National Institutes of Health to The Rockefeller University Hospital; by a training grant (AR07525) from the National Institutes of Health to the Laboratory for Investigative Dermatology; by contracts AR62269 and AR62270 from the National Institutes of Health to the Laboratory for Investigative Dermatology; by a grant from the Dystrophic Epidermolysis Bullosa Research Association (D.E.B.R.A.) of America, Inc.; and with general support from the Pew Trusts.

References

1. Carter DM, Caldwell D, Varghese M, Balin AK. Effectiveness of Bactroban ointment in chronic skin infection: report of a clinical study. In: Dobson RL, Leyden JJ, Noble WC, Price JD, eds. *Bactroban (Mupirocin): Proceedings of an International Symposium.* Amsterdam: Excerpta Medica; 1985: 228–234.
2. Caldwell D, Carter DM, Lin A, Varghese M. Topical mupirocin in epidermolysis bullosa: safety and efficacy of long-term treatment. In: Wood C, eds. *Proceedings of the Royal Society of Medicine;* Round Table Series, Number 4. Oxford: Alden Press; 1986: 12–26.
3. Lin AN, Caldwell D, Varghese M, Pratt L, Balin A, Carter DM. Efficacy of long term mupirocin therapy in epidermolysis bullosa and its effect on growth and lifespan on cultured fibroblasts. *J Invest Dermatol.* 1986;87:152.
4. Rahman M, Noble WC, Cookson B. Mupirocin-resistant *Staphylococcus aureus* (letter). *Lancet.* 1987;2:387.
5. Moy J, Caldwell-Brown D, Lin AN, Pappa KA, Carter DM. Mupirocin-resistant *Staphylococcus aureus* after long-term treatment of patients with epidermolysis bullosa. *J Am Acad Dermatol.* 1990;22:893–895.
6. Bauer EA, Eisen AZ. Recessive dystrophic epidermolysis bullosa: evidence for increased collagenase as a genetic characteristic in cell culture. *J Exp Med.* 1978;148:1378–1387.
7. Eisenberg M, Stevens LJ, Schofield PJ. Epidermolysis bullosa: new therapeutic approaches. *Austr J Dermatol.* 1978;19:1–8.
8. Bauer EA, Tabas M. A perspective on the role of collagenase in recessive dystrophic epidermolysis bullosa. *Arch Dermatol.* 1988;124:734–736.
9. Bauer EA, Cooper TW, Tucker DR, Esterly NB. Phenytoin therapy of recessive dystrophic epidermolysis bullosa: clinical trial and proposed mechanism of action on collagenase. *N Engl J Med.* 1980;303:776–781.
10. Cooper TW, Bauer EA. Therapeutic efficacy of phenytoin in recessive dystrophic epidermolysis bullosa. *Arch Dermatol.* 1984;120:490–495.
11. Lin AN., Stern RB, Caldwell-Brown D, Carter DM, collaborators. Phenytoin for recessive dystrophic epidermolysis bullosa. *J Invest Dermatol.* 1989;92:472.

12. Winberg J-O, Real C, Gedde-Dahl Jr T, Bauer EA. Collagenase expression in skin fibroblasts from families with recessive dystrophic epidermolysis bullosa. *J Invest Dermatol.* 1989;92:82–85.

13. Kero M. Epidermolysis bullosa in Finland: clinical features, morphology and relation to collagen metabolism. *Acta Derm Venereol (Stockh).* 1984; Suppl 110:1–51.

14. Kero M, Palotie A, Peltonen L. Collagen metabolism in two rare forms of epidermolysis bullosa. *Br J Dermatol.* 1984;110:177–184.

15. Fine J-D, Johnson L. Efficacy of systemic phenytoin in the treatment of junctional epidermolysis bullosa. *Arch Dermatol.* 1988;124:1402–1406.

16. Rogers RB, Yancey KB, Allen BS, Guill MF. Phenytoin therapy for junctional epidermolysis bullosa. *Arch Dermatol.* 1983;119:925–926.

17. Guill MF, Wray BB, Rogers RB, Yancey KB, Allen BS. Junctional epidermolysis bullosa: treatment with phenytoin. *Am J Dis Child.* 1983;137:992–994.

18. Bergfeld WF, Orlowski JP. Epidermolysis bullosa letalis and phenytoin (letter). *J Am Acad Dermatol.* 1982;7:275–276.

19. Winer MN, Orman JM. Epidermolysis bullosa: a suggestion as to possible causation. *Arch Dermatol Syphilol.* 1945;52:317–321.

20. Thompson RG, Leedham CL, Hailey H. Epidermolysis bullosa hereditaria. *South Med J.* 1949;42:647–653.

21. Hall-Smith SP, Daunt FO'N. Recurrent bullous eruption of feet: report of a case. *Lancet.* 1948;1:66–67.

22. Kumar K, Kumar R. Epidermolysis bullosa dystrophica et albo-papuloidea Pasini in an Indian: a case report. *Dermatologica.* 1973;147:137–143.

23. DesGrosseilliers J-P, Brisson P. Localized epidermolysis bullosa: report of two cases and evaluation of therapy with glutaraldehyde. *Arch Dermatol.* 1974;109:70–72.

24. Tkach JR. Treatment of recurrent bullous eruption of the hands and feet (Weber-Cockayne Disease) with topical aluminum chloride (letter). *J Am Acad Dermatol.* 1982;6:1095–1096.

25. Jennings JL. Aluminum chloride hexahydrate treatment of localized epidermolyis bullosa. *Arch Dermatol.* 1984;120:1382.

26. Younger IR, Priestley GC, Tidman MJ. Aluminum chloride hexahydrate and blistering in epidermolysis bullosa simplex. *J Am Acad Dermatol.* 1990;23:930–931.

27. Niemi K-M, Kero M, Kanerva L, Mattila R. Epidermolysis bullosa simplex: a new histologic subgroup. *Arch Dermatol.* 1983;119:138–141.

28. Rosset M. Epidermolysis bullosa in the newborn. *Can Med Assoc J* 1956;75:507–509.

29. Silver HK. Epidermolysis bullosa hereditaria letalis: report of a case surviving for two and a half years. *Arch Dis Child.* 1957;32:216–219.

30. Moynahan EJ. Epidermolysis bullosa affecting the buccal and pharyngeal mucosa. *Proc R Soc Med.* 1963;56:885–888.

31. Fattah AA. Epidermolysis bullosa hereditaria letalis (Herlitz). *Dermatologica.* 1966;133:475–481.

32. Pearson RW, Potter B, Strauss F. Epidermolysis bullosa hereditaria letalis: clinical and histologic manifestations and course of the disease. *Arch Dermatol.* 1974;109:349–355.

33. Schachner L, Lazarus GS, Dembitzer H. Epidermolysis bullosa hereditaria letalis: pathology, natural history and therapy. *Br J Dermatol.* 1977;96:51–58.

34. Walther T. Epidermolysis bullosa hereditaria letalis: a review and report of two own cases. *Ann Ped Int Rev Pediatr.* 1953;180:382–392.
35. Leland LS, Hirschl D. Epidermolysis bullosa hereditaria letalis in newborn twins: report of two cases with failure to respond favourably to cortisone. *Am J Dis Child.* 1954;87:321–327.
36. Henderson AT. Epidermolysis bullosa hereditaria letalis: report of a case failing to respond to cortisone. *J Pediatr.* 1955;46:186–191.
37. Roberts MH, Howell DRS, Bramhall JL, Reubner B. Epidermolysis bullosa letalis: report of three cases with particular reference to the histopathology of the skin. *Pediatrics.* 1960;25:283–290.
38. Lowe LB. Hereditary epidermolysis bullosa. *Arch Dermatol.* 1967;95:587–595.
39. Bergenholtz A, Olsson O. Epidermolysis bullosa hereditaria letalis: a survey of the literature and report of 11 cases. *Acta Derm Venereol (Stockh).* 1968;48:220–241.
40. Oakley CA, Wilson N, Ross JA., Barnmetson RStC. Junctional epidermolysis bullosa in two siblings: clinical observations, collagen studies and electron microscopy. *Br J Dermatol.* 1984;111:533–543.
41. Gill S. Epidermolysis bullosa dystrophica with peculiar mutilation of hands. *Israel Med J.* 1961;20:11–12.
42. Taft EH. Dystrophic epidermolysis bullosa. *Austr. J. Dermatol.* 1969;10:189–190.
43. Tidman MJ, Marsden RA. Severe dominant dystrophic epidermolysis bullosa. *Br J Dermatol.* 1985;113(Suppl 29):80–81.
44. Drury RE, Prieto Jr A. Epidermolysis bullosa dystrophica. Report of two cases within a family group. *Oral Surg Oral Med Oral Pathol.* 1964;18:544–551.
45. Caldiera Jde B, Costa MHL. Epidermolysis bullosa hereditaria: clinical trial with fluocinonide FAPG 0.05% in five cases. *Acta Derm Venereol (Stockh).* 1972; Suppl 67:88–90.
46. Enell H, Lindeas K. Epidermolysis bullosa hereditaria dystrofica. I. Treatment with cortisone. *Acta Derm Venereol (Stockh).* 1953;33:488–496.
47. Katz J, Gryboski JD, Rosenbaum HM, Spiro HM. Dysphagia in children with epidermolysis bullosa. *Gastroenterology.* 1967;52:259–262.
48. Moynahan EJ. The treatment and management of epidermolysis bullosa. *Clin Exp Dermatol.* 1982;7:665–672.
49. Koob TJ, Jeffrey JJ, Eisen AZ. Regulation of human skin collagenase activity by hydrocortisone and dexamethasone in organ culture. *Biochem Biophys Res Commun.* 1974;61:1083–1088.
50. Severin GL, Farber EM. The management of epidermolysis bullosa in children: effective topical steroid treatment. *Arch Dermatol.* 1967;95:302–309.
51. Wilson HD. Treatment of epidermolysis bullosa dystrophica by alpha tocopherol. *Can Med Assoc J.* 1964;90:1315–1316.
52. Ayres Jr S, Mihan R. Pseudoxanthoma elasticum and epidermolysis bullosa: response to vitamin E (tocopherol). *Cutis.* 1969;5:287–294.
53. Ayres Jr S, Mihan R. Vitamin E (tocopherol): a reappraisal of its value in dermatoses of mesodermal tissues. *Cutis.* 1971;7:35–45.
54. Sehgal VN, Sanyal RK. Vitamin E therapy in dystrophic epidermolysis bullosa (letter). *Arch Dermatol.* 1972;105:460.
55. Sehgal VN, Vadiraj SN, Rege VL, Beohar PC. Dystrophic epidermolysis bullosa in a family: response to vitamin E (tocopherol). *Dermatologica.* 1972;144:27–34.

56. Michaelson JD, Schmidt JD, Dresden MH, Duncan C. Vitamin E treratment of epidermolysis bullosa. Changes in tissue collagenase levels. *Arch Dermatol.* 1974; 109:67–69.
57. Bonnetblanc JM, Bouquier JJ. Response to pipamperone in case of epidermolysis bullosa herpetiformis. *Lancet.* 1986;1:1327–1328.
58. Kahn S, Trieger N. Epidermolysis bullosa hereditaria letalis: a case report with special emphasis on oral manifestations. *J Oral Med.* 1976;31:32–35.
59. Haber RM. Reply to the editor (letter). *J Am Acad Dermatol.* 1988;18:142–143.
60. Unger WP, Nethercott JR. Epidermolysis bullosa dystrophica treated with vitamin E and oral corticosteroids. *Can Med Assoc J.* 1973;108:1136–1138.
61. Trent WG. Epidermolysis bullosa. *Arch Dermatol.* 1976;112:256.
62. Harper JI, Copeman PWM. Pretibial epidermolysis bullosa: the use of homograft skin dressings. *Br J Dermatol.* 1983;109(Suppl 24):60–62.
63. Ayres Jr S, Mihan R. Letter to the Editor. *Dermatologica.* 1973;146:61.
64. Ayres Jr S, Mihan R. Vitamin E treatment of dermolytic bullous dermatosis (letter). *Arch Dermatol.* 1974;109:99.
65. Ayres Jr S. Epidermolysis bullosa controlled by vitamin E. *Int J Dermatol.* 1986;25:670–671.
66. Fine J-D. Reply to Dr. Ayres (letter). *Int J Dermatol.* 1986;25:671.
67. Reed WB. Vitamin E treatment of dermolytic bullous dermatosis (letter). *Arch Dermatol.* 1975;111:524.
68. Smith EB, Michener W. Vitamin E treatment of dermolytic bullous dermatosis: a controlled study. *Arch Dermatol.* 1973;108:254–256.
69. Adams RH, Main RA, Marsden RA. A controlled study of vitamin E treatment in epidermolysis bullosa. *Br J Dermatol.* 1975;93(Suppl 11):10.
70. Briggaman RA, Paller AS, Pessar A. Epidermolysis bullosa. In: Provost TT, Farmer ER, eds. *Current Therapy in Dermatology.* Philadelphia: BC Decker; 1985:70–75.
71. Shubailat G, Oumeish OY, Amr SS. Epidermolysis bullosa dystrophica triggered by sun exposure. *Ann Plast Surg.* 1983;10:239–243.
72. Baer TW. Epidermolysis bullosa hereditaria treated with antimalarials. *Arch Dermatol.* 1961;84:503–504.
73. Marrero L, Enriquez S, Bolat I. Epidermolysis bullosa simplex. *Arch Dermatol.* 1962;86:163.
74. Dorsey CS. Dystrophic epidermolysis bullosa treated with chloroquine. *Arch Dermatol.* 1959;79:122.
75. Bauer EA, Seltzer JL, Eisen AZ. Inhibition of collagen degradative enzymes by retinoic acid in vitro. *J Am Acad Dermatol.* 1982;6:603–607.
76. Cooper TW, Tabas M, Bauer EA. Retinoic acid in recessive dystrophic epidermolysis bullosa: in vitro effects on collagenase and preliminary therapeutic trials. In: Saurat JH, eds. *Retinoids: New Trends in Research and Therapy.* New York: S. Karger, 1985:219–224.
77. Tabas M, Spraker MK. Report on the first national epidermolysis bullosa conference November 29 to December 1, 1984. *Pediatr Dermatol.* 1985;3:79–82.
78. Fritsch P, Klein G, Aubock J, Hintner H. Retinoid therapy of recessive dystrophic epidermolysis bullosa (letter). *J Am Acad Dermatol.* 1983;9:766–777.
79. Bauer EA, Seltzer JL, Eisen AZ. Retinoic acid inhibition of collagenase and gelatinase expression in human skin fibroblast cultures. Evidence for a dual mechanism. *J Invest Dermatol.* 1983;81:162–169.

80. Adreano JM, Tomecki KJ. Epidermolysis bullosa simplex responding to isotretinoin (letter). *Arch Dermatol.* 1988;124:1445–1446.
81. Tidman MJ, Wells RS, MacDonald DM. Epidermolysis bullosa simplex (Dowling-Meara). In: Wilkinson DS, Mascaro JM, Orfanos CE, Albers J, eds. *Clinical Dermatology, The CMD Case Collection, World Congress of Dermatology.* Stuttgart: Schattauer, 1987:16–17.
82. Crikelair GF, Hoehn RJ, Domonkos AN, Binkert B. Skin homografts in epidermolysis bullosa dystrophica: case report. *Plast Reconstr Surg.* 1970;46:89–92.
83. Furue M, Ando I, Inoue Y, Tamaki K, Oohara K, Kukita A. Pretibial epidermolysis bullosa; successful therapy with a skin graft. *Arch Dermatol.* 1986;122:310–313.
84. Harper JI, Copeman PWM. Pretibial epidermolysis bullosa: the use of homograft skin dressings. *Br J Dermatol.* 1983;109(Suppl 24):60–62.
85. Rhymes Jr R, Hardin JC, Metts Jr D, Krantz R. Dystrophic epidermolysis bullosa: extra-articular ankylosis treated with oral skin grafts: report of a case. *J Oral Surg Anesth Hosp D Serv.* 1963;21:63–67.
86. Skivolocki W, Harris BH, Boles Jr ET. A new method for skin grafting a burned patient who has epidermolysis bullosa. *Plast Reconstr Surg.* 1974;53:355–357.
87. Carter DM, Lin AN, Varghese MC, Caldwell D, Pratt L, Eisinger M. Treatment of junctionaol epidermolysis bullosa with epidermal autografts. *J Am Acad Dermatol.* 1987;17:246–259.
88. Lin AN., Carter DM, Caldwell-Brown D. Wound healing and cultured epidermal autografts in epidermolysis bullosa. In: Priestley GC, Tidman MJ, Weiss JB, Eady RAJ, eds. *Epidermolysis Bullosa: A Comprehensive Review of Classification, Management and Laboratory Studies.* Crowthorne: Dystrophic Epidermolysis Bullosa Research Association; 1990:152–155.
89. McGuire J, Birchnall N, Cuono C, Moellmann G, Kuklinska E, Langdon R. Successful engraftment of allogeneic keratinocyte cultures in recessive dystrophic epidermolysis bullosa. *J Invest Dermatol.* 1987;88:506.
90. Schofield OMV, Cassella J-P, Navsaria HA, Leigh IM, Mayou BJ, Eady RAJ. Cultured keratinocyte allografts indystrophic epidermolysis bullosa: preliminary observations. *Br J Dermatol.* 1990;123(Suppl 37):66.
91. Brogden RN, Pinder RM, Sawyer PR, et al. Bufexamac: a review of its pharmacological properties and therapeutic efficacy in inflammatory dermatoses. *Drugs.* 1975;10:351–356.
92. Fine J-D, Johnson L. Evaluation of the efficacy of topical bufexamac in epidermolysis bullosa simplex: a double-blind placebo-controlled crossover study, *Arch Dermatol.* 1988;124:1669–1672.
93. Golub LM, McNamara TF, D'Angelo G, Greenwald RA, Ramamurthy NS. A non-antibacterial chemically-modified tetracycline inhibits mammalian collagenase activity. *J Dent Res.* 1987;66:1310–1314.
94. White JE. Minocycline for dystrophic epidermolysis bullosa (letter). *Lancet.* 1989;1:966.
95. Keller L. Silver nitrate therapy in epidermolysis bullossa hereditaria of the newborn. *J Pediatr.* 1968;72:854–856.
96. Husz S, Olah J, Korom I, Szekeres L, Kemeny E, Dobozy A. Cyclosporine for dystrophic epidermolysis bullosa (letter). *Lancet.* 1989;2:1393–1394.
97. Crow LL, Finkle JP, Gammon WR, Woodley DT. Clearing of epidermolysis bullosa acquisita with cyclosporine. *J Am Acad Dermatol.* 1988;19:937–942.

98. Fine J-D, Tamura T, Johnson L. Blood vitamin and trace metal levels in epidermolysis bullosa. *Arch Dermatol.* 1989;125:374–379.
99. Cunningham-Rundles S, Bockman RS, Lin AN, Giardina PV, Hilgartner MW. Physiological and pharmacological effects of zinc on immune response *Ann NY Acad Sci.* 1990;587:113–122.
100. Weismann K. Dystrophic epidermolysis bullosa treated unsuccesfully with oral zinc (letter). *Arch Dermatol Res.* 1985;277:404–405.
101. Ikeda S, Manabe M, Muramatsu T, Takamori K, Ogawa H. Protease inhibitor therapy for recessive dystrophic epidermolysis bullosa: in vitro effect and clinical trial with camostat mesylate. *J Am Acad Dermatol.* 1988;18:1246–1252.
102. Hashimoto I, Katabira Y, Mitsuhashi Y, Nomura K, Hanada K. Treatment of epidermolysis bullosa with PUVA therapy. In: Orfanos CE, Stadler R, Gollnick H, eds. *Dermatology in Five Continents: Proceedings of the XVII World Congress of Dermatology, Berlin, May* 24–29, 1987. Berlin: Springer-Verlag; 1988:1173.
103. Matsuoka LY, Safai B. Resolution of epidermolysis bullosa following oophorohysterectomy (letter). *J Am Acad Dermatol.* 1980;3:205–206.
104. Zackheim HS. Failure of human growth hormone to benefit dystrophic epidermolysis bullosa (letter). *Arch Dermatol.* 1983;119:537.
105. Haber RM, Ramsay CA, Boxall LBH. Assessment of a treatment for epidermolysis bullosa (letter). *Can Med Assoc J* 1984;131:10–14.
106. Haber RM, Ramsay CA, Boxall LBH. Epidermolysis bullosa: assessment of a treatment regimen. *Int J Dermatol.* 1985;24:324–328.
107. Katz SI, Bauer EA, Lazarus GS, McGuire Jr JS, Briggaman RA, Sulica V. Mr. Kozak's regime for epidermolysis bullosa (letter). *J Am Acad Dermatol.* 1983;8:565–566.

23
Nursing Aspects of Epidermolysis Bullosa: A Comprehensive Approach

DOROTHEA CALDWELL-BROWN, SHEILA GIBBONS, and MIGDALIA REID

Although much has been written, in this text and elsewhere, about diagnostic classification, mode of inheritance, and clinical manisfestations of epidermolysis bullosa (EB),[1-5] relatively little has been said about wound care for affected individuals. This points to the need for more clinical research in this area. This chapter focuses on our experiences with wound care, and prevention and management of common complications of EB; we provide a general overview of clinical problems and guidelines for delivering comprehensive care.

While medical scientists investigate the myriad complexities of EB in search of the molecular defects, effective therapies, and possible cures, clinicians, patients, and their caregivers must grapple with numerous challenges in managing the disease. For many patients, quality of life depends on nursing care that must extend beyond bandaging wounds. Because EB involves multiple organ systems such as gastrointestinal, musculoskeletal, ophthalmological, respiratory, and genitourinary, an array of medical services is required and nurses are often obliged to coordinate these services.[6] At our respective university hospitals, we have observed that with family support and access to improved therapeutics, overall health has greatly increased for these patients.

Blistering is a feature common to all forms of EB. Depending on subtype, lesions appear in a localized, generalized, or inverse pattern of distribution, and morbidity ranges from mild seasonal blisters that heal without scarring to nonhealing wounds that result in disfigurement. In some cases, lifethreatening complications such as sepsis, squamous cell carcinomas, and malnutrition may occur. There is also marked clinical variability within each subtype.[2] Blister activity tends to decrease with advancing age,[7] but areas chronically wounded and scarred in early life are more likely to blister throughout the patient's life. Scarring can also occur in "nonscarring" (simplex) forms of EB if wounds become infected. The long-term effects of early intervention are being monitored prospectively by the National EB Registry. However, quality skin care that begins in infancy is thought to be of utmost importance in minimizing complications of EB.

Skin Care

Protection against mechanical trauma is a prime objective in caring for EB patients. In general, friction and rubbing can cause blisters and erosions in areas vulnerable to breakdown whereas direct presssure may be tolerated. Suggestions for trauma protection include egg crate padding, water or air mattress, sheepskin, or some other soft material. Dressings and other materials such as athletic protectors (e.g., knee pads) or commercially available shoulder pads can be used to shield bony prominences and body parts that are prone to friction such as elbows, knees, and feet. However, dressings must be applied so as not to impede mobility or development. A hydrocolloid gel dressing such as Duoderm, a thick gelatinous pad, may be used prophylactically in patients with EB simplex whose lesions are localized to hands and feet. Because its adhesive backing may cause trauma upon removal, Duoderm is left in place for up to several days, until it gradually peels away, and it is not indicated in scarring forms of EB.

Pruritus is a common complaint, particularly at night. Avoidance of overheating and dry skin can help allay itching and lessen blister formation. An air-conditioned home environment is recommended to provide a cool environment, which seems to decrease blistering. Oatmeal baths, open wet soaks, and emollients are soothing therapies for mild itching. Treatment with systemic hydroxyzine or diphenlhydramine may be indicated in protracted cases.[7,8]

Patients with moderate to severe disease require special considerations with regard to routine medical, nursing, and surgical procedures such as blood pressure and cardiac monitoring, urine collections from infants and young children, venesection, parenteral therapy, preoperative preparations, and mask-delivered anesthesia. Table 23.1 provides guidelines for select clinical procedures. These guidelines are adopted at The Rockefeller University Hospital and Stanford University Hospital.

Although trauma prevention can never entirely protect an EB patient from developing lesions, it can markedly reduce the incidence of blisters and limit the severity of associated complications. However, a clear distinction must be made between providing a safe environment that allows for optimum development versus an overly restrictive lifestyle that may result in physical and psychological debilitation. Patients and their caregivers need to accept the chronic nature of this disease so as not to assign blame or guilt when blisters occur and, that given proper instruction and supervision, wounds can be managed satisfactorily.[7,9]

Wound Care

No single approach to managing EB wounds has proved totally effective. There exists a wide variety of topical agents and primary wound coverings that are nonadherent and effective in promoting healing. Some examples of

TABLE 23.1. Special precautions to minimize cutaneous trauma during select clinical procedures.

Procedure	Suggestions
Blood pressure (BP) monitoring	Apply dressing under BP cuff
Electrocardiogram monitoring	Use a nonadhesive plastic film such as Omiderm (which does not interfere with electrical conduction[27]) as a barrier between the patient's skin and the adhesive of the electrode pads
Urine collections (young children)	Wring out cloth diaper; Do not apply urine bags containing adhesives
Blood drawing	To cleanse skin, allow alcohol or betadine swab to remain in place for 5 min without rubbing; place tourniquet over padding to protect skin. Or, apply direct pressure on vein using thumb in a parallel position to skin
Parenteral therapy	Cut a piece of hydrocolloid dressing (Extra Thin Duoderm or Resolve) into a horseshoe shape and put dressing with adhesive backing side in contact with skin. Start the IV between the legs of the horseshoe bandage and tape the tubing onto the dressing. Secure IV with roller gauze. Or, place a snug-fitting piece of tube gauze such as Bandnet on extremity adjacent to IV and secure with tape to tube gauze
Preoperative preparations: operating room, table, surgical drapes, and surgical scrub	Operating room table should be well padded. Sheepskin covered by a table-sized burn pad such as Exudry (which has a double layer of meshed material to minimize friction) is advised. If positioning with pillows is necessary for patients with joint contractures, place Exudry pad between pillow and patient's skin
	Sterile sheets of nonadherent mesh (Exudry Mesh or N-terface) are placed under sterile drapes to protect exposed skin from friction. Fold mesh over edge of drape and secure with clamps as usual. Adhesive drapes are contraindicated
	Apply antimicrobial solution to surgical site. Allow to remain on skin for 5 min then irrigate to rinse. Repeat this process 3 times
Mask-delivered anesthesia	Protect skin on face from possible shearing with a nonadhesive polyurethane film, such as Omiderm (which adheres to any damp surface and is easily removed by rewetting). Or, apply copious amount of petrolatum to face before applying mask

primary dressings include the following: Allevyn, Biobrane, Second Skin, Exudry, Omiderm, and Telfa. As tape is potentially damaging if applied directly to skin, outer dressings are used to hold the primary dressings in place. These dressings are typically made of soft woven or elasticized roller or tubular gauze that conforms to body contours; examples of such dressings include Kling, Kerlix, Conform, Bandnet, and Surginet.

Choice of dressings must be guided by the patient's diagnosis, areas of involvement, condition of wounds, availability of supplies, cost, ease of application, and personal preference. Thus, care must be "tailored" to the individual. It is not unusual for a patient with generalized involvement to present with multiple wounds in various stages of healing and to require more than one type of dressing. For example, a patient may present with dry crusty wounds on the posterior aspect of the neck and oozing wounds on the feet. One may consider applying a moist dressing, such as Second Skin, to the neck in order to minimize crusting, and Exudry, a thick pad that absorbs moisture, to the feet.

Creative dressing techniques and devices are required for treating difficult areas such as the face and digits (these are wrapped separately in cases at risk for psuedosyndactyly).[7, 9] Figures 23.1–23.4 depict the hand of a patient with junctional EB to illustrate a bandaging technique for keeping fingers separate. When dressings are applied to flexural areas, care must be taken to preserve full joint motion.

Daily skin care of patients with moderate to severe involvement can be labor intensive and compliance may be inversely related to the pain and difficulty a patient experiences. Pain is more frequently reported upon removal of dressings when wounds become exposed to air. Thus, one aims to minimize wound exposure by completing care in an expeditious manner. Some patients with extensive infection and/or erosions may require analgesic

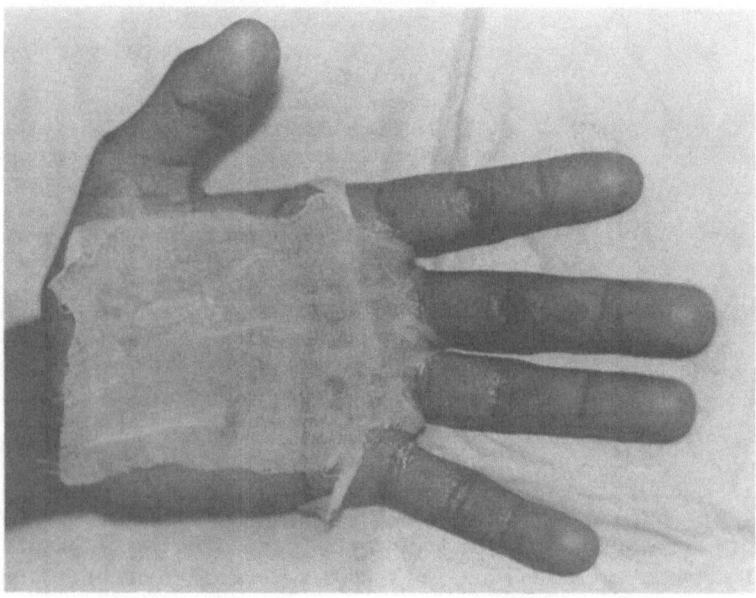

FIGURE 23.1. Petrolatum gauze is cut at one end into five long strips and placed on the palm of the hand.

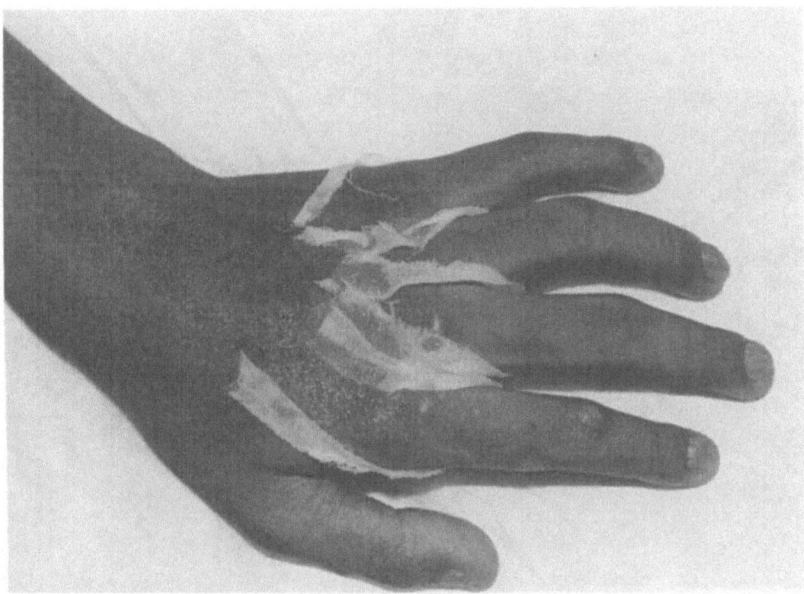

FIGURE 23.2. Individual strips of petrolatum gauze are drawn through the interdigital web spaces to the dorsum of the hand.

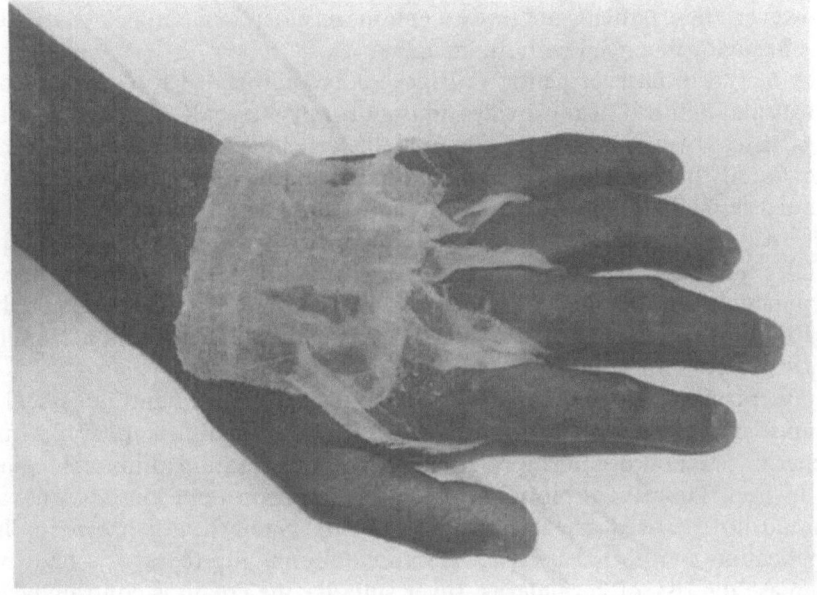

FIGURE 23.3 Petrolatum gauze is placed on the dorsum of the hand over the strips.

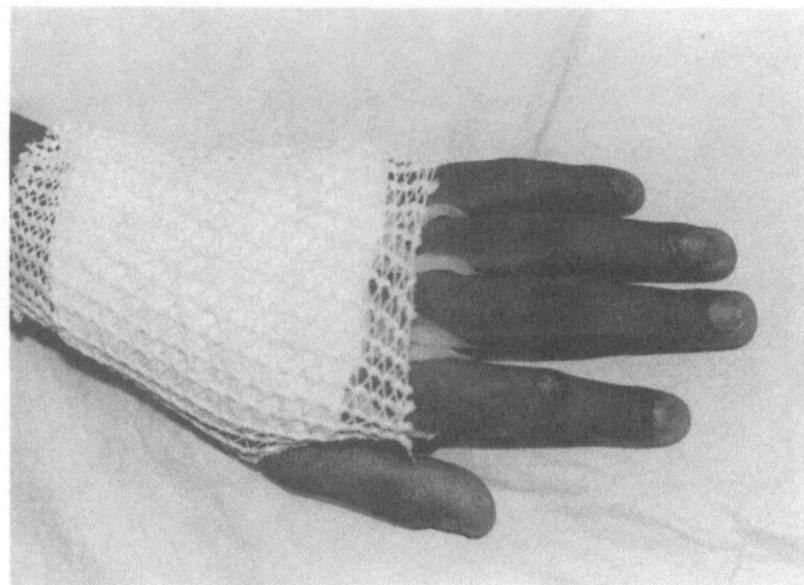

FIGURE 23.4. Sponge dressings are placed over the petrolatum gauze on both hand surfaces. These are held in place by a tubular net bandage with a cut-out area to anchor net on thumb.

medication at an appropriate time interval in advance of the dressing change. However, these patients are rare exceptions as most, including newborns, can be effectively managed without analgesia.

A daily tub bath or gentle whirlpool is recommended to cleanse skin of crusts and debri. It also provides an opportunity to soak off adherent dressings, assess overall skin condition, and exercise limbs. After the bath, excess moisture is blotted from the skin with a soft bath sheet or towel; for badly eroded skin a hair dryer on low/cool setting may be useful. Next, blisters are slit open with a sterile hypodermic needle or iris scissors to drain fluid that, if left intact, may spread and lead to further erosion of the blister base.[7,9,10] A puncture-type opening is less effective as the hole will quickly seal and fluid reaccumulate.[9] After draining blisters, antibacterial ointments are applied and covered with primary and outer dressings.

The prophylactic and chronic use of any single topical antibiotic such as mupirocin requires monitoring by health professionals for possible emergence of resistant organisms.[11] An alternating or rotating antibiotic regimen is advised. Topical antibiotics are generally applied to open lesions only and should not be used as lubricating ointments. Some health providers limit application to infected lesions.[9] Because sulfonamide therapy is known to increase the risk of kernicterus, silver sulfadiazine cream is contraindicated in newborns up to 8 weeks of age.[12] Antibiotic creams or ointments containing neomycin are not recommended because of the potential for sensitization with long-term use.

Patients/caregivers are taught basic aseptic techniques (i.e., handwashing before and after dressing changes, clean set-up, and proper handling of sterile instruments). Stricter sterile measures, including masks, gowns, drapes, etc. are unnecessary, except in institutional settings where there is significant risk for nosocomial infections.

Because universal blood precautions mandate medical personnel to wear gloves when engaged in wound care, it is recommended that rubber gloves be lubricated so as to avoid possible trauma to skin.

Wound Complications

Skin Infections

Skin infections complicate wound healing and may lead to scarring in forms of EB that would not otherwise scar. Patients with extensive blistering are at constant risk for infection because they often have open wounds that become colonized with bacteria.[13,14] However, with careful attention wounds can heal despite bacterial colonization. Oral antibiotics are used on a short-term basis when indicated for infection.

Wounds that are recalcitrant to therapy may require evaluation for underlying complications such as osteomyelitis;[7] those that develop a warty texture or are unusually slow to heal are examined and biopsied to rule out squamous cell carcinoma.[14-16]

Systemic Infections

Sepsis is a serious complication and may result in death, particularly in infancy.[8] Therefore, we recommend the prophylactic use of topical antibiotic agents for newborns and that they be closely monitored with frequent bacteriologic studies. Poststreptococcal glomerulonephritis may be seen in patients as a complication of frequent beta-hemolytic streptococcal infections involving the skin. Renal failure secondary to amyloidosis has also been reported.[17] Because of the potential for kidney complications in these patients, we recommend regular biochemical monitoring of renal function.

Scarring

Scarring is common in (but not limited to) dystrophic forms of EB and may cause everted eyelids (ectropion), decreased mouth opening (microstomia), restricted tongue movement (ankyloglossia), joint contractures, decreased muscle function, webbing of digits (pseudo-syndactyly) with resorption of bone, and abnormal posture causing decreased intercostal muscle function.

Physical and occupational therapy are indicated to increase physical endurance, prevent or minimize contractures, aid ambulation, and to enable independence in activities of daily living.[18] Hand splints (paddle, functional, and dynamic) and other orthopedic devices may be used as prophylactic or rehabilitive measures. Orthopedic or plastic surgery may also be beneficial for those with impaired joint function.

The larynx may be involved with blistering and scarring in some forms of junctional EB and to a lesser extent in dystrophic forms of EB. Laryngeal involvement is typically evident in early childhood and can manifest as respiratory distress (i.e., stridor, audible breathing sounds, retractions, etc.), abnormal cry/voice, and/or feeding difficulties. Any one of these important signs warrants further medical evaluation in consultation with an otolaryngologist. Other scarring complications common in junctional EB include meatal stenosis of the ear, which can result in chronic ear infections and meatal stenosis of the external genitalia.

Health Maintenance

Immunizations

It is advised that infants and children be followed by a primary care practitioner who can provide routine health care. Every child should receive vaccines according to the recommendations of the American Academy of Pediatrics unless there is a specific reason to defer.[19] Fears of causing untoward skin reactions from vaccinations are unjustified as patients suffer no unusual effects. However, we do not recommend zoster immune globulin for EB patients in general. In our experience, EB patients tend to handle varicella (chicken pox) without any serious sequelae.

Skin Assessment

Skin assessments are performed with the patient undressed and all dressings removed. Observations are made for location of lesions, signs of discomfort, degree of healing, extent of scarring, signs of infection, nutritional status, and unusual lesions (hyperpigmentation, warty growths, etc.).

Development

Patients are assessed for normal progress in attaining developmental milestones and abnormalities in posture, range of motion (including face and tongue movements), and gait. Early identification and treatment of developmental delays and disorders of movement may help prevent permanent impairment.

To help preserve oral functions, parents/caregivers are advised to encourage affected infants to imitate simple facial exercises such as smiling, opening eyes, opening mouth, tongue protrusion, etc. Gentle stretching of the corners of the infant's mouth is also recommended. Older children are encouraged to lick suitable food items such as ice cream pops.

Proper alignment of the spine is an important goal for maintaining normal intercostal muscle function, particularly for cases at risk for scarring. We recommend that infants be propped in an upright position when placed in an infant's seat. This can be accomplished by placing a rolled towel at the small of infant' s back. Patients who are ambulatory are encouraged to walk with shoulders back and head up.

Sensory stimulation through touch is especially important in the emotional and cognitive development of babies and young children and can be aided by gently stroking and patting the skin.

Because the skin is the outer self we present to the world, it can become a social and emotional handicap when marred by lesions or damaged by trauma, particularly if patients are allowed to lead sheltered lives. A restrictive home environment may further diminish self-esteem and prevent the development of social skills. We encourage parents/caregivers to foster a positive self-image through repeated interactions and socialization with peers in the community and involvement with church groups, EB support groups if available, other social agencies, and school programs. Children with EB learn how to protect themselves from injury, and after a period of time, their friends and classmates will accept them as individuals and learn how to interact safely with them.

Parents/caregivers are urged to place their affected children in "normal" school programs with appropriate support services. Two federal laws, Public Law 94–142 (1975) and Public Law 99–457 (1986), mandate educational services for all children with handicaps beginning in infancy through post-school activities (including postsecondary education, vocational training, adult services, etc.[20,21]). A pamphlet entitled "Coping with Epidermolysis Bullosa in the Classroom: An informed and Sensitive Home/School Partnership makes the Difference" is available for a nominal fee from the Dystrophic Epidermolysis Bullosa Research Association of America (D.E.B.R.A.).[a]

Nutrition

Because of denudation of skin and mucosal lesions in the mouth and elsewhere in the gastrointestinal tract, which causes dysphagia, esophageal dysmotility, strictures, web formations, malabsorption, and constipation, and problems with dentition, patients are at severe risk for malnutrition. Poor nutrition retards growth, delays sexual maturation, and complicates wound healing.

[a] D.E.B.R.A. of America, Inc., 141 Fifth Avenue, New York, NY 10010 (212) 995–2220.

Dietary supervision is initiated as soon as the disease is evident and before problems occur. Oral feedings may proceed despite blisters in the mouth. Parents who desire to breastfeed affected infants are supported in their efforts. Nursing mothers are encouraged to initiate milk flow before placing the child at the breast. For bottle-fed infants, preemie nipples are recommended as these are soft and potentially cause less trauma to the oral mucosa.

Nutritional assessments entail analysis of hematologic, biochemical, dietary intake, and anthropometric data. An updated growth chart reveals at a glance the general trends of a child's nutritional status. Intervention may include a variety of dietary supplements that are rich in calories, iron, vitamins, protein, and fiber depending on the patient's needs.

A referral to a hematologist is indicated for cases where anemia is not corrected by dietary manipulations. Patients with gastrointestinal complications are managed in conjunction with a gastroenterologist. Temporary or long-term use of gastrostomy feeding may be indicated in pediatric and adult patients who are unable to maintain normal weight.

Dental

Referral to the pediatric dentist (pedodontist) is initiated with the eruption of primary teeth.[22,23] Because high caloric diets are typically rich in carbohydrates (which can further increase risk for dental caries), prophylactic counseling and therapy are indicated. It is not unusual for adult patients with microstomia to be referred to pediatric dentists who are better equipped to treat small mouths.

Eyes

Ocular complications of EB include corneal erosions, corneal scarring, lacrimal duct obstruction, blepharitis (inflammation of the eyelid), symblepharon (eyelid attachment to eyeball), and cicatricial ectropion (everted eyelid). All of these problems are associated with rubbing and trauma. Prophylactic measures involve protecting eyes from irritants, such as wind, dry heat, and bright lights and the use of ocular lubricants such as Lacrilube, which may prevent or reduce trauma associated with dry eyes. One of us has observed (S.G., unpublished) an increase in the incidence of corneal erosions in two patients with recessive dystrophic EB in association with the prophylactic use of atropine before surgery. Prompt treatment of eye infections may reduce risk of scarring. Referral to the ophthalmologist is initiated as early as possible in the newborn period and follow-up visits are planned accordingly.

Family Assessment

Each patient must be assessed in relation to his or her family's physical, emotional, and social resources. Unaffected siblings (and others in the household) are often deprived of the attention they would otherwise receive and may be at risk for psychological distress.[24,25] As with many other chronic disorders, family dysfunction can further complicate the disease. In addition to the psychological stress and grief experienced with giving birth to an affected child, parents must manage the daily care requirements of EB patients, which are physically demanding. Parents/caregivers are compelled to be proficient in areas that are normally the domain of health professionals. Thus, they are advised to maintain their nutrition, obtain adequate rest (including respite breaks), and distribute tasks in order to prevent exhaustion.

In our experience, those patients who make "healthy" adjustments to their disease are those whose families are empowered with knowledge, energy, motivation, and psychological and social supports.

Genetic Counseling

Adult patients and parents of affected children must be informed of the heredity of EB and the chances that their subsequent children may be similarly affected.[26] However, counseling must be based on an accurate diagnosis and conducted by one with expertise in EB.

Social Services

Because EB can cause severe physical, emotional, and financial hardships for affected persons and their families, referrals to the social worker are a necessary component of comprehensive care. The social worker can help patients and their families in identifying sources of financial support, educational, vocational, and rehabilitative services, and in obtaining other supportive services such as visiting nurse services and psychological counseling.

Other Services

The Dystrophic Epidermolysis Bullosa Research Association of America (D.E.B.R.A.), founded in 1980, provides information and guidance to families with EB, serves in an advocacy capacity before congress and governmental agencies, initiates and supports local self-help groups, publishes two informational newsletters, sponsors conferences for families and professionals, publishes and distributes educational literature on various matters pertaining to patients, and supports EB research. D.E.B.R.A. has also produced a videotape entitled "Living with Epidermolysis Bullosa," which provides advice on caring for patients and parental insights on managing the disease. Independent D.E.B.R.A. organizations also exist in Australia, England, Israel, New Zealand, and South America.

The National EB Registry was established with federal funds in 1986 under the leadership of D. Martin Carter, M.D., Ph.D., at The Rockefeller University in New York. The Registry contains a comprehensive data base of demographic and disease characteristics. It consists of four regional EB Clinical Centers; these are located at The Rockefeller University in New York City, Stanford University in Palo Alto California, University of North Carolina at Chapel Hill, and the University of Washington School of Medicine in Seattle. Patients undergo comprehensive dermatologic examinations at the centers and may be referred for additional medical evaluations; emphasis is placed on establishing accurate diagnoses.

Administrators of the Registry endeavor to define EB better, determine the national incidence and prevalence, promote research, and improve patient care. For more information about the Registry and how to enroll patients, contact The National Epidermolysis Bullosa Registry, The Rockefeller University, 1230 York Avenue, New York, New York, 10021-6399, Telephone (212) 570-8280, Fax (212) 570-8232.

Acknowledgments. The authors wish to thank Alex Buenaventura, R.N., Charge Nurse, and Patricia Gilleaudeau, B.S.N., Dermatology Nurse Specialist, at The Rockefeller University Hospital and Nancy Burns, R.N., Staff Nurse at Stanford University Hospital, for their assistance and support in the preparation of this manuscript.

Supported in part by a General Clinical Research Center grant (M01-RR00102) from the National Institutes of Health to The Rockefeller University Hospital; by a training grant (AR07525) from the National Institutes of Health to the Laboratory for Investigative Dermatology; by contracts AR62269 and AR62270 from the National Institutes of Health to the Laboratory for Investigative Dermatology; by a grant from the Dystrophic Epidermolysis Bullosa Research Association (D.E.B.R.A.) of America, Inc.; and with general support from the Pew Trusts.

References

1. Bauer ER, Gedde-Dahl T, Eisen AZ. The role of human collagenase in epidermolysis bullosa. *J Invest Dermatol.* 1977;68:119–124.
2. Gedde-Dahl T Jr. Clinical heritability in epidermolysis bullosa: speculations on causation and consequence for research. *J Invest Dermatol.* 1984;86:91–93.
3. Fine J Epidermolysis bullosa clinical aspects, pathology and recent advances in research. *Int J Dermatol.* 1986;25:143–157.
4. Lin AN, Carter DM. Epidermolysis bullosa: when the skin falls apart. *J Pediatr.* 1989;114:349–355.
5. Fine J, Bauer ER, Briggaman RA, et al. Revised clinical and laboratory criteria for subtypes of inherited epidermolysis bullosa: a consensus report by the subcommittee on diagnosis and classification of the national epidermolysis bullosa registry. *J Am Acad Dermatol.* 1991;24:119–135.
6. Foster P. Nursing care and management of epidermolysis bullosa. In: Priestley GC, Tidman MJ, Weiss JB, Eady RAJ, eds. *Epidermolysis Bullosa: A Comprehen-*

sive Review of Classification Management and Laboratory Studies. Crowthorne, England: DEBRA; 1990:37–39.

7. Pessar A, Verdicchio JF, Caldwell D. Epidermolysis bullosa: the pediatric dermatological management and therapeutic update. In: Callen JP, Dahl MV, Golitz LE, Schachner LA, Stegman SJ, eds. *Advances in Dermatology.* vol 3. Chicago: Year Book Medical Publishers; 1988:99–120.

8. Briggaman RA, Paller AS, Pessar A. Epidermolysis bullosa. In: Farmer ER, Provost TT, eds. *Current Therapy in Dermatology.* St Louis: CV Mosby; 1985:70–75.

9. Gibbons S. Care of epidermolysis bullosa patients: a nursing challange. *Derm Nurs.* 1990;2:195–214.

10. Hurwitz S. Bullous disorders of childhood. In: *Clinical Pediatric Dermatology.* Philadelphia: WB Saunders; 1981:323–330.

11. Moy JA, Caldwell-Brown D, Lin AN, Carter DM. Emergence of mupirocin-resistant *Staphylococcus aureus* in chronic wounds of patients with epidermolysis bullosa. *J Am Acad Dermatol.* 1990;22:893–895.

12. Fligner CL, Jack R, Twiggs GA, et al. Hyperosmolality induced by propylene glycol: a complication of silver sulfadiazine therapy. *JAMA.* 1985;253:1606–1609.

13. Caldwell D, Carter DM, Lin A, Varghese M. Topical mupirocin in epidermolysis bullosa: safety and efficacy of long-term treatment. In: Wood C, ed. *Round Table No. 4.* London Proceedings of the Royal Society of Medicine; 1986:12.

14. Leyden JJ. Pyoderma pathophysiology and management. *Arch Dermatol.* 1988;124:753–755.

15. Goldberg GI, Eisen AZ, Bauer EA. Tissue stress and tumor promotion: possible relevance to epidermolysis bullosa. *Arch Dermatol.* 1988;124:737–741.

16. Tidman MJ. Skin malignancy in epidermolysis bullosa. In Priestley GC, Tidman MJ, Weiss JB, Eady RAJ, eds. *Epidermolysis Bullosa: A Comprehensive Review of Classification Management and Laboratory Studies.* Crowthorne England: DEBRA; 1990:156–160.

17. Mann JFE, Zeier M, Zilow E. The spectrum of renal involvement in epidermolysis bullosa dystrophica hereditaria: report of two cases. *Am J Kidney Dis.* 1988;11:437–441.

18. Hough F. Physiotherapy for epidermolysis bullosa. In: Priestley GC, Tidman MJ, Weiss JB, Eady RAJ, eds. *Epidermolysis Bullosa: A Comprehensive Review of Classification Management and Laboratory Studies.* Crowthorne England: DEBRA, 1990:81–83.

19. American Academy of Pediatrics: *Report of the committee on infectious diseases, Red book* 1991. 22nd ed. Evanston Il1.

20. Gallagher JJ, Trohanis PL, Clifford RM. *Policy Implementation and PL 99–457.* Baltimore: Paul H. Brookes 1989.

21. Community Alliance for Special Education (CASE). Revised by Protection and Advocacy, Inc. (PAI): *Special Education Rights and Responsibilities.* 2nd ed. San Francisco; 1989.

22. Nowak AJ. Oropharyngeal lesions and their management in epidermolysis bullosa. *Arch Dermatol.* 1988;124:742–745.

23. Wright JT. Comprehensive dental care and general anesthetic management of hereditary epidermolysis bullosa. *Oral Surg Oral Med Oral Pathol.* 1990;70:573–578.

24. Landsdown R, Nabarro E. The psychology of epidermolysis bullosa. In: Priestley GC, Tidman Mj, Weiss JB, Eady RAJ, eds. *Epidermolysis Bullosa: A Comprehensive Review of Classification Management and Laboratory Studies*. Crowthorne England: DEBRA; 1990:18–20.
25. Meyer DJ, Vadasy PF, Fewell RR. *Living with a Brother or Sister with Special Needs*. Seattle: University of Washington; 1987.
26. Atherton DJ. Counselling in epidermolysis bullosa. In Priestley GC, Tidman MJ, Weiss JB, Eady RAJ, eds. *Epidermolysis Bullosa: A Comprehensive Review of Classification Management and Laboratory Studies*. Crowthorne England: DEBRA; 1990:13–17.
27. Barak M, Hershkowitz S, Rod R, Dior S. The use of a synthetic skin covering as a protective layer in daily care of low birth weight infants. *Eur J Pediatr*. 1989; 148:665–666.

Index